W9-AEV-189

DATE DUE			

 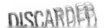

Lymphocytes

a practical approach

TITLES PUBLISHED IN
THE
PRACTICAL APPROACH
SERIES

Affinity chromatography

Animal cell culture

Biochemical toxicology

Biological membranes

Carbohydrate analysis

Centrifugation (2nd Edition)

DNA cloning

Drosophila

Electron microscopy in molecular biology

Gel electrophoresis of nucleic acids

Gel electrophoresis of proteins

H.p.l.c. of small molecules

Human cytogenetics

Human genetic diseases

Immobilised cells and enzymes

Iodinated density-gradient media

Lymphokines and interferons

Microcomputers in biology

Mitochondria

Mutagenicity testing

Neurochemistry

Nucleic acid and protein sequence analysis

Nucleic acid hybridisation

Oligonucleotide synthesis

Photosynthesis: energy transduction

Plant cell culture

Prostaglandins and related substances

Spectrophotometry and spectrofluorimetry

Steroid hormones

Teratocarcinomas and embryonic stem cells

Transcription and translation

Virology

Lymphocytes

a practical approach

Edited by
G G B Klaus

National Institute for Medical Research, The Ridgeway,
Mill Hill, London NW7 1AA, UK

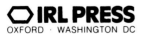 **IRL PRESS**
OXFORD · WASHINGTON DC

IRL Press Limited
PO Box 1,
Eynsham,
Oxford OX8 1JJ,
England

©1987 IRL Press Limited

British Library Cataloguing in Publication Data

Lymphocytes : a practical approach. – (Practical
  approach series)
  1.   Lymphocytes
  I.   Klaus,G.G.B.   II.   Series
  611'.0185   QP95

ISBN 1-85221-018-4 (hardbound)
ISBN 1-85221-019-2 (softbound)

Printed by Information Printing Ltd, Oxford, England.

Preface

Cellular immunology only came of age a mere 25 years ago, with the demonstration by James (now Sir James) Gowans and his coworkers that lymphocytes are the mediators of immunological responses. Until then the function of these numerous, widely distributed, but morphologically uninteresting cells was unknown. Even then it took some years before the full degree of heterogeneity of the cellular components of the lymphoid system became appreciated. This era yielded evidence for the division of labour between T and B cells, and the subsequent subdivision of these broad compartments into functional subpopulations of cells gradually emerged from the combined efforts of a growing body of immunologists. With this knowledge came the increasing awareness of the importance of cell–cell interactions in the initiation and control of immune responses, involving not only lymphocytes proper, but also a variety of accessory cells, which are needed to process and/or to present antigens to the actual protagonists in the immunological arena.

The desire to untangle the complex network of interacting and differentiating cells which are found in the sites of immune responses *in vivo* inevitably stimulated the development of novel methods. Thus, increasingly sophisticated procedures have evolved for the purification of lymphocyte and accessory cell subpopulations, together with culture and assay systems for measuring the growth and effector functions of both T and B cells *in vitro*. A major advance was the discovery that subpopulations of lymphoid cells can be distinguished by the array of marker molecules which they display on their surfaces, and the advent of monoclonal antibodies has markedly accelerated progress in this field.

This volume contains a collection of chapters dealing with various aspects of the study of lymphocytes *in vitro*. These cover methods for preparing lymphocytes and accessory cells from various sources, and for characterizing lymphocyte subpopulations, both in cell suspensions and in tissue sections. Other chapters deal with techniques for culturing and cloning lymphocytes and for measuring their differentiated effector functions, whether these be antibody secretion, or the capacity to kill virus-infected target cells. Most of the volume concerns the biology of lymphocytes. However, enormous strides have also been made in understanding the molecular biology of these cells. It therefore seemed appropriate to also provide the reader with a flavour of some of the contemporary methods being used for characterizing the surface molecules which lymphocytes use for communicating with their environment.

Although the last 25 years have produced an impressive body of knowledge about these fascinating cells, it is clear that many questions about the induction and regulation of immune responses remain unanswered. Hopefully this volume will provide a useful compendium of procedures which can be applied to answering at least some of these questions.

Gerry G.B.Klaus

Contributors

P.L.Amlot
Department of Immunology, Royal Free Hospital, Pond Street, London NW3 2QG, UK

M.H.Brown
Imperial Cancer Research Fund Laboratories, Lincolns Inn Fields, London WC2A 3PX, UK

S.Cobbold
Department of Pathology, University of Cambridge, Tennis Court Road, Cambridge CB2 1QP, UK

D.H.Crawford
Department of Virology, Royal Postgraduate Medical School, Ducane Road, London W12 0HS, UK

A.A.Davies
Imperial Cancer Research Fund Laboratories, Lincolns Inn Fields, London WC2A 3PX, UK

D.W.Dresser
Division of Immunology, National Institute for Medical Research, Mill Hill, London NW7 1AA, UK

S.Funderud
The Norwegian Radium Hospital, Montebello, 0310 Oslo, Norway

G.Gaudernack
The National Hospital, Oslo, Norway

K.S.Gilbert
Division of Immunology, National Institute for Medical Research, Mill Hill, London NW7 1AA, UK

A.S.Hamblin
Department of Immunology, St. Thomas' Hospital Medical School, London SE1 7EH, UK

S.V.Hunt
Sir William Dunn School of Pathology, South Parks Road, Oxford OX1 3RE, UK

G.Janossy
Department of Immunology, Royal Free Hospital, Pond Street, London NW3 2QG, UK

S.C.Knight
Division of Rheumatology, Clinical Research Centre, Northwick Park, Middlesex HA1 3UJ, UK

T.Lea
The National Hospital, Oslo, Norway

I.Lefkovits
Basle Institute for Immunology, Grenzacherstrasse 487, Basle, Switzerland

D.W.Mason
MRC Cellular Immunology Unit, Sir William Dunn School of Pathology, South Parks Road, Oxford OX1 3RE, UK

K.H.G.Mills
Division of Immunology, National Institute for Medical Research, Mill Hill, London NW7 1AA, UK

K.Nustad
The Norwegian Radium Hospital, Montebello, 0310 Oslo, Norway

A.O'Garra
Division of Immunology, National Institute for Medical Research, Mill Hill, London NW7 1AA, UK

W.J.Penhale
MRC Cellular Immunology Unit, Sir William Dunn School of Pathology, South Parks Road, Oxford OX1 3RE, UK

J.D.Sedgwick
MRC Cellular Immunology Unit, Sir William Dunn School of Pathology, South Parks Road, Oxford OX1 3RE, UK

P.Stenstad
SINTEF, NTH, Trondheim, Norway

P.M.Taylor
Division of Immunology, National Institute for Medical Research, Mill Hill, London NW7 1AA, UK

D.B.Thomas
Division of Immunology, National Institute for Medical Research, Mill Hill, London NW7 1AA, UK

J.Ugelstad
SINTEF, NTH, Trondheim, Norway

F.Vartdal
The Norwegian Radium Hospital, Montebello, 0310 Oslo, Norway

H.Waldmann
Department of Pathology, University of Cambridge, Tennis Court Road, Cambridge CB2 1QP, UK

E.V.Walls
Department of Virology, Royal Postgraduate Medical School, Ducane Road, London W12 0HS, UK

Contents

3. FRACTIONATION OF LYMPHOCYTES BY IMMUNO-
    MAGNETIC BEADS 55
    Steinar Funderud, Kjell Nustad, Tor Lea, Frode Vartdal, Gustav
    Gaudernack, Per Stenstad and John Ugelstad

4. IMMUNOFLUORESCENCE AND IMMUNOHISTO-
    CHEMISTRY 67
    George Janossy and Peter Amlot

Abbreviations

AET	2-amino ethylisothiouronium bromide hydrobromide
AIDS	acquired immunodeficiency syndrome
ALL	acute lymphocytic leukaemia
AML	acute myeloid leukaemia
AMP	2-amino-2 methyl-1-propanol
AO	acridine orange
AP	alkaline phosphatase
APAAP	immuno-alkaline phosphatase-anti-alkaline phosphatase
APC	antigen-presenting cells
ARS	AIDS-related syndromes
ATCC	American Type Culture Collection
BCDF	B cell differentiation factor
BCGF	B cell growth factor
BCIP	5-bromo-4-chloro-3-indolyl phosphate
BHK	baby hamster kidney
BL	Burkitt's lymphoma
BLCL	B lymphoblastoid cell lines
BrdU	bromodeoxyuridine
BSA	bovine serum albumin
BSE	biotin succinimide ester
BSF	B cell-stimulatory factor
BSS	balanced salt solution
CD	Cluster of differentiation
CFT	complement fixation test
CML	cell-mediated lympholysis
CLL	chronic lymphocytic leukaemia
Con A	concanavalin A
CSF	colony-stimulating factor
CTL	cytotoxic T cells
DAB	3,3'-diaminobenzidine
DABCO	diazo-bicyclooctane
DMSO	dimethyl sulphoxide
DNP	2,4-dinitrophenyl
DTT	dithiothreitol
EB	ethidium bromide
EBNA	Epstein–Barr virus nuclear antigen
EBV	Epstein–Barr virus
EDF	eosinophil differentiation factor
EDTA	ethylene diamine tetraacetic acetate
ELISA	enzyme-linked immunosorbent assay
Endo F	endo-β-N-acetylglucosaminadase F
Endo H	endo-β-N-acetylglucosaminadase H
EP	endogenous pyrogen
FACS	fluorescence-activated cell sorter
FCS	fetal calf serum
FDC	follicular dendritic cell(s)
FITC	fluorescein isothiocyanate

HBSS	Hank's balanced salt solution
Hepes	N-2-hydroxyethyl piperazine-N'-2-ethane sulphonic acid
HEV	high endothelial venules
HLA	human leucocyte antigen
HPGF	hybridoma/plasmacytoma growth factor
HRP	horseradish peroxidase
IEF	isoelectric focusing
IF	immunofluorescence
IHC	immunohistochemical
IL	interleukin
KLH	keyhole limpet haemocyanin
LAK	lymphokine-activated killer
LDA	limiting dilution analysis
LEM	leukocyte endogenous mediator
LGL	large granular lymphocyte
LPS	(bacterial) lipopolysaccharide
MAb	monoclonal antibody
MCGF	mast cell growth factor
MEM	minimal essential medium
MHC	major histocompatibility complex
MLR	mixed leukocyte reaction
Mops	3-(N-morpholino)propanesulphonic acid
NEPHGE	non-equilibrium pH gradient electrophoresis
NIP	nitro-iodo-phenacetyl
NK	natural killer
NP-40	Nonidet P-40
OPD	o-phenylenediamine
ORBC	ox red blood cells
PBL	peripheral blood lymphocytes
PBMC	peripheral blood mononuclear cells
PBS	phosphate-buffered saline
PE	phycoerythrin
PEC	peritoneal exudate cells
PFC	plaque-forming cell(s)
PHA	phytohaemagglutinin
PLL	poly-L-lysine
PMA	phorbol myristic acetate
PMSF	phenylmethylsulphonyl fluoride
POL	polymerized flagellin (from *Salmonella* spp.)
PPD	purified protein derivative
PWM	pokeweed mitogen
RBC	red blood cells
RIA	radioimmunoassay
SDS-PAGE	sodium dodecyl sulphate-polyacrylamide gel electrophoresis
SKSD	streptokinase/streptodomase
SRBC	sheep red blood cells
Tc	cytotoxic T cell
T_h	helper T cell
TBS	Tris-buffered saline
TCA	trichloroacetic acid

TCGF	T cell growth factor
TRF	T cell replacing factor
TDL	thoracic duct lymphocytes
TdT	terminal deoxynucleotidyl transferase
TG	thioglycollate
TEMED	N,N,N',N'-tetramethylethylenediamine
TNBS	trinitrobenzyl sulphonic acid
TNP	2,4,6-trinitrophenyl
TPA	12-O-tetradecanoyl phorbol-13-acetate
TRITC	tetramethylrhodamine isothiocyanate
VDU	visual display unit
ZIPP	zones of inhibited phage plaques

CHAPTER 1

Preparation of lymphocytes and accessory cells

SIMON V.HUNT

1. GENERAL CONSIDERATIONS

1.1 Sources of lymphoid cells

This chapter starts (Section 1) with some general comments on the different kinds of lymphocytes and accessory cells that can easily be obtained. Sections 2 and 3 are concerned with how to get cells from sources which respectively are already in suspension or need disrupting to get them into suspension. The follow-up steps are considered in Section 4 for simple purifications (see also Chapter 2 for rosetting, panning, etc.), while Section 5 is about cell counting. Useful compendia of immunological methods are to be found in refs 1−3.

1.1.1 Primary lymphoid organs

In the adult the bone marrow and the thymus are the main sites of generation of new lymphocytes and these organs contain immature as well as mature components (reviewed in 4). The mature fraction, is in the minority (say 5−10%). The immature cells are destined either to mature or to die. Large, dividing ('blast') cells can be found in this immature population but the small cells predominate. Neither organ is on the main pathway of re-circulation of small peripheral lymphocytes, so mature cells do not re-enter in significant numbers because of this kind of migration. However, marrow does contain some mature, immunocompetent small lymphocytes that have been in the periphery and returned. The T cell component of marrow can be eliminated, if necessary, by antibody-mediated cytotoxicity (Chapter 2). Conversely, reports of B cell contamination of the thymus partly reflect accidental inclusion of parathymic lymph nodes, which lie immediately adjacent. These may become particularly significant after intraperitoneal (i.p.) immunization, which drains to these nodes. It should be clear that if mature T and B lymphocytes are wanted, it is best to go to the peripheral, secondary lymphoid tissues and separate T from B. Only use primary lymphoid organs if the study of the maturation process itself, or some other equally good reason, demands it.

In adolescence, when the primary lymphoid organs are at their maximum cellularity, marrow may contain up to 30−50% lymphocytes. The mature B cells from marrow can be identified and isolated by their surface Ig: in mice about 15% of nucleated cells are B cells, and a roughly equal proportion pre-B cells, while in rats the figures are around 5% B and 25% pre-B. Cocktails of monoclonal antibodies that specifically stain (or leave unstained) only the pre-B cells have been described for mouse and rat

1

(5,6), to permit their isolation by bulk depletion methods (Chapter 2).

The thymus of young animals is almost wholly lymphoid. There are rare dendritic cells, epithelial cells, macrophages and a few other cell types, such as thymic nurse cells (see 7−9). The thymus varies in size according to age, stress and strain of animal. In 'nude' animals it is congenitally absent. Among the thymocytes in a young active thymus the total mature cells may be no more than 10%. These are about equally divided between those bearing only the CD4 antigen, that is with the phenotype of T helper cells, or bearing CD8, the antigen associated with recognition of major histocompatibility complex (MHC) class I antigen (T cytotoxic/suppressor phenotype). A very small population bears neither of these antigens.

The great majority of thymic lymphocytes carry both these CD4 and CD8 markers. The thymic medulla contains predominantly the singly-marked cells, and the cortex the double stainers. In old age, or after exposure of an animal to stress or to injection of hydrocortisone, the thymic cortex shrinks. Enriched mature thymocytes from mice or rats have been traditionally obtained by giving 0.1 mg of cortisone acetate per g body weight 24−48 h previously. Such cortisone-resistant thymocytes have many of the properties of peripheral T cells. However, it should be remembered that they have been exposed to substantial doses of steroid, which may have a direct effect on them. Also it is possible that cortisone may cause selective destruction of a subset of cells within those that bear the mature phenotype. A recent study has cast doubt on the ortho-dox equation of cortisone-resistant cells with medullary thymocytes (10). As with bone marrow, if you want mature cells then go to the periphery.

Fetal liver is a primary lymphoid organ *in utero*, being the main site of haemopoiesis in the last week of gestation in mice and rats, and from week 6 onwards in man. Although some pre-B cells can be found they are so outnumbered by other cell types that this is not a preferred source. Its main value is as a source of extremely potent haemopoietic stem cells (11,12). If taken early in gestation these are uncontaminated by mature T lymphocytes, in contrast to the bone marrow. This makes it especially useful when setting up MHC-incompatible allogeneic radiation chimeras, since the problems of graft-versus-host disease are avoided.

1.1.2 Secondary lymphoid organs

Spleen, lymph nodes, Peyer's patches and tonsil (with other mucosal-associated lym-phoid tissue) are the places to find immunocompetent lymphocytes. They are physiologically interconnected by the migration of the majority if not all small lym-phocytes. Each re-circulating lymphocyte travels up the thoracic duct every 24−48 h. A few lymphocytes may remain sessile in the secondary lymphoid tissues, unaffected by thoracic duct drainage. Lymphoblasts do not re-circulate unless they first differen-tiate into small lymphocytes (reviewed in 13).

Cell yields from these organs vary considerably depending both on induced and background levels of immunization. Thus, specific-pathogen-free animals have much smaller organs. The ratio of T cells to B cells is characteristically different in the dif-ferent organs. Lymph nodes contain the most T cells (55−80%, comparable with thoracic duct lymph), spleen is intermediate (40% among lymphocytes) and Peyer's patch has the fewest (~30%). Obviously, it is best to go for the most enriched source if either of these subpopulations is needed.

2

1.1.3 *Lymphoid cell lines*

Cell lines have the general advantages of reproducibility and ease of scaling up, especially with human material. In practice, much care should be taken to monitor that no unwanted variant or contaminant creeps in. In many cases if surface antigenic profiles, delineated by panels of monoclonal antibodies, are compared between the cell lines and normal tissue cells, then a leukaemia or lymphoma can be assigned to its normal cellular counterpart (14,15). Cell lines are particularly valuable for biochemical studies of molecules of naturally low abundance (secreted or cell-bound) if overproducing variants can be selected, and for examining cellular metabolism. Lines established from normal T cells are discussed in Chapter 6.

1.2 Suspensions from solid organs

Most lymphoid tissues can be dissociated with relatively little difficulty, since the cells are not tightly bound to each other by tight junctions or by substantial amounts of connective tissue. Simply crushing or teasing a lymphoid organ releases large numbers of lymphocytes with reasonable viability. But it should be remembered that minor populations that selectively resist these simple isolation procedures may be missed, and what may be minor in number may nonetheless be major in importance (e.g. accessory cells, Section 1.3, or thymocyte sub-populations). Also, there may be cell types which are more or less fragile, and which succumb more or less readily to mechanical trauma (e.g. lymphoblasts are reputed to survive less well than small lymphocytes). The comparative difficulty of obtaining lymphoid cells from other sites may focus too much attention on the central processes in the immune response, and too little on the afferent and efferent arcs. Important areas like the whole mucosal immune system (gut, mammary gland, female reproductive tract, salivary gland, bronchi), or the effector cells of graft rejection (skin, kidney, heart) or of autoimmune processes (nervous system, endocrine organs) need further exploration of their lymphoid content. *Table 1* indicates where to look for methods for isolation of cells from some of these non-lymphoid organs.

Lymphoid organs are not simply bags of lymphocytes awaiting puncturing to release them (see 26,27). They have:

(i)   capsules;
(ii)   stromal cells;
(iii)   endothelial cells of different kinds (notably the columnar cells of the so called

Table 1. Cell preparations from non-lymphoid organs (for lymphoid cells except where stated).

Organ	Species	Reference
Kidney	human	16
Kidney	rat	17
Heart	rat	18
Skin (Langerhans cells)	human	19
Skin (Langerhans cells)	mouse	20,21
Salivary gland	mouse	22
Intestine (mast cells)	rat	23
Intestine (macrophages)	rat	24
Spinal cord	rat	25

high endothelial venules, HEV, in the lymph node paracortex); and
(iv)   accessory cells (Section 1.3).

The spleen also contains red pulp, which serves as a reservoir of all blood cells, as well as being the sites of antibody formation by plasma cells, and of antigen trapping by macrophages. Spleen cell suspensions therefore contain red and white blood cells of all kinds as well as lymphocytes.

Releasing cells from lymphoid organs becomes ultimately a compromise between simplicity and speed on the one hand, and viability and full recovery on the other. The main decision is whether to use enzyme digestion. It is quicker without enzymes, and cells do not have to be raised to 37°C, so the handling medium can be kept simple (Section 1.4.1). Enzymes may also destroy cell surface molecules. On the other hand, tougher organs give higher yields of lymphocytes following 20−60 min in collagenase, or collagenase plus the neutral protease Dispase. We routinely treat Peyer's patches, fetal liver, tissues from irradiated animals and sometimes tissue from very old animals in this way. DNase may help to prevent entrapment and loss of still living cells by strands of DNA derived from dead cells (in thymus and young bone marrow, in particular). Enzymes are essential for releasing dendritic cells: their long processes are too fragile to withstand mechanical disaggregation and entrapped lymphocytes must be freed as gently as possible. In the gentlest protocols of all, for preparing follicular dendritic cells (FDC), collagenase is administered intravenously (i.v.) 30 min before killing the animal (28), or it may be perfused through an isolated spleen.

Purely mechanical disruption can be performed with varying degrees of vigour. Chopping the organ into large fragments, followed by teasing with watchmaker's fine-pointed forceps, is the most gentle method, but needs patience and may easily leave important cells in the residue. Grinding the organs through stainless steel or plastic mesh, or homogenizing with a loose-fitting glass tissue grinder, or squashing between two frosted glass microscope slides may give up more cells but at the expense of viability. The methods in Section 3 and *Table 6* are based on our own practice using young adult rats, but in any situation out of the ordinary it will be worth preliminary experimentation with other methods.

1.3 Accessory cell heterogeneity

The need for non-lymphoid cells to help lymphocytes make immune responses *in vitro* was first shown 20 years ago (29). Since then, adherence, buoyant density, radioresistance and surface markers like Fc receptors and MHC class II antigens have been used to enrich accessory cells. Broadly, they can be divided into macrophages and dendritic cells, though each of these can be further subdivided into categories based on physiological state, for example degree of macrophage activation, or on histological location. In particular, FDC which are found in the primary and secondary follicles of peripheral lymphoid tissues, should be distinguished from other kinds of dendritic cells (Section 1.3.3). This is not the place for a detailed review of a still highly controversial field where the relationships between the different kinds of accessory cells are under active scrutiny (reviewed in 27,30).

As a broad generalization, the properties of phagocytosis and adherence often go hand in hand. However, adherence can only be usefully employed as long as it can be reversed by some gentle method, for example treating cells with trypsin is likely to cause at least transient trauma to the cell's physiology. The nature of the substratum is crucial. It was a useful discovery in work on human macrophages for instance when it was shown that the microexudate left on plastic surfaces by confluent growth of baby hamster kidney (BHK) cells provides a foothold for adherent cells that could subsequently be released by EDTA alone (31).

1.3.1 *Macrophages*

Macrophages both process antigen and dispose of it finally. Conceptually at least, and perhaps also in fact, antigen presentation is a separate process, often performed by other cell types (e.g. dendritic cells, B cells). Macrophages also secrete a large variety of locally active products (32), such as cytokines, enzymes, prostaglandins, colony-stimulating factors, etc. They are ubiquitous, and arise from bone marrow myeloid cells by way of blood monocytes. There are a few macrophages normally *resident* in the peritoneum, in alveoli and in milk or colostrum, all of which can be useful sources. However, the sterile exudate inducible in the peritoneal cavity by injection of materials such as proteose peptone or Brewer's thioglycollate generates, after 3−5 days, large numbers of *inflammatory* cells widely used in many protocols. Live bacterial vaccines (BCG or *Corynebacterium parvum*) engender *activated* macrophages within 10−21 days. The chief precaution in these preparations is to get rid of contaminating granulocytes. This is easy since macrophages adhere, and granulocytes do not to any great extent. Some contamination with mast cells, fibroblasts and lymphocytes may also occur. Tissue macrophages, though often abundant, for example the Kupffer cells of liver, are more difficult to obtain pure, because of the problems of dispersing cells from solid organs.

Macrophage populations vary. For instance, the different macrophage populations mentioned above exhibit different characteristics [e.g. increased expression of MHC class II upon activation (33), microbicidal capacity (34), secreted proteins (35)]. There may be 'natural' variations in the degree of activation of apparently unstimulated macrophages according to the condition of the animal colony. Peritoneal macrophages bear the antigens MRC OX43 (rats; 36) and OKM5 (humans; 37), but tissue macrophages do not, so peritoneal macrophages may not be typical of all macrophages. Peritoneal macrophages bear the CD4 antigen in rats, while those from bronchi do not (38). More subtle differences may also exist between macrophages located within different regions of lymphoid tissue. Thus, in the lymph node, macrophages of the medullary sinus, of the superficial cortex beneath the subcapsular sinus, and of the germinal centre have different histological or surface features which may reflect different functions (39). Blood monocytes, which are widely used in work on human cells, are developmentally less mature than their tissue counterparts. These kinds of variation must of course be taken into account when planning an experiment.

1.3.2 *Dendritic cells*

It is convenient to group together accessory cells whose chief feature is the capacity to present antigen to T cells. These include 'veiled' and non-lymphoid cells of peripheral lymph, Langerhans cells of the epidermis, 'interdigitating' cells of the paracortex of lymph nodes and cells called simply 'dendritic' from blood and Peyer's patches. It is

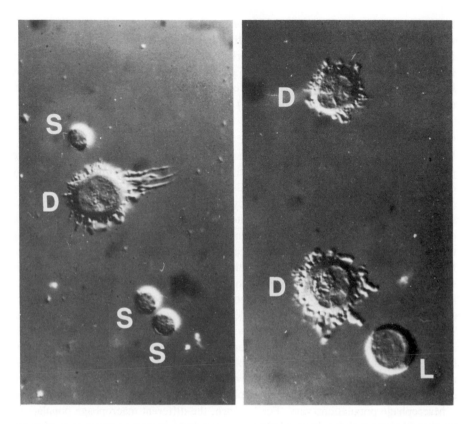

Figure 1. Lymphocytes and non-lymphoid accessory cells from the thoracic duct of mesenteric lymph-adenectomized rats. Live cells have settled on the glass slide. See Section 1.3.2. Note the fine processes of the dendritic cells (D), compared with the featureless small lymphocytes (S) and large lymphoblast (L). (1300×, Nomarski interference optics).

uncertain though how their accessory cell activity correlates with cells identified histologically, if and how these cell types are related to each other and how physiologically relevant antigen is handled and processed before presentation by dendritic cells. Heterogeneity is rife here as elsewhere in cellular immunology.

The non-phagocytic dendritic cell found in mouse spleen by Steinman *et al.* (40,41) is extraordinarily potent in a variety of antigen presentation assays. These cells are so rare (<1%), that they can only be cleanly isolated by fairly lengthy purification procedures. Cell for cell, no other cell type from an organ source is as stimulatory to T cells. Mouse spleen is a good source: the frequency of dendritic cells in adherence-fractionated spleen is quite high (up to 40%). This points the way to a simple, if impure preparation (note the exception here to the rule correlating phagocytosis with adherence). A monoclonal antibody to dendritic cells exists, 33D1 (42), which helps distinguish them from macrophages and FDC (by cytotoxicity only; it is a weak staining antibody). They also lack the macrophage antigen F4/80 (43). 33D1 and polyclonal antisera against the F4/80 antigen (though not the monoclonal, which is not cytotoxic) can be employed in complement-mediated cytolysis procedures as described in Chapter

2. During purification these markers should be followed, together with the characteristic morphology seen in phase contrast or interference microscopy (*Figure 1*).

Dendritic cells are also found in afferent lymph, especially from the skin. They are filtered by lymph nodes and do not escape in efferent lymph. A reasonable hypothesis is that these cells come from Langerhans cells of the skin, or from MHC class II positive cells of the gut (Peyer's patches or lamina propria), which can also be isolated and shown to function in antigen-presenting assays. From the practical point of view they can only be obtained in species large enough to permit direct access to afferent lymph (sheep, pigs, etc.), or where substantial numbers of lymph nodes can be extirpated to prevent filtration by the node, and then collecting the modified 'efferent' lymph, as in the rat several weeks after mesenteric lymphadenectomy (44). The great advantage of lymph as a source of accessory cells is that the cells are already in suspension. They still need purification from residual lymphocytes, and may themselves be heterogeneous as judged by surface markers (sub-populations carrying CD4, Thy-1, MRCOX2 in the rat, ref. 45).

1.3.3 *Follicular dendritic cells*

FDC trap and retain antigen − antibody complexes on their surfaces. This requires complement component C3, so presumably occurs via their abundant C3 receptors (CR1 and CR2). They are not phagocytic, do not internalize antigen and lack lysosomes. Like other accessory cells they are radioresistant (doses up to 10 Grays), but controversy surrounds the question of their ontogeny, whether from a haemopoietic source or from some autochthonous, stromal origin. Their very extended and delicate processes particularly entrap B cells, and there is a convincing case that in the mouse they stimulate B memory cells in germinal centres (46). Their role in stimulating primary immune responses is not well explored. It is in dispute whether they display MHC class II (28,47), so they are not considered prime candidates for antigen presentation to T cells.

Being so intimately connected with lymphocytes they are especially hard to obtain pure and undamaged. They are presumed to be sessile cells. Hence they must be obtained by very gentle disruption of whole organs (lymph node or spleen). Their purification is best monitored by pre-labelling them with fluorescein-conjugated aggregated IgG (or antigen − antibody complexes), injected i.v. 3 days before organs are harvested. Aggregates taken up by macrophages are degraded by 48 h and the label eliminated, leaving only FDC labelled (28). The markers distinguishing FDC from other accessory cells are: lack of 33D1 (mouse); possession of R4/23 (human, 49) and CR1 and CR2 (28). Their isolation from human tonsil is described in ref. 48.

1.3.4 *Myelomonocytic cell lines*

Most macrophage-related cell lines derive from tumours, for example, WEHI-3 and J774 in BALB/c mice. Different lines show phenotypes of cells at varying stages of maturing (i.e. some more monocyte-like, others more differentiated). Some lines have grown out as permanent derivatives of long-term bone marrow or macrophage cultures with repeated re-feeding (see 50−52 for reviews). As with lymphoid lines, stability of phenotype may be a problem. The P388 line started as a lymphoma (and doubtless many sublines still are): but the presumed derivative P388D1 has macrophage-like properties. The difference is probably an interesting reflection of the ability of some cells initially to switch phenotype *in vitro* (53). The point is to be extremely careful about the exact origin of the line, and to repeatedly look for signs of drift by comparison with frozen stocks of the original.

1.4 Handling conditions

We generally assume that what is good for a cell *in vivo* should be good for it *in vitro*. But the body's buffering systems, mainly bicarbonate-based, and nutrient complexities are hard to mimic. Fortunately, small lymphocytes are relatively metabolically inactive, especially at 4°C. They then will survive treatments for 24 h in simple phosphate-buffered media functionally intact. The more active large lymphocytes are more fussy. A simple purification of small lymphocytes (54), in which small lymphocytes differentially survive from among a mixture with large, is incubation for 24 h in rather unfavourable medium. Therefore no fixed universal rules can be drawn up for all cell types, and what follow are broad generalizations.

1.4.1 *Temperature*

For manipulations lasting a few hours, suspensions of peripheral lymphocytes in balanced salts solutions (BSS) tolerate room temperature well. The conventional view is that extended procedures lasting overnight are better done at $0-4°C$. However, in a study of the effect of temperature during collection of thoracic duct lymphocytes (55), monitoring their migratory ability as a test of function, cooled lymphocytes migrated less well than those collected over 4 h at room temperature. This effect was transitory. Nevertheless many protocols call for removal of organs from the body immediately into ice-cold medium. Certainly both bone marrow and thymus lose viability rapidly, unless the organs go straight into ice-cold medium. Perhaps the most important guide is that *changes* in temperature are widely assumed to be damaging, so a refrigerated centrifuge is a necessity except for very simple procedures.

For incubations at 37°C, a suitably buffered nutritious medium should be used. The particular medium is to the experimenter's choice. For rat cells we use RPMI 1640 with 5% newborn calf serum, or better, DA rat serum for incubations of $2-3$ days as in lymphocyte stimulation assays.

1.4.2 *pH, tonicity, nutrients*

The normal pH of the blood is 7.4. Handling media for cells may be buffered with phosphate, which provides a strong buffering without change of pH due to exposure to air. For culture, the relatively high [phosphate] cannot be tolerated: either bicarbonate-buffered Hanks' BSS, Earle's BSS, or minimal essential medium (MEM), or RPMI 1640, or HEPES + bicarbonate (Iscove's modified MEM) are used instead. These buffers lose CO_2 to the air gradually and the cultures are therefore incubated in an atmosphere of 5% CO_2 in air. Another non-bicarbonate buffer used with macrophages in particular is α-morpholinopropane sulphonic acid (α-MOPS).

There is wide variation in the tonicity of serum. The following equivalent [NaCl] were measured [mmol/l: (56)]: human and monkey, 147 (= physiological saline), rat

153, mouse and chick 168, fetal calf 170. It is obvious that one single medium formulation for all these species will not suit each exactly. But how much this matters in practice has not been systematically investigated for lymphocytes. One case where tonicity does matter is in isopycnic centrifugation. Small alterations in tonicity have a substantial effect on cell density (56).

As suggested previously, the choice as to how rich the medium should be depends largely on the temperature and on the cell type. The simplest medium contains inorganic salts (Dulbecco's 'A' = phosphate-buffered saline, PBS, see Appendix). This may have Ca^{2+} and Mg^{2+} added (Dulbecco's 'B' to make DAB). Most workers consider it essential to add protein (5% newborn calf serum or 0.2% bovine serum albumin, BSA) to reduce non-specific binding to the surfaces of containers. Where cessation of metabolic activity is required (for instance, to prevent capping during labelling with antibodies), it is common practice to work in the presence of sodium azide (3 – 10 mM) at 4°C, but azide is not included in room temperature or 37°C media. DAB with 0.2% BSA and 3 mM NaN_3 is our day-to-day handling medium. BSS is slightly grander, containing glucose and phenol red. To permit growth, amino acids, vitamins and reducing agents are needed, as in MEM and its various modifications.

In the protocols given in this chapter, no particular recommendations are made as to which of these media may be best. They are simply grouped under the generic title 'nutritious media' to distinguish them from the simple salts solutions. Formulations are listed in commercial catalogues (Flow, GIBCO, etc). With the exception of the fully defined media, growth factors present in serum (and likely to vary from batch to batch) are necessary.

1.4.3 *Mechanical damage; centrifuging*

All cells are susceptible to shear forces, especially those with processes like dendritic cells. This must be why grinding organs gives lower viabilities compared with teasing. To resuspend a pellet of lymphocytes, for example after centrifuging, suck them up and down in a small volume of medium that can be almost entirely contained within the Pasteur pipette. Then all the cells pass through the narrowest part of the tube before more medium is added. Do not introduce air since the bubbles trap cells in the high-shearing environment of a thin film. For adherent cells avoid scraping cells with a rubber policeman, unless poor viability is of no consequence (see Section 4.4).

To pellet cells, centrifuge for 7 – 10 min at 300 g in the usual 10 cm long tube. Recovery from denser media (e.g. the cells harvested from a density gradient, Section 4.3) may need a harder spin. High g forces are not intrinsically damaging to cells. They survive several thousand g in self-forming density gradients, provided they remain in suspension. Only if they pellet to the bottom and become compressed is damage caused.

2. CELLS FROM BODY FLUIDS

2.1 **Blood**

Peripheral blood, obtained by cardiac puncture in mice and rats, and from veins in larger animals and man, is the most accessible source of lymphocytes, and also con-

Table 2. Preparation of blood mononuclear cells.

1.	Prepare the gradient. Add about 3 ml of Metrizoate−Ficoll (Appendix) mixture to a 10−15 ml capped centrifuge tube. *Equilibrate to room temperature.* (4°C will not work).
2.	Take blood. Decant into a conical flask containing a dozen 2 mm glass beads and swirl orbitally and gently in the palm of the hand until they no longer clink (5−10 min) because of the clot (N.B. human blood is a biohazard).
3.	Dilute the cell suspension with an equal volume of handling medium (PBS or BSS) at room temperature.
4.	Transfer carefully as an overlay to the gradient. Use a Pasteur pipette with its end bent to 90° (heat over a small flame), cut off with a diamond knife just past the bend. This helps stop mixing with the gradient. (Alternatively, start with the suspension in a clean centrifuge tube and introduce Metrizoate−Ficoll as the underlay).
5.	Centrifuge at 1500 *g*, 15 min, room temperature (brake off during deceleration to minimize swirling).
6.	The pellet contains red cells and granulocytes. The interface contains mononuclear cells. Aspirate and discard the supernatant to just above the turbid interface. Aspirate and keep the interface, sweeping over the whole area. Cells stuck to the walls can be dislodged by gentle scraping with the pipette tip. Transfer to a new tube.
7.	Dilute with a >4-fold excess of medium, mix well. Handling from now on can be at 4°C. Centrifuge at 300 *g* for 10 min to collect the PBMC.

tains accessory cells. Human blood contains $5-10 \times 10^6$/ml leukocytes and 1000-fold more erythrocytes. About 30% of leukocytes are lymphocytes and $1-3$% monocytes (referred to jointly as peripheral blood mononuclear cells, PBMC). The rest are granulocytes. Remove platelets by defibrination. Employing the anti-coagulants citrate or heparin leaves them in suspension and platelets may cause clumping of leukocytes.

Boyum (57) established the routine density-gradient procedure (*Table 2*) for rapid preparation of PBMC by centrifugation from whole blood in good yield (~ 50% of theoretical, i.e. just over 10^6/ml of blood). Older methods (reviewed in refs. 58,59) employ sedimentation in gelatin or dextran, but these give lower purities. These 1000-fold purifications work because the giant polymers in the separation media (Ficoll, dextran, or gelatin in Plasmagel) cause the formation of high-density rouleaux. Erythrocytes in these rouleaux pellet to the bottom, along with granulocytes which are presumably dense because of their granules.

Dendritic cells can be isolated from human PBMC. Present in very low concentrations, $(1-2 \times 10^3$/ml) they can be obtained by adherence and overnight culture, much like mouse spleen (Section 4.4.3), except they stick not quite so strongly. Then follows cytolysis with a monoclonal antibody cocktail against monocytes, T cells and B cells (41). The purity should be $65-80$%.

Among PBMC, T cells form the majority (~ 70%). They can be enriched by nylon wool adherence purification (Section 4.4), by rosette depletion of B cells, or by rosette enrichment of 'E$^+$ cells' [those that bind sheep erythrocytes treated with 2-aminoethylisothiouronium bromide hydrobromide (AET)]. A protocol for E-rosette enrichment is given in (60). Monocytes may be removed by Percoll step gradient centrifugation (61), thus avoiding adherence which may affect some T cells.

2.2 Lymph

Afferent lymph contains lymphocytes from tissues and organs which originated from the blood. These are relatively few (62) by comparison with the 10- to 20-fold greater numbers that enter lymph nodes via the HEV. Afferent lymph also contains macrophages and dendritic cells, which are virtually undetectable in efferent lymph. The efferent lymphatics from the nodes below the diaphragm merge at the cisterna chyli. From this chamber a single large trunk passes anteriorly adjacent to the aorta to enter the left subclavian vein. This is the thoracic duct. It carries prodigious quantities of lymphocytes, both small, non-dividing cells (T and B) that form part of the re-circulating pool, and lymphoblasts.

Over 3 or 4 days more than 80% of the re-circulating pool can be drained through a thoracic duct fistula. The proportion of T cells is usually 55 − 85%. As drainage proceeds this proportion diminishes, because T lymphocytes have a faster modal re-circulation tempo. Collections of lymph after say 4 days therefore contain predominantly B lymphocytes (63). Concomitantly the proportion of large lymphocytes rises from about 5% to 15 − 30%. If the duct is cannulated carefully, with minimal haemorrhage, the lymph is barely contaminated with any other cell types. Very occasional phagocytic cells may be found, which probably result from inflammatory reactions due to surgery.

For the first 24 h after cannulation the yields of thoracic duct cells are roughly as follows: mouse, $100 - 150 \times 10^6$ (63); rat, $300 - 600 \times 10^6$; guinea-pig $300 - 400 \times 10^6$ (64); rabbit $2 - 3 \times 10^9$ (65); dog (66); sheep (67) and man (68). (The references cited give details of operative techniques.) These figures can vary widely, depending in particular on the immune status of the individual, and whether the animal is specific-pathogen-free or conventional.

For thoracic duct cannulation of rats (Section 2.2.1) preferably use male rats around 250 g, which have the least fat. Lewis rats are reputedly difficult to cannulate. Cannulate first thing in the morning to ensure milky and therefore visible lymph following night-time feeding and also to maximize the time for post-operative observation. This is important because the main reason for technical failure is clotting in the cannula before lymph flow is well established. Remove clots quickly, preferably by gentle suction with a syringe, or by twirling them round a nylon monofilament. An i.v. cannula maintains a high fluid flow, which again helps to prevent clotting. An overnight collection may give more than 100 ml of lymph (although the cellular output is independent of the volume of lymph). With experience, surgery takes 25 − 30 min and can be done without the aid of a microscope. A good operating light, ideally a fibreoptic 'cold light' illuminator, is essential and a heated operating table desirable. The preparation can be maintained if necessary for a week or so, if the rat is cleaned, fed and watered twice daily and kept in a quiet, warm environment.

2.2.1 *Cannulation of the thoracic duct in rats (58)*

This procedure requires a Personal Licence under the Animals (Scientific Procedures) Act in the UK. The author has made a videotape, which is available on application. Materials marked (#) are as shown in *Figure 2*.

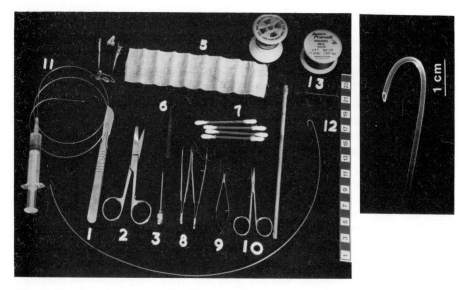

Figure 2. Typical instruments for thoracic duct cannulation. See Section 2.2.1 (**1**) Scalpel. (**2**) Blunt-nosed scissors. (**3**) Trochar (14-gauge needle). (**4**) Retractor (eye speculum modified with flange, Weiss cat. no. B3) (**5**) Cotton gauze. (**6**) Blunt dissector (home-made from a glass rod, fire-smoothed tip). (**7**) Cotton buds. (**8**) Dagger forceps. (**9**) Iridectomy scissors (Vanna's miniature spring scissors, Weiss cat. no. B1053). (**10**) Bow scissors (Weiss cat. no. B1048) (**11**) I.v. cannula (see Appendix) with syringe. (**12**) Thoracic duct cannula (see Appendix: inset shows detail). (**13**) Ligature silk (5/0) and suture silk (3/0) and ligature threader on handle (bent needle). Scale in cm.

(i)   Anaesthetize the animal with freshly evaporated ether. Shave the left abdomen dorsally as far as the spine. Insert a tail vein cannula (Appendix) (11 #); hold the needle in place with splint of three strips of 25 mm Sellotape. Infuse 3−4 ml of DAB 1 (Appendix) over about 20 sec. Clamp the infusion line to prevent backflow of blood and hence clotting. Keep the animal warm.

(ii) Swab the skin with 70% ethanol. Make a sub-costal incision (~3 cm) at the lower margin of the left ribs (scalpel 1 #) and extend this laterally to fully expose the left kidney (blunt-nosed scissors 2 #). Do this for both skin and muscle layers. Gently free the kidney on its vascular stalk (gently tear fascia with cotton buds 7 #) and swing it over away from the underlying psoas muscle. Absorb any small amount of blood.

(iii) Thrust the trochar (3 #) through the psoas at a shallow angle posteriorly to exit the skin about 3 cm caudally from the entry point. Pass the cannula (Appendix) (12 #) straight end first, withdraw the trochar quickly past the bend in cannula to avoid distorting it. Fill the cannula with DAB 1. Check that it can lie naturally flat with the tip pointing caudally parallel and right next to the aorta. Re-make the cannula and/or re-align the trochar direction if not.

(iv) Restrain the hindlimbs, extended. Restrain the left forelimb extended across high and to the right (the rat's) of the chest to bring the operation site into easy view. Pack the wound with saline-moistened gauze (5 #) to keep the kidney and intestines out of the way (retractor 4 #).

(v)   Gently open up the gutter between the aorta and the psoas over 10−15 mm lengthwise (cotton buds; no sharp instruments). The thoracic duct will spring into view with its milky contents. Continue blunt-dissecting, first on the psoas side up towards the diaphragm so that at least 5 mm or more of the duct is free (glass dissectors 6 #). Probe (glass dissector) between the aorta and duct and tear very gently to isolate the duct. Do not puncture the duct at this stage. Keep probing one side then the other of the duct until there is a continuous gap beneath the duct and up to the left of the aorta. Extend the gap to 3−4 mm using the natural spring of blunt-tipped forceps as they open.

(vi)   Pass 5/0 silk with a bent needle (13 #) under the duct, and tie loosely. Pass two ties of 3/0 silk, one through the psoas near the exit of the cannula, one high up at the tip of the bend. Avoid the nerve.

(vii) Encourage the duct to inflate. If necessary block it next to the diaphragm (gentle pressure with a cotton bud) and pump (cotton bud) over the cisterna chyli lower down. Make an incision across about 1/3 of the width of the uppermost face of the duct (iris scissors 9 #). Lymph should visibly emerge, the duct will collapse and the hole must be visible. Enlarge if not. It should be possible to move one's gaze from the operation site and find the hole again without difficulty.

(viii) Grasp the filled cannula with forceps (8 #). Introduce the tip without force into the hole. 2−3 mm should penetrate, almost horizontally. If the tip meets resistance and does not slip cleanly in, withdraw and try again. Going too superficially enlarges the hole (soon so much that it is beyond use); going too deep can tear the whole duct right across. Keep trying if unsuccessful initially, though with practice it should go in first time. It is possible to try making a fresh incision about 2 mm lower down, though this is difficult with a collapsed duct. When satisfied, tug the cannula outside the rat gently downwards to hold it naturally in place. It should not spring out. Monitor the flow (drip from end). No air should enter the cannula; if it does, but otherwise looks all right, then the tip has gone too deep and needs re-insertion.

(ix)   Tighten the ties, double knotted. Check that there are no leaks, and that the flow is maintained.

(x)   Remove the packing, replace the organs (note especially that the spleen does not get twisted). Suture (two layers 13 #).

(xi)   Transfer the rat to a Bollman cage (89). The rat is slightly excitable after recovering consciousness but soon settles, particularly if kept warm and quiet by placing a lid over the cage. The bars must not compress the rat, nor be loose enough to permit it to turn round.

(xii) Start i.v. infusion of DAB 1 (4 ml/h for first 6 h then at half that rate). Offer 0.15 M NaCl in the drinking water to encourage high fluid intake for the first 50 ml, thereafter tap water. Provide food *ad libitum*. Monitor frequently for clots (see text).

(xiii) Collect into sterile DAB 20 (Appendix: 5 ml in 100 ml conical flask) when a steady flow is established, clot-free. Flow is maintained simply by the pressure differential between the rat and the end of the cannula (~15 cm).

Table 3. Mesenteric lymphadenectomy[a].

1.	Anaesthetize the rat, e.g. with ether.
2.	Shave the abdomen, swab with 70% ethanol. Make a midline incision. Identify the junction between the small and large intestine and expose this over sterile drape (*Figure 3*). Using dagger forceps to grasp just beneath the closest end of the lymph node chain, gently tear the lymphatics and mobilize the node free of the fat. Try to remove tissue in one long chain. Control bleeding with cotton buds.
3.	Repair and suture the wound in two layers (skin and muscle). Avoid strangulation of the gut. No special post-operative care is necessary. Allow 6 weeks for recovery of lymphatic connection.

[a]This procedure requires a Personal Licence under the Animals (Scientific Procedures) Act in the UK.

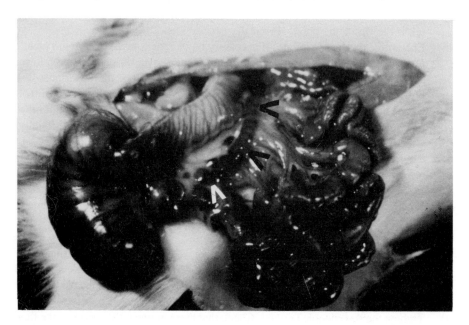

Figure 3. Mesenteric lymph node chain exposed for excision.

2.2.2 *Mesenteric lymphadenectomy*

By removing the mesenteric lymph nodes of a rat and allowing their afferent and efferent lymphatics to rejoin over a few weeks, it is possible to recover thoracic duct lymph derived from the gut wall that has not been filtered by a node, and so still contains dendritic cells (*Figure 1*). The thoracic duct of course conveys lymph derived from sources other than just the gut (see *Figure 4*), and intestinal lymph itself contains lymphocytes, so 95−99% of the cells are still lymphocytes. These may be diminished by sublethal irradiation (5 Gy) on the morning of surgery. Dendritic cells are radioresistant, at least in rats, but small lymphocytes are extremely radiosensitive. The frequency of dendritic cells may then rise to 30%, with the same absolute output as in unirradiated controls ($0.15-2 \times 10^6$/h) for the first 3 days; thereafter the ouput from irradiated rats declines. The procedure in *Table 3* follows that of Pugh *et al.* (44). Post-

Table 4. Peritoneal lavage[a].

1.	Kill the donor (cervical dislocation); or fully anaesthetize by a route not involving the peritoneum. Restrain in the supine position, limbs fully extended. Swab the skin with 70% ethanol.
2.	Inject the appropriate volume (up to 5 ml per fully-grown mouse; 10−15 ml per rat; 50 ml per guinea-pig) of PBS containing 20 U/ml heparin (23-gauge needle).
3.	Massage the abdomen for 1−2 min.
4.	*Either*
	(i) make a small skin incision in the abdominal wall just below the xiphisternum to expose (but not puncture yet) the muscle. Insert a 22-gauge needle a short distance through the muscle, bevel down. Aspirate the fluid while holding the muscle as elevated as possible.
	Or
	(ii) with an assistant to lift the abdominal wall, cut through the skin and muscle making a hole sufficiently wide to admit a fine semi-rigid plastic tube (e.g. PVC, 1.5−2 mm internal diameter) attached to a syringe. Aspirate from different parts of the cavity. Some workers like to use a tube with a side exit at the tip, rather than straight out at the end. Either way 80−90% of the inoculated liquid should be recovered.
5.	Suture with two ligatures if the animal is to recover.

[a]If performed on living animals this procedure requires a Personal Licence under the Animals (Scientific Procedures) Act in the UK.

operative mortality should be less than 10% and can be less than 1%.

2.3 Peritoneal lavage

Four kinds of peritoneal cell populations should be distinguished:

(i) 'Peritoneal wash', taken from a normal animal by simply rinsing the cavity with saline (*Table 4*). This provides 'resident', non-activated macrophages (Section 1.3.1) polymorphs and some other cells. A typical mouse (e.g. PO strain, conventionally reared) yields approximately 10^7 cells, of which 25−35% are macrophages. Rats and guinea-pigs give similar numbers, though in guinea pigs more than 95% may be macrophages.

(ii) 'Elicited' peritoneal cells. These are harvested from animals injected with casein hydrolysate, thioglycollate medium, proteose peptone or other inflammatory stimulus 16−24 h before collection. The yield is about 2×10^7 per mouse; 2×10^8 per rat; 5×10^8 per guinea-pig: they contain 70−90% neutrophils. This then is not a good source of macrophages.

(iii) 'Inflammatory' peritoneal exudate (PEC). As (ii), but taken 3−4 days after thioglycollate or equivalent. Mice and rats yield $1−2 \times 10^7$ per animal, with over 65% macrophages. A guinea-pig may produce approximately 5×10^7 cells.

(iv) 'Activated' peritoneal exudate obtained later following i.p. injection of bacterial or parasitic vaccines. One protocol is to inject 0.7 mg of *C. parvum* vaccine (Wellcome) per 100 g body weight and harvest at day 10. This should give $1−2 \times 10^7$ per rat or mouse with 70−95% macrophages.

In all cases the cell viability ought to be virtually 100%.

Table 5. Bronchial lavage.

1.	Arrange a reservoir containing about 50 ml of PBS about 75 cm above the working surface. Attach via a 3-way stopcock to (a) a 10 ml syringe, (b) tubing, outside diameter 2−3 mm (for a rat). *Completely* fill with PBS (no bubbles).
2.	Under ether or other anaesthetic, exsanguinate the animal either by aortic cannulation (rats; expose and clamp the aorta temporarily while PP50 polypropylene tube is inserted) or nicking the inferior vena cava (mice). Bleeding out minimizes blood contamination.
3.	Open the chest, partially remove the ribs. Expose the trachea. Tie the lavage tube in place.
4.	Fill the lungs under gravity (5−10 ml). Flush in and out three times (syringe); eject from the syringe into a container. Re-fill and flush twice more.

For i.p. injections it is essential to avoid puncturing abdominal organs: monitor for possible contamination by gut contents (look for microorganisms) or by blood. It is instructive for the novice to follow the fate of a small amount of dye injected i.p. (e.g. Indian ink). For injections into living animals (especially larger ones) it may be advisable to use ether anaesthesia because of the muscle-relaxing effect. This allows the progress of the needle tip through the skin and then through the muscle to be felt.

2.4 Bronchial lavage and other sources

Mature macrophages can be recovered by flushing the airways (*Table 5*). Yields should be approximately 5×10^5 for a mouse, $1-5 \times 10^6$ for a rat, with around 80−90% phagocytic cells and high viability. Rat macrophages can also be obtained from the gastro-intestinal tract (24). Human macrophages can be prepared from breast milk as adherent cells from microexudate-treated plates (Section 4.4). The cellular content of milk collected within the first 10 days after parturition averages 2×10^5/ml, with quite a wide range, of which about 40% are adherent cells (69). A method for growing human bone marrow in culture to generate abundant macrophages has recently been described (70).

3. CELLS FROM SOLID ORGANS

3.1 Spleen

In most species the spleen is the largest single aggregate of secondary lymphoid tissue in the body. In neonates the spleen serves a primary haemopoietic and lymphopoietic function as well, but even in mice and rats, very immature at birth, this is finished by 3 weeks of age. The total lymphoid content reaches adult levels at 8−10 weeks of age. As a guide the cell yield from a mouse is $5-10 \times 10^7$ and rat, $2-4 \times 10^8$. Expect about 2×10^5 nucleated cells per mg fresh wet weight, with a viability of 70−80%. By no means all the available cells are recovered even with the most assiduous teasing. If the total cell-associated radioactivity is compared before and after dissociating a rat spleen (cells labelled as immigrants with ^{51}Cr) only about 1/3 is found with the cells after washing (unpublished results, not using enzymes). The rest is in the supernatant, released from damaged cells, or in the splenic residue. The mouse has fewer blood cells in the spleen and it is correspondingly more lymphoid with fewer granulocytes.

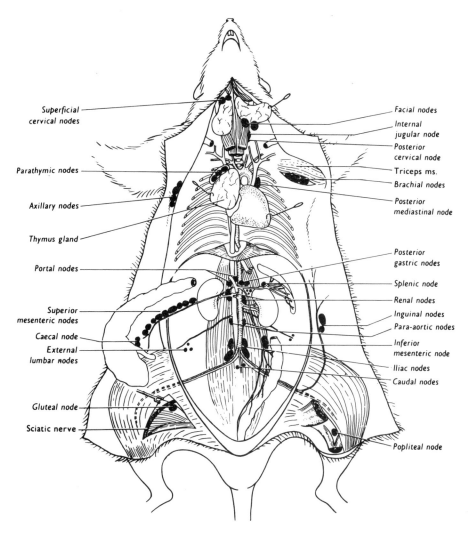

Superficial cervical nodes
Parathymic nodes
Axillary nodes
Thymus gland
Portal nodes
Superior mesenteric nodes
Caecal node
External lumbar nodes
Gluteal node
Sciatic nerve

Facial nodes
Internal jugular node
Posterior cervical node
Triceps ms.
Brachial nodes
Posterior mediastinal node
Posterior gastric nodes
Splenic node
Renal nodes
Inguinal nodes
Para-aortic nodes
Inferior mesenteric node
Iliac nodes
Caudal nodes
Popliteal node

Figure 4. Lymph nodes of the rat (88).

3.2 **Lymph nodes**

What lymph nodes lack in size, they make up for in numbers (*Figure 4*). The mesenteric nodes and the cervical nodes are generally the biggest. The superficial cervical nodes are also readily accessible for biopsy. Worthwhile numbers of cells can also be obtained from the axillary, brachial, inguinal and popliteal nodes. To find lymph nodes, inject trace amounts of indian ink sub-cutaneously (s.c.) and leave for a couple of days; or pontamine sky blue (5% in distilled water, injected i.p. at 1 ml/100 g body weight 10−14 days before dissection) also works. The popliteal node in particular has been used to assay a local graft-versus-host reaction following injection of alloantigenic cells to the hind footpad (71). To expose this node lay the animal prone, extending the hind leg straight at the knee (use your knuckle behind the joint). Cut the skin from the ankle to the hip and expose the muscle. Open the popliteal fossa by cutting quite shallow

Table 6. Dispersion to single cell suspensions.

la and lb are alternatives. See Section 1.2.

1a. Teasing. Use a flat or concave plastic or glass dish, with watchmaker's forceps. Use tissues prepared as in Section 3.8. Hold fast a chunk at a time with one pair of forceps and use the other to stroke the cells out. Alternatively, use the curved edge of blunt forceps rather than sharp points to expel the cells. Continue until the fragments can be broken no further.

1b. Grinding. Express tissue chunks through stainless steel mesh (14 strands mm^{-1}) or a plastic tea strainer, using a syringe plunger or the pestle or a glass homogenizer. Alternatively, use a stainless steel tube about 20 mm in diameter to which is fused the mesh, with a concentric stainless steel plunger to force the fragments through without them escaping round the edges (these are trickier to clean). Rinse the mesh.

2. Enzyme digestion. (Optional for lymphocyte preparations from normal spleen, lymph nodes, thymus. Strongly recommended for Peyer's patch, fetal liver, or all tissues from irradiated or aged animals. Mandatory for FDC.) Chop the tissue (scalpel or scissors) to fragments about 2 mm^3. For the gentlest procedures on lymph nodes make only a single tear in the capsule with needles.

   Transfer to a tube in about 1 ml of nourishing medium containing collagenase (1−8 mg/ml). Incubate in a capped tube for 30 min, triturating gently at 10 and 20 min through a wide-bore pipette to assist disintegration. Neutral protease such as Dispase [2 units/ml, or up to 75 times this (73)] and DNase (0.1 mg/ml) may also be added.

in the fascia between the muscle groups: this causes the node to spring up superficially.

The yield of lymph node cells in a young adult mouse may be $3-5 \times 10^7$, in a rat, $1-1.5 \times 10^8$ ($\sim 0.5-1 \times 10^6$ cells per mg wet weight, with viability of $80-85\%$).

3.3 Tonsil

Tonsil is sufficiently tough that it should be enzyme-digested (usually collagenase), not teased, for maximum cell recovery (*Table 6*).

3.4 Gut-associated lymphoid tissue

Peyer's patches are embedded at intervals along the whole length of the small intestine. There may be up to 30, and their dispersion makes it rather tedious to use this source, since each needs to be dissected from the gut wall before enzyme digestion. They are quite difficult to keep sterile, because of the proximity of the gut contents. Roughly 10^6 cells can be expected from each patch, with greater than 95% viability. Of all the secondary lymphoid tissue sources they have the highest fraction of B cells ($\sim 70\%$). In herbivores the appendix is very enlarged. One rabbit may yield $3-5 \times 10^9$ cells and the organ can be subdivided simply by a stripping technique into a fraction highly enriched for germinal centre cells (72).

3.5 Thymus

The thymus of rats and mice of about 6 weeks old is highly cellular (2×10^8 per mouse; 10^9 per rat in most strains other than PVG) but soon shrinks to, say, a quarter of this by 16 weeks. Thymocytes are delicate, and slightly rough handling will soon lead to an ever-growing gelatinous clump of dead cells entrapping live cells. Inclusion of DNase in handling media can minimize this, but if it happens, it is best to remove the lump rather than to try to break it up. With care, viabilities of $85-90\%$ are achievable. Preparation of thymic 'nurse' cells needs the most careful handling, including digestion rather than teasing.

It is vital to avoid accidentally including the parathymic lymph nodes when removing a thymus. They drain the peritoneum and so can be highlighted by i.p. injection of indian ink. They should be left behind during the dissection rather than cleaned from the organ after excision, when they may be more difficult to identify. If they are mixed in, then of course the thymocytes become contaminated with peripheral B and T cells.

3.6 Fetal liver

The liver changes its cellular composition and its size dramatically according to gestational age. The earliest liver (day $10-11$ in mouse; day 12 in rat) is haemopoietic, with high frequencies of cells that phenotypically resemble pluripotential stem cells (30% Thy-1$^+$ in rat), but in very small numbers (10^4). Very rapidly the erythroid compartment expands and dilutes the stem cells, and this predominates until late gestation in rodents. Pre-B cells appear after day 16, along with myeloid cells. The liver becomes simple to dissect with the unaided eye after about day 15, so this is probably the best stage to use it as a source of haemopoietic stem cells. It should not then be contaminated with T cells.

Re-population of irradiated hosts with this source shows that these stem cells may be different in quality from adult marrow stem cells, in that they continue to overgrow marrow stem cells long after the cell transfer. The yield from a 16-day liver (rat) is around 2×10^7 cells, and there may be $8-14$ fetuses per pregnancy. Collagenase digestion is recommended to improve yield and viability, which should be greater than 90%.

3.7 Bone marrow

Bone marrow contains a mixture of every blood cell type. It is a big organ ($\sim 1-3 \times 10^7$ nucleated cells per g body weight in different species including man). In the young adult, myeloid cells are abundant, especially in animals maintained conventionally, which have a higher granulocyte content than specific-pathogen-free animals. The lymphocytes can be roughly purified from granulocytes and erythroid cells by separation on Metrizoate–Ficoll, analogous to blood (Section 2.1). More precise purifications depend on using appropriate monoclonal antibodies with a depletion method (Chapter 2). The maximum proportion of lymphocytes occurs in younger animals, about 3 weeks in rodents. It may reach 70% or so, though the absolute number continues to increase until about 6 weeks, by which time the frequency is on the decline. The proportion of stem cells is always tiny, ($<<1\%$), so that their complete purification is a formidable problem.

Extraction of marrow from the long bones, the commonest source, is never complete, and the combined content of the femora, tibiae and humeri represents only about 1/3 of all skeletal marrow. Without taking special precautions the flushing procedure (Section 3.9) probably differentially removes axial marrow to some extent, leaving behind the endosteal marrow. This may discriminate against stem cells and perhaps progenitors. Marrow is also left behind at the extremities of the long bones. In mice the overall recovery has been estimated at $60-90\%$, in rats $35-40\%$. In short, what

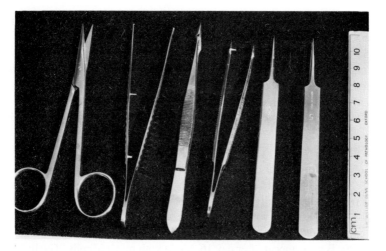

Figure 5. Typical dissecting kit for standard dissection. Note fine-pointed watchmaker's forceps (right) for teasing lymphoid organs.

is flushed from marrow by standard procedures may not be fully representative of marrow *in situ*.

Marrow lymphocytes from adolescent animals are fragile like thymocytes, so cell clumping can occur with marrow suspensions that are left to stand. Thus, for day-long sorts on the fluorescence-activated cell sorter (FACS) we suspend marrow cells in isopycnic Percoll (70%) to inhibit their aggregation.

The yields from one femur of a young adult animal are approximately as follows: mouse $2-4 \times 10^7$; rat $1-2 \times 10^8$; guinea pig $3-5 \times 10^8$. One femur contains $6-8\%$ of the total body marrow. Viability should be greater than 85%: poor viabilities correlate with the 'warm ischaemic' time between killing the animal and flushing the marrow cavity. It helps to have an assistant to try to minimize this.

3.8 Cells from lymphoid organs of rodents

(See *Figure 5* for standard dissecting instruments)

(i)   Kill the animal, by cervical dislocation or ether overdose.

(ii)   Flood the fur with 70% alcohol.

(iii)   Pin out on a dissecting board, belly up.

(iv)   Make a midline incision, jaw to pubis, using blunt-nosed, sharp-bladed scissors. Hold the skin with toothed forceps. Pull back the skin (use fingers) both sides and pin. (Do not cut the muscles yet).

(v)   For the remaining stages work aseptically if cells are to be cultured.

(vi)   For the cervical lymph nodes (*Figure 4*), locate the chain of three or four superficial nodes on each side. Like most nodes, they are partially embedded in fat. Distinguish the slightly yellowish, encapsulated nodes from the softer whiter fat (and from the much larger, slightly pink salivary glands, which they partially overlie). With blunt dissection pull at the tissue immediately around a node, tear its connecting vascular stalk and transfer immediately to rinse in medium in a small Petri dish. Do not crush the node. Collect all nodes in a second dish.

(vii)   Repeat for the deep ('posterior') cervical nodes (one or two on each side).

(viii)   For the mesenteric lymph nodes (including the caecal node), make a midline incision in abdominal muscle. Pin it back. Find the chain of nodes surrounded by fat, starting at the ileo−caecal junction, running parallel to the ileum (*Figure 3*). Dissect as in (vi) as a continuous string if possible. Avoid haemorrhage.

(ix)   For the spleen, distinguish the small, bright red spleen below the stomach to the animal's left from the much larger, more purple liver. With dagger forceps grasp and tear along its length the connective tissue and vascular stalk attaching to the hilum of the spleen. Rinse and transfer as in (vi). Weigh if necessary. Cut into 6−8 chunks (rat only).

(x)   For Peyer's patches, excise the whole of the small gut. Cut into 15 cm lengths. Flush the contents with ice-cold saline. Patches stand out as white blebs often with obvious follicles. Cut around the patch (scalpel or sharp scissors). Transfer to a rinse dish then to a test tube (say 1 ml of medium). Use enzymes (see *Table 6*): teasing alone is inadequate.

(xi)   For the thymus, cut the diaphragm and ribs up both sides and remove the whole sternum. Identify the thymus (white, flat, bilobed). Remove (blunt dissection) the parathymic lymph nodes embedded in connective tissue immediately adjacent. Grasp the posterior edge of the thymus (forceps), raise and free round the edges (scissors). Continue right until clear of the trachea. Avoid haemorrhage. Transfer through a rinse dish to a Petri dish.

(xii)   For fetal liver, grasp the cervix below the junction of the uterine horns with forceps. Cut below the forceps and pull out the V-shaped horns. Cut the Fallopian tubes. Transfer to a 9 cm Petri dish and rinse. Count fetuses; note malformations. Slit the uterus along its length (sharp scissors). Isolate (blunt dissection from uterine wall) and transfer sacs intact to a fresh dish. Slit the membranes, pull out the fetus, decapitate, cut the umbilical vessels and allow to bleed. Transfer through a rinse dish to a dissection dish (use forceps or wide bore fire-polished Pasteur pipette).

(xiii)   Identify the liver (red) and distinguish it from the heart and spleen (>day 16). Tear the abdominal wall (watchmaker's forceps), remove the liver, detach remnants of the gut. Transfer through a rinse to a test tube (say 1 ml of medium) for enzyme digestion.

3.9 Bone marrow cell preparation

(i)   Kill the animal by cervical dislocation. Soak the limbs in 70% ethanol.

(ii)   With the animal prone, cut the Achilles tendon (scalpel). Disarticulate the ankle joint (scissors). Cut off the foot.

(iii)   Cut the dorsal skin from ankle to hip. Reflect the skin (fingers).

(iv)   Cut the remaining muscle insertions at the ankle (scalpel). Break the fibula. Pull back the lower limb muscles.

(v)   Turn the animal over. Cut across the knee joint (scalpel). Disarticulate the knee.

Catch the lip of the epiphysis with bone forceps and twist it off cleanly, bringing the muscle with it. Clean the remaining surface contamination (should be very little), store the tibia on ice until able to flush it.

(vi)   Dissect the muscles from the femur to access the hip joint. Cut the ligaments and muscle insertions at the upper end. Disarticulate the hip joint to gain the femur intact. Again lift away the epiphysis at the knee by twisting with bone forceps. Clean the upper end of femur coarsely free of muscle. Store on ice until ready for flushing.

(vii)   Repeat with the other hindlimb.

(viii) For the forelimb, cut the skin from the scapula to the elbow. Disarticulate the elbow (scissors). Dissect the humerus free of muscle and cut through the shoulder. Cut the epiphysis at the elbow, removing most of the muscle. Clean the humerus and store it on ice, ready for flushing. Repeat with the other side.

(ix)   Cut about 2 mm off the ankle end of the tibia, head of femur from femur, and (flattened) head of humerus (bone forceps) to expose the cavity. Puncture the cavity at each end of each bone with a 23-gauge needle (rat) or 25-gauge needle (mouse).

(x)   Thrust a syringe (5 ml, fresh needle) into each of these cut ends, that is, the opposite ends to the former epiphyses. Check there is a tight junction with the surrounding bone. Hold the bone with forceps over a wide-mouthed container. Rapidly squirt approximately 1 ml of medium (DAB or BSS containing 5% FCS or 0.2% BSA) to expel the marrow plug. Reverse the bone and flush in the opposite direction. Repeat twice more, eventually pushing the needle along the endosteal (inner) surface. Blow out residual liquid with air.

(xi)   When all bones are complete, aspirate the clumps into and out of a syringe with a 21-gauge needle to disperse the cells.

3.10 Final stages common to all methods of dispersion

(i)   For lymphocytes: resuspend the cells thoroughly by repeated aspiration into a Pasteur pipette (they settle quickly). Filter through a single layer of lens tissue, cotton bandage, or a small plug of absorbent cotton wool in a filter funnel over a test tube. Rinse the sample dish or tube and wash the rinse liquid through the filter.

(ii)   Centrifuge. Remove the supernatant by vacuum aspiration from the top downwards (leave 2–3 mm liquid) to remove the fatty layer (particularly prominent with bone marrow).

(iii)   Add about 1 ml of medium to the pellet and aspirate in and out of the pipette until no visible lumps remain. Dilute to 10–15 ml and aspirate with the pipette to distribute the cells evenly. Discard clumps that will not disperse. Repeat (ii) and (iii) (one 'wash') up to three times, according to the particular protocol.

(iv)   Accessory cell sedimentation (may also be employed for lymphocytes). For each 5 ml of suspension, layer over 0.5 ml of 2% BSA (or introduce the albumin as an underlay). Leave to stand for 5 min. Recover the upper layer, leaving lumps behind. (Do not do this when the aim is to collect clusters, e.g. FDC).

(v)   Wash.

4. SIMPLE PURIFICATIONS

4.1 **Dead cells**

4.1.1 *Viability tests*

It is hard to know when a cell has irrevocably died. The true test would be whether its function can recover to normal. Dye-exclusion tests (*Table 7*) reflect the intactness of the plasma membrane. They were validated originally by a correlation between the efficiency of cloning of certain cell lines *in vitro* and the percentage of cells able to exclude dye. Whether normal lymphocytes would show a corresponding correlation for their function is unproven. In addition, subsets of cells in a mixed population may be more or less fragile. So finding that the bulk population has a satisfactory viability does not necessarily mean that a particular subpopulation is equally viable. Regard the viability score as a rough index of cell health rather than an accurate percentage.

Dye exclusion can be done by keeping the dye either out or in. Some dyes cannot penetrate the membrane of live cells, for example, trypan blue, eosin Y, nigrosin. Dead cells therefore become stained. Propidium iodide, a DNA stain, has also been used in two-colour immunofluorescence on the FACS (74). Trypan blue is perhaps the commonest: it must be read as soon as the cells have settled, since after 5 min, more lymphocytes begin to take up dye.

Alternatively, other dyes are retained only by live cells, for example fluorescein diacetate. It stains (fluoresces) when inside the cell because esterases liberate free fluorescein, which cannot escape from intact cells. This is the basis for micro-cytotoxicity testing as in HLA typing.

4.1.2 *Removal of dead cells*

Dead cells are more sticky than live ones. This is the basis of the separation described below which is done in low ionic strength medium (75) to minimize electrostatic ef-

Table 7. Viability testing.

Trypan blue

1. In a microtitre well or small tube, mix 10 μl of cell suspension at $\sim 10^7$/ml with 10 μl of Trypan blue solution (Appendix). Resuspend with a pipette tip.

2. Without delay, run into a haemocytometer chamber (*Table 8*). Allow 1 min for the cells to settle.

3. Within the next 3 min score more than 100 cells for blue (dead) versus unstained (live). Ignore erythrocytes.

Fluorescein diacetate

1. Freshly dilute stock fluorescein diacetate (Appendix) 10 μl in 1 ml of DAB.

2. To 50 μl of cell suspension in DAB or BSS ($\sim 3 \times 10^6$/ml) add 5 μl of diluted fluorescein diacetate. Mix well. Leave to stand at room temperature for 15 min. Centrifuge and carefully remove all the supernatant.

3. Perform a cytotoxicity test if wanted, for example, on microscale under oil (1 μl per reaction).

4. Score in a haemocytometer, or under oil with a fluorescence microscope set up for fluorescein optics. Live cells fluoresce green.

fects. It is quick, effective (>95% pure live cells) and gives good recoveries (>85%), but does not remove erythrocytes. Cells that have died in culture are also not removed by this procedure. Non-viable cells are also less dense, so they sediment less quickly. However, spinning a cell suspension over Metrizoate−Ficoll (Section 2.1), or over BSA (76) paradoxically takes them with the red cells to the pellet. Interface cells are therefore recovered with high viability with some loss of live cells. Dead cells also give a smaller low-angle light scatter signal in a FACS (Chapter 2), so can be gated out electronically during analysis or sorting. However, using the FACS simply to remove dead cells is extravagant and inefficient.

(i)   Siliconize all glassware by immersion in 'Siliclad' (Appendix), or dichloro-dimethyl silane (5% in $CHCl_3$) and thoroughly rinse.
(ii)   Loosely pack a siliconized Pasteur pipette with 5−10 mm of absorbent cotton wool.
(iii)   Dilute the cell suspension (up to 6×10^8/ml, maximum capacity ~2×10^8 per column) 0.75 vol. with 8 vols of isosmotic sorbitol (0.308 M dissolved in water for the mouse), plus 1.25 vol. of 0.308 M glucose.
(iv)   Drip cells slowly through the column and rinse with sorbitol−glucose medium.

4.2 Lysis of erythrocytes

A few red cells generally do no harm and may even be helpful markers, for example when tiny numbers of lymphocytes are being centrifuged. However, some cell fractionation procedures are limited by total cell numbers (FACS sorting, 1 g sedimentation, for instance). Red blood cells may also interfere with cell labelling studies (e.g. by ^{51}Cr for instance), so in these cases they are worth getting rid of, particularly from bone marrow or spleen. Erythrolysis may also be useful after rosetting (Chapter 2).

Two methods are commonly used. One is to spin over Metrizoate−Ficoll, as in Section 2.1 above. The other is to lyse in isotonic ammonium chloride solution (77) as described below. Some workers suspect the high $[NH_4^+]$ may cause damage and prefer to use flash lysis in water (mix concentrated cell suspension with 10 vols of water for 10 sec; rescue without further delay with 10 vols of 2× concentrated medium).

(i)   Prepare Tris-buffered NH_4Cl (Appendix). Equilibrate to room temperature.
(ii)   Centrifuge the cells at 20°C. Resuspend 3×10^8 cells in 1 ml of NH_4Cl solution. Leave to stand for 10 min at room temperature.
(iii)   Dilute with greater than 5-fold excess medium, mix well. Centrifuge.
(iv)   Repeat if lysis is incomplete.

4.3 Density gradient separation

A protocol is included here because it forms part of most methods for preparing dendritic cells. For a thorough discussion of separating cells by refined isopycnic methods see (78). The density-cum-aggregation method using Metrizoate−Ficoll has already been described (Section 2.1). Other gradient materials include metrizamide, colloidal silica and albumin. With all these methods the distinction between rate sedimentation and equilibrium density (isopycnic) centrifugation should be kept clear. In the first, all the cells are less dense than the medium and so will sooner or later sediment right through. In the second, the medium is sufficiently dense to support the cells, however long they are spun. Separation is achieved by imposing a gradient, (stepped, linear or more fancy) and spinning to equilibrium. The gradient may either be prepared in advance (more common), or generated during centrifugation (in the case of colloidal silica).

Metrizamide is a derivative of metrizoate, which is highly water-soluble and simple to prepare as the underlay of a step gradient. At 14.5 g of metrizamide plus 100 ml of medium (79), it has been used to give a quick, one-step purification of accessory cells from mouse lymph node cells and for recovering dendritic cells from afferent lymph (Section 2.2.2). It is relatively expensive (about five times the cost of either Percoll or BSA).

Colloidal silica (Percoll, Pharmacia) contains silica particles coated with polyvinylpyr-rolidone to render them non-toxic, in suspension. Dense solutions of very low viscosity can be made from this stock, appropriately diluted with concentrated medium to maintain isotonicity; it is simple to handle and relatively inexpensive. There are many applications. Self-generating Percoll gradients have been used to isolate antigen-presenting cells from human blood, and of dendritic cell−T cell clusters from mouse Peyer's patch (41).

Albumin is rather more awkward to handle. It needs extensive dialysis and neutralization if bought as the crude 'Fraction V' powder, and is slow to dissolve. Pre-treatment is avoidable by obtaining commercial 30% or 35% solutions. It is viscous at the high concentrations, so it is difficult to generate continuous gradients in conventional gradient makers, and it also takes cells longer to reach their isopycnic point in a gradient. Nonetheless it is widely used, especially in step gradients. See (80,81) for detailed protocols of isopycnic centrifugation.

The method given below is a cut-down procedure for initial purification, before the adherence step, in dendritic cell purification from mouse spleen (41). From 4×10^8 spleen, expect $2-3 \times 10^7$ low density cells, with dendritic cells concentrated 10- to 15-fold. It is essential to optimize conditions (especially the BSA density) for other species and other sources. The following modifications apply to the isolation of mouse FDC (47): lower step, 1.060 g/ml, 6 ml; upper step, 1.030 g/ml, 3 ml; overlay $2-4 \times 10^8$ enzyme-digested lymph node cells; spin at 8500 g, 4°C, 60 min and harvest 1.03/1.06 interface).

4.3.1 *Albumin density step centrifugation*

(41, modified by J.Austyn, personal communication).

(i)   Prepare BSA solution, density 1.08 g/ml. Dissolve 10.0 g of BSA (Sigma, Fraction V) in 18.6 ml of PBS + 2.9 ml of 1 M NaOH + 6.5 ml of distilled water by leaving to stand for 48 h at 4°C without stirring. The refractive index should be 1.385. Filter through a 0.45 μm filter with a pre-filter. Store in sterile aliquots at 4°C.

(ii) Suspend the cell pellet in this albumin, 10^8/ml. Transfer to a swinging-bucket centrifuge tube. Overlay with medium containing 10% newborn calf serum. Centrifuge at 10 000 g for 20 min, 4°C.

(iii)   Recover the interface cells, floating over the 1.08 g/ml layer. Wash twice.
(iv)   The cells in the pellet can be used as a lymphocyte source, though still con-
       taminated with accessory cells.

4.4 Adherence

What makes some cells stick to solid surfaces and others not? Intuitively one might
expect ionic forces to be important, since most cells have a net negative charge at
physiological pH, yet the commonly used substrates discussed below are neutral (cross-
linked dextran or Sephadex) or hydrophobic (polystyrene and siliconized glass). Paradoxically, untreated glass is acidic, not basic, and so might be expected to repel cells, yet
it is the classically used substrate. Perhaps the high dielectric constant of most media
is sufficient to minimize electrostatic interaction. The metabolic activity of the cells
has a major influence, and thus the temperature and nature of the medium help to determine adherence. Shortman (82) distinguished 'physical' from 'active' adherence, the
latter needing the cell to metabolize normally and therefore only becoming operative
at 37°C.

The adherence procedures described here are done at 37°C. Generalizations are
sometimes difficult because of species differences (rat versus mouse dendritic cells for
instance). In broad terms, however, the following hierarchy of cell types applies, in
order of decreasing adherence: macrophages > dendritic cells = antibody-forming
cells > B lymphocytes > T lymphocytes = erythrocytes. Dead and damaged cells
tend to be very sticky, perhaps because of adherent DNA they release.

4.4.1 *Macrophages*

To use 'active' adherence to enrich for macrophages, which are amongst the stickiest
of cells because of their habit of rapidly flattening on surfaces, it is not difficult to
get rid of the unwanted, non-adherent cells. More difficult is to recover the wanted
population without damage. On a hydrophobic surface the degree of adherence seems
to correlate in the mouse with the amount of expression of the antigen Mac-1 (Crocker
and Gordon, personal communication).

The protocol in Section 4.4.3 is based on experiments with peritoneal cells (resident
and inflammatory). It should apply also to spleen and lung Mac-1$^+$ macrophages and
bone marrow monocytes, but not bone marrow macrophages or Kuppfer cells, which
are Mac-1$^-$. It is very simple, and manipulates the divalent cation concentration to
release the cells. It is especially valuable after culture of macrophages (up to 7 days),
when the cells are relatively less sticky and often float off. With tissue culture plastics
both mouse peritoneal cells and human blood monocytes stay firmly stuck unless the
surface has been coated with the 'micro-exudate' from the BHK cell line (31; commercially available as 'ECM plates', International Biotechnologies Inc.). After incubation
on this surface adherent cells can be recovered in good yield (>80%), with greater
than 95% viability and 90% pure judged by phagocytosis and spreading. Plastics can
also be coated with gelatin or collagen (83). Macrophages can be removed with a 'rubber policeman' (10−20 mm length of glass rod encased in silicone rubber tubing), trypsin (with or without 0.1−3 mM EDTA) or lignocaine (10−15 mM), but here the
viabilities and yields can be expected to be lower. 'Non-stick' surfaces [poly-tetrafluoro-

ethylene, 'Teflon', (84) and 'poly-HEMA' (85)] have also been tried. With the latter the degree of adhesiveness can be varied by altering the concentration in alcoholic solution as the plates are prepared.

Typical yields from peritoneal cells after 1 h attachment:

	Resident	Inflammatory	
	Mouse	Rat	Mouse
Plated $\times$ 10^{-6}	50	20	10
Recovered $\times$ 10^{-6}	5	5	5

(About 95% of the adherent cells are recovered in >95% viability).

4.4.2 *Dendritic cells*

There are two broad routes to preparing dendritic cells, either from solid organs then purifying, or from thoracic duct lymph of lymphadenectomized animals. The advantage of the latter is that it is a freshly prepared suspension that has received minimal treatment *in vitro*. This must be weighed against the surgical intervention required to prepare the animals. For mouse spleen and lymph node, and for human blood (86), the Steinman-based methods rely on the sequence adherence, then non-adherence after overnight culture. Because the cells are rare, it is simpler to initially purify the low density cells (ϱ <1.08) on a BSA gradient (Section 4.3). Then the adherence step can be done in a single dish, since otherwise 10 times as many cells have to be handled. For mouse Peyer's patch, and for all rat sources, dendritic cells are non-adherent immediately after isolation. Klinkert *et al.* (87) describe the rat methods in detail.

A neat way to remove macrophages, which may depend on either phagocytosis or on adherence, is to incubate the cells with carbonyl iron (Appendix) and remove those cells attached to the iron with a magnet. Incubate 5×10^7 cells in nourishing medium (Section 1.4.2) with approximately 200 mg of thoroughly washed and autoclaved iron powder for 45 min (resuspending every 5 min). A simple bar magnet will then rapidly deplete the phagocytic cells. For complete removal of the finest iron particles use a stronger, horseshoe magnet. Expect a yield of 30−50% of the non-adherent cells from mouse spleen (3).

4.4.3 *Plate method for dendritic cells*

Use tissue culture grade plastic (polystyrene). Macrophages adhere very firmly to this, mouse dendritic cells adhere initially then detach.

(i)   Suspend the cells in nourishing medium containing 1−10% FCS or 0.2% BSA at approximately 2.5×10^6/ml. Add 10 ml per 45 mm Petri dish (40 ml per 85 mm dish; 1 ml per well of 24-well cell culture plate). Incubate 1−3 h at 37°C (CO_2 incubator unnecessary). Pipette gently with a wide-bore Pasteur pipette to wash away non-adherent cells. Examine microscopically to monitor, especially around the edges where cells concentrate because of the meniscus effect.

(ii) Re-culture on normal plates in medium with 5% FCS in a humidified CO_2 incubator for 18 h. Detach the dendritic cells, now less adherent, by gentle pipetting as in (i). Separate the dendritic cells from macrophages by either Fc rosetting or re-adhering macrophages as in (i) using fresh medium.

(iii)   Fc rosetting. Count the cells. Suspend them at about 5×10^6/ml. Add an equal volume 1% erythrocyte−anti-erythrocyte (EA) suspension (Appendix). Mix well. Centrifuge gently (150 g, 5 min, 4°C). Leave to stand for 20 min at 4°C. Gently resuspend. Centrifuge over Metrizoate−Ficoll (Section 2.1), or dense BSA (Section 4.3, $\varrho = 1.080$). Aspirate the layer that floats (dendritic cells, Fc receptor negative).

4.4.4 *Plate method for macrophages*

The aim here is to recover the adherent fraction. Use a surface to which macrophages stick less strongly (not tissue culture plastic). Bacteriological grade polystyrene (untreated) is simplest and cheapest. Alternatives are discussed in Section 4.4.1.

(i)   Incubate the cell suspension as in Section 4.4.3(i) for 1 h.
(ii)   Gently aspirate away the non-adherent fraction using medium containing Ca^{2+} to rinse.
(iii)   Briefly and gently rinse once or twice with PBS (Ca^{2+} and Mg^{2+}-free), add the same PBS containing 5 mM glucose and leave at 37°C for 15 min. Macrophages often detach spontaneously; any still adherent may be taken off with gentle pipetting. Avoid mechanical recovery or EDTA if possible.

4.4.5 *Column method for depletion of adherent cells*

Columns can consist of glass beads, glass wool (Appendix), Sephadex G-10 (Pharmacia) or a variety of other substrates (Section 4.4).

(i)   Half fill a syringe barrel (equipped with an outlet tap) with the substrate (50 ml syringe for cell loads of 10^8-10^9; 10 ml for loads of $<10^8$). Equilibrate with nourishing medium containing 10% FCS or 0.4% BSA at 37°C. N.B. cover the column — bicarbonate-buffered media rapidly go alkaline.
(ii)   Introduce the cell suspension ($\sim 1.5 \times 10^8$/ml) in the same medium plus protein as an overlay. Allow the cells to enter the column bed. Rinse the cells in with an equal volume of pre-warmed medium. Adjust the flow-rate to a trickle so that the first cells emerge in about 10 min. Collect the effluent. Rinse with two further volumes of warmed medium, at the same flow-rate.

4.4.6 *Nylon wool columns for T cells*

(i)   Boil or autoclave 0.6 g of wool from a Leuko-Pak filter in four changes of distilled water. Pack to 5 ml in a 10 ml syringe barrel with an outlet tap. Equilibrate in nourishing medium at 37°C for 30 min. Eliminate air bubbles. Rinse with two column volumes of medium.
(ii)   Load the cells (10^8 in 1 ml of medium with 5% FCS). Allow to penetrate the column with a further 0.5 ml rinse. Cover. Incubate at 37°C for 30−40 min. Elute at about 1 drop/sec with 20 ml of pre-warmed medium.

5. CELL COUNTING

Cells in suspension sediment very rapidly. Immediately before sampling for any reason, including for counting, mix by gentle pipetting. This is obvious but vital.

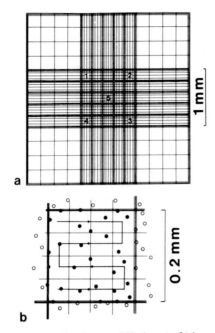

Figure 6. Standard haemocytometer ruling (improved Neubauer). (**b**) is a magnified view of the square 1 (length of side 0.2 mm) in (**a**) and is the field of view seen typically under a 40× objective. A scanning pattern is suggested (filled circles count). Chamber depth is normally 0.1 mm. See *Table 8*.

Table 8. Use of the haemocytometer.

1.	Rinse the chamber in medium, water, then alcohol or acetone. Dry. Moisten two parallel sides of a coverslip; immediately press down these edges hard on each side of the counting chamber trough. Look for Newton's rings (interference-generated colours between slip and slide). The coverslip should not move even if the slide is inverted.
2.	The optimal cell concentration is 10^7/ml, but the scorable range is from 2×10^5 to 4×10^7. Dilute in medium, trypan blue or Turk's as appropriate, to these final concentrations. Mix well.
3.	Transfer to one half of the chamber. Run in sufficient to cover the semi-chamber area, but not flood the surrounding trough.
4.	Place on a horizontal surface to allow the cells to settle (~1 min).
5.	Under ×10 or ×40 objective, count at least 200 cells according to pattern (*Figure 6b*). Score only those cells wholly inside the area or touching the upper and left borders of the squares.
6.	Calculate the concentration. Standard chamber depth is 0.1 mm. One square (i.e. whole of *Figure 6b*) has sides of 0.2 mm, area 0.04 mm^2. Multiply the total counts in 25 such squares (i.e. the whole of central area) by 10^4 to get concentration in 10^6/ml. Do not forget factor for dilution if performed.

5.1 Haemocytometer

This is the simplest, cheapest and most informative way of enumerating cells. Their morphology, gross microbial contamination, debris, proportion of red cells, etc., can be monitored by inspecting the cells themselves, rather than watching electronic blips on a screen. Both live and dead cells can be scored using the dye-exclusion test (*Table*

29

7). The disadvantage of rather poor statistical precision by comparison with an electronic counter is unlikely to be serious in most immunological applications.

For many purposes, the cells can be counted in the medium in which they are suspended. Erythrocytes can be identified by their smaller size, their highly refractile circumference and sometimes by their reddish tinge. If a definitive nucleated cell count is required, dilute the cell suspension in Turk's solution, which lyses erythrocytes with acetic acid and stains nuclei purple.

5.2 Electronic particle counting

The Coulter counter draws a known volume of diluted cell suspension $(5-100 \times 10^3/\text{ml};$ 10 ml or more needed) through a hole (usually 50 μm) across which an electrical potential is maintained. As a cell passes, it increases the electrical resistance by an amount proportional to its volume. The voltage spike is amplified and those above a definable threshold are counted. It can therefore discriminate cells according to their size. Erythrocytes can thus be gated out electronically provided they are not in excessive concentration. In spleen, bone marrow and blood cell counting, however, they should be lysed, by adding one drop of saponin ('Zaponin') immediately before counting.

The counting threshold should be determined in advance by preliminary calibration. For unlysed cells we use greater than 30 μm^3 for total cells (red and white); greater than 120 μm^3 for lymphocytes and a rather arbitrary greater than 290 μm^3 for large lymphocytes. After Zaponin treatment nucleated cells are scored as greater than 30 μm^3. These values can be obtained by noting the threshold corresponding to the edge of the plateau, as counts on a given suspension are graphed against the incrementing threshold. They can be cross-checked against a haemocytometer count.

Sometimes cells pass through together within the resolving time of the machine. This coincidence increases as a square function of the cell concentration. The raw count must therefore be corrected according to the table supplied by the manufacturers. Background should be subtracted if low counts are recorded (<5000). Note that Zaponin addition may increase background due to tiny air bubbles generated while mixing it in. Let these float to the surface before taking a count.

6. ACKNOWLEDGEMENTS

I thank my colleagues in the Department for their comments, especially Paul Crocker, Jonathan Austyn, Gordon Macpherson and David Chao. Data from many D.Phil. theses have stiffened some of the numbers (including S.Highnam, S.Hirsch, A.Robinson); I am especially grateful to Chris Pugh for generously allowing me to publish *Figures 1* and *3*. *Figure 4* is reproduced from (88) by kind permission of Cambridge University Press, and *Figure 6* is from ref. 1 by kind permission of Blackwell Scientific Publications.

7. REFERENCES

1. Hudson,L. and Hay,F.C. (1976) *Practical Immunology*. Blackwell's Scientific Publications, Oxford.
2. Weir,D.M., Blackwell,C., Herzenberg,L.A. and Herzenberg,L.A., eds (1986) *Handbook of Experimental Immunology*. 4th edition, Blackwell Scientific Publications, Oxford.
3. Mishell,B.B. and Shiigi,S.M. (1980) *Selected Methods in Cellular Immunology*. W.H.Freeman, San Francisco.

4. Osmond,D.G. (1985) *J. Invest. Dermatol.*, **85**, (Suppl. 1) 2s.
5. Coffman,R.L. (1983) *Immunol. Rev.*, **69**, 5.
6. Opstelten,D., Deenen,G.J., Rozing,J. and Hunt,S.V. (1986) *J. Immunol.*, **137**, 76.
7. Wekerle,H., Ketelsen,U-P., and Ernst,M. (1980) *J. Exp. Med.*, **151**, 925.
8. Ritter,M.A., Sauvage,C.A. and Cotmore,S.F. (1981) *Immunology*, **44**, 439.
9. Kyewski,B.A. (1986) *Immunol. Today*, **7**, 374.
10. Reichert,R.A., Weissman,I.L. and Butcher,E.C. (1986) *J. Immunol.*, **136**, 3529.
11. Micklem,H.S., Ford,C.E., Evans,E.P., Ogden,D.A. and Papworth,D. (1972) *J. Cell. Physiol.*, **79**, 293.
12. Hunt,S.V. and Fowler,M.H. (1981) *Cell Tissue Kinet.*, **14**, 445.
13. Ford,W.L. (1975) *Prog. Allergy*, **19**, 1.
14. Abbas,A.K. (1982) *Adv. Immunol.*, **32**, 301.
15. Greaves,M.F. (1986) *Science*, **234**, 697.
16. von Willebrand,E. and Hayry,P. (1978) *Cell. Immunol.*, **41**, 358.
17. von Willebrand,E., Soots,A. and Hayry,P. (1979) *Cell. Immunol.*, **46**, 309.
18. Tilney,N.L., Strom,T.R., Macpherson,S.G. and Carpenter,C.B. (1975) *Transplantation*, **20**, 323.
19. Morhenn,V.B., Wood,G.S., Engelman,E.G. and Oseroff,A.R. (1984) *J. Invest. Dermatol.*, **81**, (Suppl.1), 127s.
20. Sullivan,S., Bergstresser,P.R., Tigelaar,R.E. and Streilein,J.W. (1985) *J. Invest. Dermatol.*, **84**, 491.
21. Schuler,G. and Steinman,R.M. (1985) *J. Exp. Med.*, **161**, 526.
22. Oudghiri,M., Seguin,J. and Deslauriers,N. (1986) *Eur. J. Immunol.*, **16**, 281.
23. Lee,T.D.G., Shanahan,F., Miller,H.R.P., Bienenstock,J. and Befus,A.D. (1985) *Immunology*, **55**, 721.
24. Sminia,T. and Jeurissen,S.H.M. (1986) *Immunobiology*, **171**, 72.
25. Burns,J., Rozenzweig,A., Zweiman,B., Moskowitz,A. and Lisak,R. (1984) *J. Immunol.*, **132**, 2690.
26. Weiss,L. and Greep,R.O. (1983) *Histology*. 5th edition, McGraw Hill.
27. Fossum,S. and Ford,W.L. (1985) *Histopathology*, **9**, 465.
28. Humphrey,J.H., Grennan,D. and Sundaram,V. (1984) *Eur. J. Immunol.*, **14**, 859.
29. Mosier,D.E. and Coppleson,L.W. (1968) *Proc. Natl. Acad. Sci. USA*, **61**, 542.
30. Sorg,C. and Bowers,W.E. (1984) *Immunobiology*, **168**, 133.
31. Ackerman,S.K. and Douglas,S.D. (1978) *J. Immunol.*, **120**, 1372.
32. Werb,Z., Banda,M.J., Takemura,R. and Gordon,S. (1986) In *Handbook of Experimental Immunology*. Weir,D.M., Blackwell,C., Herzenberg,L.A. and Herzenberg,L.A. (eds), Blackwell Scientific Publications, Oxford, p. 471.
33. Beller,D.I., Kiely,J-M. and Unanue,E.R. (1980) *J. Immunol.*, **124**, 1426.
34. Nathan,C.F. and Root,R.K. (1977) *J. Exp. Med.*, **146**, 1648.
35. Werb,Z. and Chin,J.R. (1983) *J. Exp. Med.*, **158**, 1272.
36. Robinson,A.P., White,T.M. and Mason,D.W. (1986) *Immunology*, **57**, 231.
37. Talle,M.A., Rao,E., Westberg,E., Allegar,N., Makowski,M., Mittler,R.S. and Goldstein,G. (1983) *Cell. Immunol.*, **78**, 83.
38. Robinson,A.P., White,T.M. and Mason,D.W. (1986) *Immunology*, **57**, 239.
39. Dijkstra,C.D., Dopp,E.A., Joling,P. and Kraal,G. (1985) *Immunology*, **54**, 589.
40. Steinman,R.M., Kaplan,G., Witmer,M.G. and Cohn,Z.A. (1979) *J. Exp. Med.*, **149**, 1.
41. Steinman,R.M., Voorhis,W.C.van and Spalding,D.M. (1986) In *Handbook of Experimental Immunology*. Weir,D.M., Blackwell,C., Herzenberg,L.A. and Herzenberg,L.A. (eds), Blackwell Scientific Publishers, Oxford, p. 49.1.
42. Steinman,R.M., Witmer,M.D., Nussenzweig,M.C., Gutchinov,B. and Austyn,J.M. (1983) *Transplant. Proc.*, **15**, 299.
43. Austyn,J.M. and Gordon,S. (1981) *Eur. J. Immunol.*, **11**, 805.
44. Pugh,C.W., MacPherson,G.G. and Steer,H.W. (1983) *J. Exp. Med.*, **157**, 1758.
45. MacPherson,G.G. and Pugh,C.W. (1984) *Immunobiology*, **168**, 338.
46. Klaus,G.G.B., Humphrey,J.H., Kunkel,A. and Dongworth,D.W. (1980) *Immunol. Rev.*, **53**, 3.
47. Schnizlein,C.T., Kosco,M.H., Szakal,A.K. and Tew,J.G. (1985) *J. Immunol.*, **134**, 1360.
48. Lilet-Leclercq,D., Radoux,D., Heinen,E., Kinet-Denouel,C., Defraigne,M.P., Houben-Defresne,M.P. and Simar,L.J. (1984) *J. Immunol. Methods*, **66**, 235.
49. Naiem,M., Gerdes,J., Abdulaziz,H., Stein,H. and Mason,D.Y. (1983) *J. Clin. Pathol.*, **36**, 167.
50. Ralph,P. (1986) In *Handbook of Experimental Immunology*. Weir,D.M., Blackwell,C., Herzenberg,L.A. and Herzenberg,L.A. (eds), Blackwell Scientific Publishers, Oxford, p. 45.1.
51. Minowada,J., Tatsumi,E., Sagawa,K., Lok,M.S., Sugimoto,T., Minato,K., Zgoda,L., Prestine,L., Kover,L. and Gould,D. (1984) In *Leukocyte Typing*. Bernard,A., Boumsell,L., Dausset,J., Milstein,C. and Schlossman,S.F. (eds), Springer Verlag, p. 519.
52. Reinherz,E.L., Haynes,B.F., Nadler,L.M., Bernstein,I.D., (eds) (1986) *Leukocyte Typing II*. Springer Verlag, New York, Vol. 3, p. 1.

53. Bauer,S.R., Holmes,K.L., Morse,H.C.III and Potter,M. (1986) *J. Immunol.*, **136**, 4695.
54. Gowans,J.L. and Uhr,J.W. (1966) *J. Exp. Med.*, **124**, 1017.
55. Smith,M.E. and Ford,W.L. (1983) *Immunology*, **49**, 83.
56. Williams,N., Kraft,N. and Shortman,K. (1972) *Immunology*, **22**, 885.
57. Boyum,A. (1968) *Scan. J. Clin. Lab. Invest.*, **21**, Suppl. 97, p. 77.
58. Ford,W.L. (1978) In *Handbook of Experimental Immunology.* Weir,D.M. (ed.), Blackwell Scientific Publications, Oxford, 3rd edition, p. 23.6.
59. Patrick,C.C., Graber,C.D. and Loadholt,C.B. (1976) *J. Immunol. Methods*, **11**, 321.
60. Beverley,P.C.L. (1986) In *Handbook of Experimental Immunology.* Weir,D.M., Blackwell,C., Herzenberg,L.A. and Herzenberg,L.A. (eds), Blackwell Scientific Publishers, Oxford, p. 58.1.
61. Callard,R.E. and Smith,C.M. (1981) *Eur. J. Immunol.*, **11**, 206.
62. Smith,J.B., McIntosh,G.H. and Morris,B. (1970) *J. Anat.*, **107**, 87.
63. Sprent,J. (1973) *Cell. Immunol.*, **7**, 10.
64. Dineen,J.K. and Adams,D.B. (1970) *Immunology*, **19**, 11.
65. Sanders,A.G., Florey,H.W. and Barnes,J.M. (1940) *Br. J. Exp. Pathol.*, **21**, 254.
66. Grindlay,J.H., Cain,J.C., Bollman,J.L. and Mann,F.L. (1950) *Surgery*, **27**, 152.
67. Lascelles,A.K. and Morris,B. (1961) *Q. J. Exp. Physiol.*, **46**, 199.
68. Tilney,N.L. and Murray,J.E. (1968) *Ann. Surgery*, **167**, 1.
69. Balkwill,F.R. and Hogg,N.M. (1979) *J. Immunol.*, **123**, 1451.
70. Hume,D.A., Allan,W., Goldner,J., Stephens,R.W., Doe,W.F. and Warren,H.S. (1985) *J. Leukocyte Biol.*, **38**, 541.
71. Ford,W.L., Burr,W. and Simonsen,M. (1970) *Transplantation*, **10**, 258.
72. Waksman,B.H., Ozer,H. and Blythman,H. (1973) *Lab. Invest.*, **28**, 614.
73. Monfalcone,A.P., Szakal,A.K. and Tew,J.G. (1986) *J. Leukocyte Biol.*, **39**, 617.
74. Parks,D., Hardy,R.R. and Herzenberg,L.A. (1983) *Immunol. Today*, **4**, 145.
75. von Boehmer,H. and Shortman,K. (1973) *J. Immunol. Methods*, **2**, 293.
76. Shortman,K., Williams,N. and Adams,P. (1972) *J. Immunol. Methods*, **1**, 273.
77. Boyle,W. (1968) *Transplantation*, **6**, 761.
78. Miller,R.G. (1986) In *Handbook of Experimental Immunology.* Weir,D.M., Blackwell,C., Herzenberg,L.A. and Herzenberg,L.A. (eds), Blackwell Scientific Publications, Oxford, p. 54.1.
79. Macatonia,S.E., Edwards,A.J. and Knight,S.C. (1986) *Immunology*, **59**, 509.
80. Marbrook,J. (1980) In *Selected Methods in Cellular Immunology.* Mishell,B.B. and Shiigi,S.M. (eds), W.H.Freeman, San Francisco, p. 188.
81. Raidt,D.G. (1980) In *Selected Methods in Cellular Immunology.* Mishell,B.B. and Shiigi,S.M. (eds), W.H.Freeman, San Francisco, p. 193.
82. Shortman,K., Williams,N., Jackson,H., Russel,P., Byrt,P. and Diener,E. (1971) *J. Cell Biol.*, **48**, 566.
83. Lin,H-S. and Gordon,S. (1979) *J. Exp. Med.*, **150**, 231.
84. Van der Meer,J.W.M., Bulterman,D., van Zwet,T.L., Elzenga-Claasen,I. and van Furth,R. (1978) *J. Exp. Med.*, **147**, 271.
85. Folkman,J. and Moscona,A. (1978) *Nature*, **273**, 345.
86. van Voorhis,W.C., Hair,L.S., Steinman,R.M. and Kaplan,G. (1982) *J. Exp. Med.*, **155**, 1172.
87. Klinkert,W.E.F., LaBadie,J.H. and Bowers,W.E. (1982) *J. Exp. Med.*, **156**, 1.
88. Tilney,N.L., (1971) *J. Anat.*, **109**, 371.
89. Waynforth,H.B. (1980) *Experimental Surgical Techniques in the Rat*, Academic Press, London, p. 115.

8. APPENDIX

Materials and reagents

Reagent	Preparation
Ammonium chloride solution (ACT)	Mix 9 vols of NH_4Cl (0.83% w/v in water) with 1 vol. of Tris (2.06% w/v in water, adjust pH to 7.65). Check pH is 7.2. Sterilize by membrane filtration.
Albumin, bovine	Dissolve BSA (Cohn Fraction V, Sigma) approximately 200 g in 25 mM of Tris-saline buffer, pH 7.4 (3.03 g of Tris base, 8.2 g of NaCl in 1 l of water: adjust pH)

for 24−48 h at 4°C. Adjust the pH to 7.4. Centrifuge for 45 min at 14 000 r.p.m. Discard the pellet. Dilute in the same Tris-saline buffer to 10% w/v. Check the OD_{280} of 1:100 dilution is 0.66. For BSA solutions for use at high concentration (>20%), first dialyse BSA against water extensively and freeze-dry.

Cannula, tail vein	Melt off and discard the hub of a 23-gauge × 11/4 inch needle. Insert into an approximately 40 cm polythene cannula of internal diameter 0.58 mm (Portex).
Cannula, thoracic duct	Using polythene tubing (see tail vein cannula) make a tight loop, unkinked. Warm by swift passage through a Bunsen flame to fix the bend (*Figure 2*). The bend should be a full 180°. Cut an upward-facing 45° bevel with a scalpel at the tip.
Carbonyl iron	Grade SF, particle size 4.5−5.2 μm. Wash in water, sterilize by dry heat. Do not use batches that impart colour to water.
Dulbecco's 'A' + 'B' (DAB)	To 500 ml of sterile PBS add 2.5 ml of 'B' sterile salts (Oxoid). This gives $MgCl_2$, $CaCl_2$ each at a final concentration of 1 g/l.
DAB + 1 U/ml heparin (DAB 1)	To 500 ml of sterile DAB add 500 U of preservative-free heparin.
DAB + 20 U/ml heparin (DAB 20)	To 100 ml of sterile DAB add 2000 units of preservative-free heparin.
Erythrocyte−antibody complexes (EA)	Wash sheep blood three times in saline. Mix a 5% suspension with hyperimmune rabbit anti-sheep erythrocyte serum at just sub-agglutinating dose for 20 min at 20°C. Wash three times in DAB/0.2% BSA/3 mM NaN_3. Resuspend to 10% v/v. Wash once just before use.
Fluorescein diacetate	5 mg/ml in acetone. Thaw immediately before use. Store dark, aliquotted at −20°C.
Glass beads	Diameter 450 μm is suitable [e.g. Ballotini micro range No 8 (Jencons)]. Wash with acid (concentrated HCl: concentrated HNO_3:water, 4:4:1 by vol.), rinse, wash with alcoholic KOH, rinse, siliconize with 'Siliclad', rinse and dry. For re-use, wash with saline, boil with detergent, wash with alcoholic KOH and re-siliconize.
Glass dissector	3 mm soda glass rod, drawn and bent in a flame as in *Figure 2*. Fire polish the tip. Experiment to get the best tip diameter.

Metrizoate – Ficoll (=Isopaque – Ficoll) (=Hypaque – Ficoll)	The Ficoll concentration determines the final density. For human cells, use 9% w/v to give a final density of 1.078 g/ml. For rats, make 14% w/v to give a final density of 1.087 g/ml. Prepare stock solution in distilled water by extended stirring at room temperature. Mix 10 vols of sodium metrizoate solution (32.8% w/v) (e.g. 'Isopaque', Nyegaard) with 24 vols of sterile Ficoll solution. Check the density.
Phosphate-buffered saline (= Dulbecco's 'A')	NaCl 8.0 g/l, KCl 0.2 g/l, Na_2HPO_4 (anhydrous) 1.15 g/l, KH_2PO_4 0.2 g/l (tablets, Oxoid).
'Siliclad' (= 'Sigmacote')	5% dimethyldichlorosilane in $CHCl_3$. Can be re-used many times.
Trypan blue	0.2% w/v in PBS/3 mM NaN_3 (extended stirring). Microcentrifuge before use.

CHAPTER 2

Preparation of lymphocyte subpopulations

DON W.MASON, W.JOHN PENHALE and JON D.SEDGWICK

1. INTRODUCTION

It has long been recognized that immunological responses involve interactions between different cell types that make up the immune system. The classical early experiments on T cell/B cell collaboration in the antibody response were possible only because virtually pure populations of T cells could be obtained from the thymus and T cell-free B cells from the bone marrow. However, since the demonstration that subpopulations of lymphoid cells can be distinguished by serological means, the study of functional heterogeneity within the cells of the immune system has become a major aspect of immunological research. This work has depended almost entirely on the availability of monoclonal antibodies that recognize tissue-restricted antigens. Cell fractionation procedures, involving the use of these reagents, have superseded virtually all other methods of isolating the individual cellular components of the immune system.

This chapter deals with four serological methods of cell separation, namely:

(i)   cell sorting by flow cytofluorography;
(ii)   rosetting;
(iii)   panning;
(iv)   complement-mediated lysis.

Of these (ii) and (iv) are depletion procedures, that is they remove, from a heterogeneous cell population, cells that express a certain cell membrane antigenic marker. In contrast, techniques (i) and (iii) isolate both the antigen-positive and antigen-negative subsets. Further discussion of the merits and demerits of these various methodologies will be deferred to the end of this chapter.

2. FLOW CYTOFLUOROGRAPHY AND CELL SORTING

Optical/electronic devices, that measure cell size and detect the presence of cell-bound fluorochrome-labelled antibodies, have come into widespread use over the last 10 years. They have proved to be powerful tools in the study of lymphocyte heterogeneity at both the phenotypic and functional level. Several of these flow cytofluorographs are commercially available, for example, the Becton Dickinson FACS Systems, the Coulter EPICS and the Ortho Cytofluorograf. The instruments are produced in two forms — either as analytical machines or as devices which additionally can separate subpopulations of cells on the basis of the analytical data generated. The term 'cell sorter' is commonly applied to this second type of device.

Commercially available machines differ in some aspects, particularly with regard to the method of assessing cell size or volume. Readers are referred to manufacturers' literature for details, but the following description is sufficiently general to illustrate the principles, and the advantages and disadvantages of using cell sorters to separate cell subpopulations.

2.1 Principle: analysis of cell phenotypes

A single-cell suspension, appropriately labelled with fluorochrome-conjugated antibodies to cell surface antigens, is forced through the nozzle of the machine under pressure. The cells, confined to the axis of the resultant fluid stream by a concentric sheath of cell-free fluid, pass through a laser beam which is focused onto the stream. The laser light is scattered and reflected by the cells and it also excites the fluorochromes bound to the cell membrane. The scattered and reflected light and that emitted by the excited fluorochromes is detected by a suitable arrangement of lenses, optical filters and photo-electric devices (*Figure 1*). The electrical signals generated are analysed by computer and may be processed at once, or stored for subsequent examination. When the flow

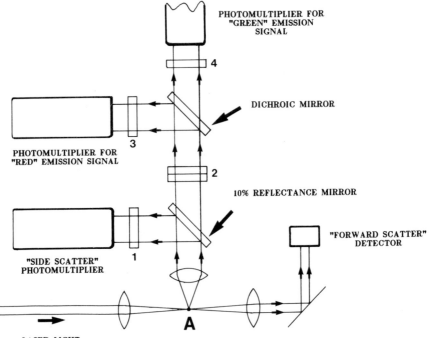

Figure 1. Optical system for a four-parameter flow cytofluorograph. The diagram shows, in schematic form, the arrangement of mirrors and optical filters for a flow cytofluorograph constructed to detect 'forward scatter', 'side scatter' and two colour fluorescence. The nozzle is above the plane of the diagram and the fluid stream, which intersects the laser beam at A, is at right angles to it. The diagram is not to scale. For a system in which the two fluorochromes are fluorescein (green) and PE (red) the following optical devices are used in the positions indicated: Position 1: neutral density filter, 2: 520 nm long pass interference filter, plus 530 nm long pass glass filter, 3: 575/25 nm band pass filter, 4: 560 nm short pass interference filter. The dichroic mirror is a 560 nm short pass. Note that interference filters vary considerably in their optical characteristics and carefully selected filters are required. Manufacturers now supply kits of filters with very good wavelength selectivity.

cytofluorograph is used to separate subpopulations of cells these electrical signals are also used to activate the cell sorting process.

For those instruments in which the intersection of the fluid stream and laser beam occurs in air (i.e. after the stream has left the nozzle assembly) four pieces of data are commonly generated.

(i) *Forward light scatter.* That is, light that is deflected out of the laser beam through a small angle. The intensity of this co-called 'forward scatter' signal is a measure of cell size. As dead cells give rise to a smaller forward scatter signal than live cells this parameter is particularly useful in discriminating between viable and non-viable cells. It also permits a clear distinction to be made between nucleated cells and mammalian erythrocytes.

(ii) *90° light scatter.* The light that is deflected, by the cells, through a large angle, depends not on cell size but rather on the heterogeneity of cell structure. Thus cells with large numbers of cytoplasmic granules or other organelles scatter more light than erythrocytes or lymphocytes.

The simultaneous measurement of forward scatter and 90° scatter (commonly referred to as 'side scatter') allows the identification of lymphocytes, monocytes and granulocytes in peripheral blood (1), and is potentially of value in the purification of subpopulations of cells from bone marrow (see below).

(iii) *Fluorescein emission.* As described in Section 2.5.1, fluorescein is readily coupled to antibodies; such conjugates can be used to label those cells that express the antigen(s) to which the antibodies specifically bind. Argon lasers have a strong emission line at 488 nm, close to the excitation maximum for fluorescein, and are most frequently used as light sources for cell sorters. The same laser beam generates the forward scatter and side scatter signals and, with the recent introduction of the fluorochrome B-phycoerythrin, it can also be used very effectively to generate a second fluorescence signal (see below).

(iv) *Phycoerythrin (PE) emission.* The chromophore B-phycoerythrin, a protein with a molecular weight of 250 000, is found in seaweed where it plays a role in photosynthesis. It is also efficiently excited by light at 488 nm, but its emission maximum occurs around 575 nm, that is at a wavelength about 50 nm longer than that for fluorescein. These characteristics, combined with its high quantum yield (i.e. the efficiency with which the fluorochrome converts the exciting radiation into emitted light), make it an ideal fluorochrome for flow cytofluorographic analyses. By suitable choice of optical filters the emission from PE can be distinguished from that from fluorescein, so that the two fluorochromes can be used simultaneously. PE is commercially available covalently linked to avidin (Serotec) and a suitable labelling protocol, using the two fluorochromes is given in Section 2.3.3. It may be noted that alternative fluorochromes to PE exist, but none has such good fluorescence characteristics in this wavelength range.

The signals generated by the four detectors can, after suitable amplification, be viewed on a visual display unit (VDU) in a variety of ways:

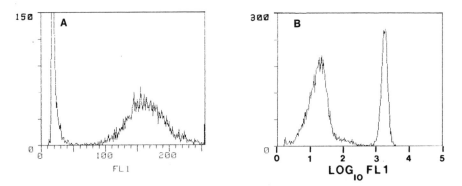

Figure 2. Advantage of logarithmic over linear displays of fluorescence histograms. Rat thoracic duct lymphocytes (TDL) were labelled with a mouse monoclonal antibody against rat CD4 antigen, washed and incubated with fluorescein-conjugated rabbit $F(ab')_2$ anti-mouse Ig. Fluorescence histograms, obtained on a Becton Dickinson FACS, are displayed: in (**A**) both ordinate (cells/channel) and abscissa (cell fluorescence brightness) scales are linear, while in (**B**) the abscissa is a logarithmic scale.

(i) The first is a simple histogram which plots, for example, cell frequency versus cell size or cell frequency versus fluorescence. Most cell sorters can convert the two fluorochrome-derived signals to logarithmic form and histograms of cell frequency versus log fluorescence are often preferable to arithmetic histograms. The latter tend to conceal heterogeneity of fluorescence of weakly positive cells, and fail to display the cell frequency of very dull cells which 'overshoot' the top end of the ordinate scale (cf. *Figure 2 A and B*).

(ii) The second form of display, which allows simultaneous viewing of data from two different sensors, generates a dot on the screen of the VDU for each cell passing through the laser beam. The position of each dot is determined by the amplitude of the signals from the two sensors selected. Such an '*X* − *Y*' dot display is illustrated in *Figure 3* where, in this case, the *X* coordinate for each dot is determined by the amplitude of the 'forward scatter' signal and the *Y* coordinate by the 'side scatter' signal.

(iii) The final display format also deals simultaneously with data from two different sensors, but generates a contour plot with each contour representing a pre-selected cell frequency (*Figure 4*). Unlike *X* − *Y* dot displays, contour plots can be generated only after all the data have been entered into the computer memory and the relevant computer programme executed. The former type of display, although less quantitative than the contour plot, is sufficient for many purposes.

In addition, so called 'isometric' displays are available: these attempt to generate a semblance of a three-dimensional view of a contour plot. In general they contribute little to the clarity of presentation of data and we have not found them to be useful.

2.2 Cell sorting

To sort the cells issuing from the nozzle of the machine into two subpopulations according to their detected characteristics, the fluid stream is first induced to break up into separate droplets by a microscopically small vertical vibration of the nozzle assembly.

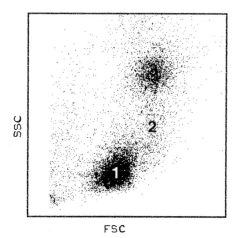

Figure 3. *'X−Y'* dot display of scatter signals generated by rat bone marrow cells. Rat bone marrow cells, depleted of erythrocytes by hypotonic flash lysis, were analysed on a FACS using 'forward scatter' (FSC) and 'side scatter' (SSC) signals to generate the *'X−Y'* dot display shown. These two parameters demonstrate the existence of three cell types: **1**, small mononuclear cells: **2**, large mononuclear cells (blasts); **3**, granulocytes.

The droplets are given an electrical charge as they form at the end of the unbroken fluid stream, by applying a charging pulse to the whole stream. The polarity of this pulse is predetermined by the experimenter. Thus, for example, droplets containing brightly fluorescent cells may be given a positive charge, and those containing dull cells a negative one. More complex sorting criteria can be chosen, which make use of all of the four parameters measured for each cell. The charged drops then pass through a transverse electric field, which is formed between two metal plates differing in potential by about 3 kV. Positively charged drops are deflected towards the negative plate and negatively charged ones towards the positive plate. The resultant diverging streams of droplets are then collected in separate tubes, while the undeflected component of the stream, formed of droplets that contain either no cells or cells whose parameters do not satisfy the chosen sorting criteria, is discarded.

2.3 Practical considerations regarding cell sorting

2.3.1 Handling cells

For cell sorting to be performed satisfactorily a number of simple rules need to be observed.

(i)   Ensure that the cell sample contains no cell debris or aggregates of dead cells. These may block the orifice of the nozzle and stop the sorting process. Alternatively, partial blockages can occur which deflect the fluid stream. Note also that some antibodies used to label cells can cause leukocyte agglutination, so that the machine registers two or more cells as a single one. Remove aggregates of dead cells by filtering the suspension through a double layer of lens tissue and dissociate agglutinated leukocytes by forcing the suspension fairly vigorously through a 25-gauge hypodermic needle. Such treatment does not significantly affect cell viability.

(ii)   Choose the right size nozzle for the cells to be separated. As a rule we use a 50 μm diameter nozzle for cells up to about 15 μm diameter and a 100 μm diameter nozzle for larger cells.

(iii)   Determine whether the fluorescence signal is a consequence of specific labelling of the cells. Run unlabelled cells through the machine first to evaluate the level of autofluorescence and follow these by a negative control sample in which an irrelevant antibody is used to label the cells. For example, with rat lymphocytes, the negative control we use is incubated with a mouse monoclonal antibody to a human complement component, followed by fluorescein-conjugated rabbit F(ab')$_2$ anti-mouse Ig

(iv)   Avoid 'capping' of the fluorescent label by keeping the cells at 4°C and/or using 10 mM sodium azide in the medium. We keep our cell suspensions cold, since 10 mM sodium azide at ambient temperature is reportedly toxic for cells.

(v)   When rare cells are being isolated, collect the deflected droplets directly into a fluid medium. Otherwise the small volume of deflected cells may dry out during sorting, since sorting runs of 6−7 h are not uncommon. When sorting rare cells it is impossible to see the deflected droplets since these are too infrequent to form a visible stream. In these circumstances it is useful to monitor the arrival of the deflected droplets at their collection point. We have developed an electronic device for this purpose and use it routinely (2).

(vi)   When harvesting the sorted cells by centrifugation of the collecting tubes, add 1% bovine serum albumin to discourage the cells from sticking to the walls of the tubes.

2.3.2 *Sterile sorting*

To sterilize the cell sorter for the separation of cells for subsequent tissue culture it is sufficient to introduce a 0.2 μm Millipore filter into the sheath fluid supply line, and to flush through this filter about 10 ml of absolute ethanol. The tube connecting the sheath fluid reservoir to the filter is clamped off and the alcohol injected, via a syringe, into a side arm situated between the clamp and the filter. The alcohol passes through the filter, along the sheath fluid line, into the nozzle assembly and then, retrogradely, through the tube that delivers the cell suspension to the nozzle. After 20 min the side arm is clamped off, the in-line clamp is removed, and fresh sheath fluid run through the system for approximately 20 min. It is not necessary to pre-filter the sheath fluid, but always make it up with 10 mM sodium azide.

2.3.3 *Labelling of cells with fluorochrome-tagged antibodies*

For many applications a 'sandwich' technique is to be preferred since such a method allows the use of unmodified hybridoma tissue culture supernatants. When two different fluorochromes are used a more complex protocol must be followed.

For single fluorochrome work, steps (ii) and (iii) of the procedure set out below are employed. For two colour applications the full protocol described has proved successful (*Figure 4*).

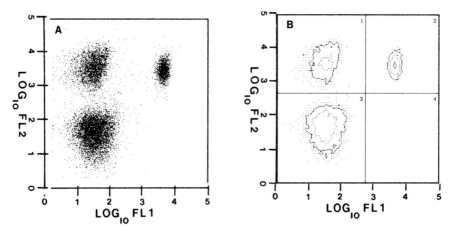

Figure 4. Comparison of '*X−Y*' dot display to contour plot. The figure shows, in (**A**) the '*X−Y*' dot display obtained from rat TDL that were labelled with mouse-anti-rat CD8 monoclonal antibody (FL1-fluorescein) and mouse anti-rat CD5 (FL2-phycoerythrin) according to the protocol in the text. The display clearly shows that the CD8-positive cells are a subset of the CD5-positive ones. In (**B**) the identical data are displayed as a contour plot. All scales are logarithmic. Laser power was 200 mW, 488 nm wavelength.

(i)   Prepare the desired lymphoid cell suspension (Chapter 1)

(ii)   Incubate cells with mouse monoclonal antibody that recognizes cell surface antigen A. Use 25 μl/10^7 cells. Wash twice.

(iii)   Incubate with fluorescein-conjugated rabbit F(ab')$_2$ anti-mouse Ig (RAM−FITC) at 20 μg/ml. Wash twice.

(iv)   Block any free mouse Ig binding sites on the RAM−FITC by incubating the cells for 20 min in 1% heat inactivated normal mouse serum.

(v)   Incubate the cells with biotin-conjugated mouse monoclonal antibody to cell surface antigen B (20 μg/ml). Wash twice.

(vi)   Finally, incubate the cells with avidin-conjugated phycoerythrin (PE−avidin) at approximately 20 μg/ml and wash twice.

All incubations are at 4°C and are for 20 min−1 h in duration. Antibody A can be in the form of tissue culture supernatant. The biotinylated antibody B is prepared, as described below, from mouse hybridoma antibody isolated, as purified immunoglobulin, from ascitic fluid. Optimum concentrations of the reagents must be determined by preliminary trial and the above figures are for guidance only. Tissue culture supernatants can usually be diluted at least 3-fold. Contrary to popular belief, antibody reaction kinetics are not particularly fast (3), but incubation times can be reduced in length if higher concentrations of reagents are used. However, the use of more concentrated reagents is wasteful so that one needs to balance time saved against expense.

Some consideration should be given as to which monoclonal antibody will be used with RAM−FITC and which one will be biotinylated for use with PE−avidin. The emission spectra for fluorochromes tend to have rather sharply defined short wavelength limits, but their longer wavelength emission often tails off rather slowly with increasing wavelength. Thus, although fluorescein has an emission maximum at around 530 nm it fluoresces up to 575 nm, where PE has its peak emission. It is not possible therefore to design an optical filter that will pass PE emission, but totally exclude that from fluorescein (the converse problem, of PE emission breaking through the fluorescein signal, is much less severe because PE emits very little in the 530 nm range). Flow cytofluorographs have electronic compensation devices that help to overcome the problem of 'green' to 'red' breakthrough, but these devices, have some limitations. Therefore, where very different labelling intensities are anticipated, it is preferable to make the 'green' (fluorescein) signal the weaker one.

For analytical purposes it is sufficient to label about 5×10^6 cells. For a cell sort lasting all day about $1-2 \times 10^8$ cells are required.

2.4 Yields, purities and sort rates

Cell sorters typically produce separated populations that are $97-99\%$ pure. Cell yields are, in our experience, never greater than 40% of the starting number and, although one can account for about half of the 60% that are lost, about 30% disappear without trace. It is probable that they get destroyed in the droplet-forming process.

A typical sorting run would produce the following set of data.

Cells labelled	1.5×10^8
Cells recovered	5×10^7
Purity of 'bright' fraction	97%
Purity of 'dull' fraction	99%
Sort rate	5.5×10^3 cells/sec
Duration of sort	7.5 h

2.5 Preparation of conjugated antibodies

2.5.1 Conjugation of purified antibodies with fluorescein isothiocyanate

(i)   Conjugation buffer. Make the following solutions in distilled water:
   A. Na_2CO_3 5.3%
   B. $NaHCO_3$ 4.2%
   C. NaCl   0.85%

(ii)   Mix 5.8 ml of A with 10 ml of B. Take 1 vol. of this mixture and add it to 9 vols of C. Adjust the pH to 9.5 by the addition of small amounts of A (if pH is too low), or B (if pH is too high).

(iii)   Transfer the purified antibody into the conjugation buffer by de-salting it on a Sephadex G-50 (Pharmacia) column pre-equilibrated with the buffer. It is important that no azide is present as this interferes with the conjugation reaction.

(iv)   Adjust the antibody concentration to $4-6$ mg/ml. (The starting concentration, before de-salting, should therefore be >10 mg/ml).

(v)   Dissolve (FITC) Isomer 1 (Nordic) to 1 mg/ml in the conjugation buffer. Add 0.3 ml to each 1 ml of antibody solution.

(vi)   Incubate in the dark for 2 h at room temperature.

(vii)   Separate the conjugated antibody (1st peak) from free FITC on a Sephadex G-50 column pre-equilibrated with phosphate-buffered saline (PBS) pH 7.4, containing 10 mM sodium azide.

(viii) Measure the OD_{495} and OD_{280} of the conjugated antibody. The ratio should be approximately 1 for optimum conjugation. Calculate the protein concentration as:

$$\frac{OD_{280} - (OD_{495} \times 0.35)}{1.4} \text{ mg/ml}$$

(ix) Store, in aliquots, at $-20°C$.

Example: 10.4 mg rabbit F(ab')$_2$ anti-mouse Ig at 6.1 mg/ml gave, after conjugation and diluting 1:10, optical densities of: $OD_{280} = 0.78$; $OD_{495} = 0.89$. Ratio $OD_{495}:OD_{280} = 1.1$. Antibody concentration = 3.36 mg/ml and total yield 9.7 mg.

This reagent gave satisfactory labelling of rat lymphocytes, pre-incubated with mouse monoclonal antibodies to cell surface antigens, at a dilution of 1:200, that is an antibody concentration of about 17 μg/ml.

2.5.2 *Biotinylation of purified antibodies*

This method is that of Dr B.Roser, Cambridge, UK.

(i) Use biotin (linker)-N-hydroxysuccinimide ester (Pierce and Warriner).
(ii) Prepare antibody in 0.1 M NaHCO$_3$ buffer, pH 8.4, at a concentration of 2−5 mg/ml.
(iii) Weigh the ester immediately before use (must be dry) and make up to 20−40 mg/ml in dimethylsulphoxide.
(iv) Add 150−200 μg of ester per 1 mg of antibody and incubate for 2 h at room temperature.
(v) Separate the conjugate on a Sephadex G-25 column pre-equilibriated with PBS containing azide. Store at $-20°C$.

3. ROSETTING

The method described has been developed from one described by Parish and Hayward (4). It has been used successfully to fractionate subpopulations of cells from a variety of single cell suspensions, including thoracic duct lymphocytes, thymocytes, splenocytes, lymph node cells and bone marrow cells.

The technique permits one to remove, from a cell population, a subset of cells reacting with a particular antibody. The latter is generally a monoclonal antibody, but immunoabsorbent-purified polyclonal antisera have been used in some instances.

3.1 **Principle**

Antibody is coupled to sheep erythrocytes (SRBC) by means of chromic chloride and the antibody-coated red cells are then mixed with the leukocyte population to be fractionated. The SRBC bind to those cells that express the relevant antigen and large aggregates form which can be spun out by centrifugation. The supernatant contains the cells that are antigen-negative. The purity of these cells is typically better than 99% (as assessed by subsequent flow cytofluorographic analysis). Yields are about 60% of theoretical, but can be increased by resuspending the cell pellet in fresh medium and repeating the rosetting and centrifugation steps. This increases the total yield to about 80%.

3.2 **Preparation of chromic chloride solution**

(i)   Dissolve 0.5 g of chromic chloride ($CrCl_3.6H_2O$) in 500 ml of 0.9% sodium chloride at room temperature.

(ii)   Adjust the pH to pH 5.0 by careful addition of 1 M sodium hydroxide.

(iii)   Repeat the pH adjustment three times each week for 3 weeks (the pH drifts downwards between intervals).

(iv)   The reagent is now ready for use. It will remain usable, if stored at room temperature, for at least 2 years, and no preservative is required.

3.3 **Preparation of antibody-coated sheep erythrocytes**

The SRBC used for rosetting are coated with rabbit anti-mouse Ig as follows.

(i)   Wash the SRBC four times with 0.85% sodium chloride (occasional batches of SRBC are not suitable because they lyse when washed in saline).

(ii)   To 10 ml of a 5% (v/v) suspension of the washed SRBC add 800 μg of immunoabsorbent-purified rabbit anti-mouse Ig and, with vigorous mixing, 400−500 μl of 0.1% chromic chloride (*all in saline*).

(iii)   Incubate at room temperature for 5 min by which time the majority of the erythrocytes will sediment down as a consequence of the agglutination produced by the chromic chloride.

(iv)   Wash the antibody-coated erythrocytes twice in PBS and once in Dulbecco's A+B medium/bovine serum albumin (DAB/BSA). A little haemolysis during the PBS washes often occurs and is of no consequence.

(v)   Resuspend the SRBC in 10 ml of DAB/BSA and use as described in the rosetting protocol.

The following points should be noted:

(i)   Rabbit anti-mouse Ig, when immunoabsorbent-purified by elution off a mouse Ig column, cross-reacts with Ig of related species such as the rat. To remove these cross-reactive specificities absorb the antiserum on an Ig column of the relevant species. Although this removes the great bulk of the cross-reactive antibody, a little remains and this can result in rosette formation between antibody-coated SRBC and, for example, rat B cells. To prevent this add 10% normal rat serum to rabbit anti-mouse Ig-coated SRBC before using them to rosette rat lymphocytes. Clearly, if the aim of the rosette depletion is to remove B cells then the cross-reactivity is actually beneficial and in this case cross-reactive antibody may be used to coat the erythrocytes.

(ii)   Chromic chloride coupling is ineffective at physiological pH, so the immunoabsorbent-purified rabbit anti-mouse Ig should either be dialysed against saline before use, or prepared in normal buffers at a protein concentration in excess of 1 mg/ml. In the latter case the amount of buffer transferred with the antibody is too little to interfere with the coupling reaction.

(iii)   This sensitization procedure is very reliable provided erythrocytes are used that do not haemolyse during the initial washes in saline. We commonly use batches that have been kept in Alsever's solution at 4°C for 2−3 weeks after delivery from the supplier.

3.4 **Method**

3.4.1 *Standard protocol*

All the steps described are carried out at 4°C.

(i)   To 10^9 washed and pelleted lymphoid cells add approximately 50 µg of monoclonal antibody. (We shall assume, in what follows, that the monoclonal antibody is of mouse origin). If the antigen-positive cells are only a minor sub-population, proportionally less antibody may be used.

(ii)   Incubate for 1 h.

(iii)   Wash the cells twice in DAB containing 0.2% BSA, or some other suitable cell handling medium.

(iv)   Resuspend in 10 ml of DAB/BSA. Retain a few million of the labelled cells for subsequent analysis (see later).

(v)   Transfer the remainder to a 20 ml screw cap bottle together with 10 ml of 5% SRBC coated with rabbit anti-mouse Ig antibody (Section 3.3). If the monoclonal antibody used in the first step is not of mouse origin, then an appropriate choice of rabbit anti-immunoglobulin must be made.

(vi)   Top up the bottle with DAB/BSA until, on replacing the cap, only 0.5 ml of air space remains above the fluid.

(vii)   Mix the contents thoroughly by rotating the bottle end-over-end on a vertical wheel for 20 min in a cold room at 4°C.

(viii) Centrifuge the bottle at 160 g for 45 sec and harvest the supernatant that contains the antigen-negative cells.

(ix)   If a high yield is important, gently resuspend the pellet with a Pasteur pipette and then top up the bottle as before. Mix end-over-end for 10 min to re-form any aggregates that may have become dissociated by the pipetting.

(x)   Centrifuge the bottle exactly as before and harvest the supernatant.

(xi)   Pool the supernatants from the two centrifugations and spin down the cells. Remove contaminating SRBC by ammonium chloride lysis or flash lysis with distilled water.

(xii)   Wash the cells in DAB/BSA and count. The yield should be 60% for the one-step process, and 80% for the two-step. Note that these yields are obtained only if the original cell suspension is essentially 100% viable. Flash lysis removes damaged and dead cells as well as SRBC. If cell viability of the starting population is significantly less than 100% then the yield will be proportionally reduced.

(xiii) Examine the purity of the harvested cells by incubating an aliquot with RAM−FITC. Determine the percentage of labelled cells either by fluorescence microscopy or flow cytofluorography.

(xiv)   Determine the percentage of antigen-positive cells in the starting population by concurrently labelling the cells retained from the pre-depletion suspension.

(xv)   If a flow cytofluorograph is not immediately available labelled cells can be kept at 4°C for several days if fixed with 1% formalin as follows. Resuspend the fluorochrome-labelled cells in 0.5 ml of DAB/0.2% BSA/10 mM sodium azide, add 0.5 ml of 2% formalin in PBS. The 2% formalin should be adjusted to pH 7.2 with a few drops/100 ml of 1 M HCl before use and can be kept as a stock solution.

45

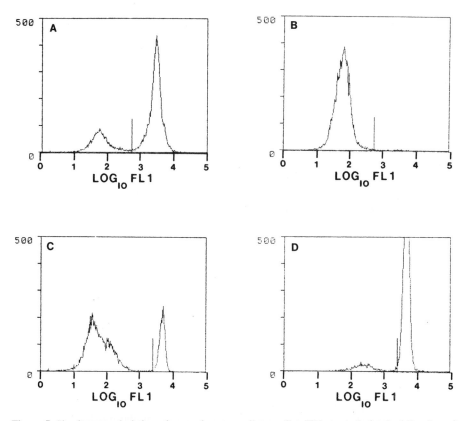

Figure 5. Simultaneous depletion of more than one cell type. Rat TDL were depleted of B cells and CD4-positive T cells by rosetting (Section 3.4.1). The lymphocytes were incubated in a mixture of monoclonal antibodies that react with rat Ig kappa chains (MRC OX-12) and two non-competing anti-CD4 monoclonals (W3/25 and MRC OX-35). Pre-depletion and post-depletion samples were examined on a Becton-Dickinson FACS and details are set out in *Table 1*. The FACS histograms show: (**A**) the pre-depletion sample labelled with MRC OX-12, MRC OX-35 and W3/25 monoclonal antibodies followed by fluorescein-conjugated rabbit F(ab')$_2$-anti mouse Ig. Cell number/channel is plotted in the ordinate and log fluorescence on the abscissa. There are 74.4% cells with brightness above that shown by the marker; (**B**) in the post-depletion sample labelled with the same antibodies, only 0.8% of cells are brighter than the marker; (**C**) in pre-depletion cells labelled with an anti-CD8 monoclonal antibody (MRC OX-8), 23.3% of cells are positive; (**D**) in the post-depletion sample labelled for CD8-positive cells, 90.8% are positive. Note that the depletion process has also enriched the 'null' population from 2.3% to 9.2%.

(xvi)   By incubating a cell population with an appropriate mixture of monoclonal antibodies it can be simultaneously depleted of more than one phenotypically distinct cell type. A typical result is shown in *Figure 5* and *Table 1*.

3.4.2 *Depletion of rare cells*

If the cell population to be removed is present at low frequency, ($<20\%$) the above procedure is modified to ensure adequate aggregate formation.

(i)   Carry out the rosetting procedure exactly as described above as far as the 20

Table 1. FACS analyses of TDL depleted of B cells and CD4-positive T cells.

Sample	Total cell number $\times 10^{-7}$	% positive cells			Observed yield Theoretical maximum yield[c]
		Ig^+ or $CD4^+$	$CD8^+$	$Null^a$	
Pre-depletion	26.4	74.4	23.3	2.3	–
Post-depletion	4.8	0.8	90.8	9.2 (calculated value $= 9.0$)[b]	71%

[a]The percentage of null cells was calculated as $100 - (74.4 + 23.3)$, i.e. 2.3%.
[b]The calculated value is $2.3 \times \dfrac{100}{(100 - 74.4)}$ i.e. 9.0%
[c]The theoretical maximum yield is that expected with no losses, i.e.
$26.4 \times 10^7 \times \dfrac{(100 - 74.4)}{100} = 6.76 \times 10^7$

     min end-over-end mixing (step vii). At this stage the monoclonal antibody-labelled cells form rosettes with the sensitized SRBC, but these rosettes are too infrequent for aggregation to occur.

(ii)   Divide the contents of the 20 ml bottle equally between two identical 20 ml bottles and add 5 ml of a 5% suspension of SRBC, coated with mouse Ig, to each. Top up the bottles with DAB/BSA leaving a 0.5 ml air bubble as before.

(iii)   Carry out a second 20 min period of end-over-end mixing. The rosettes formed in the first rosetting step co-aggregate with the RBC/RBC rosettes formed in the second step and can be removed by differential centrifugation ($160\ g$, 45 sec) as in the standard protocol.

3.4.3 *The direct method*

If monoclonal antibody is available as immunoglobulin purified from ascitic fluid, or when an immunoabsorbent-purified antibody to a cell surface antigen can be prepared, then these may be coupled directly to SRBC.

    The procedure is precisely the same as that of the standard protocol except, of course, that no incubation of the cell population with monoclonal or immunoabsorbent-purified antibody is required. This method is less suited to the simultaneous depletion of more than one cell type, and is not useful for the removal of rare cells. However, it has been used successfully in those applications that do not involve these complications (5).

3.5 **Rosetting cells for subsequent tissue culture**

The rosetting procedure can readily be carried out using conventional tissue culture sterile techniques. It is not necessary to Millipore filter the chromic chloride solution before use because of its germicidal properties.

4. SEPARATION OF LYMPHOCYTES USING PLASTIC SURFACES COATED WITH ANTI-IG ANTIBODIES ('PANNING')

This procedure is based on the observation that polystyrene surfaces can adsorb proteins and that the antigen-binding capabilities of antibodies are retained (6). Subsequently, the phenomenon has been applied to the separation of lymphocyte subpopulations (7,8).

4.1 **Principle**

A heterogeneous population of lymphocytes is allowed to settle onto the bottom of a plastic Petri dish coated with a relevant antibody. The antigen-positive cells become bound to the plastic, while the antigen-negative cells can be readily decanted off (negative selection). After gentle washing to remove non-adherent cells, the antigen-positive cells can also be recovered by more vigorous pipetting (positive selection). Recovery of the adherent population may be facilitated by the use of soluble eluting agents (see Section 4.2.1).

In practice lymphocytes are usually pre-incubated with a subpopulation-specific monoclonal antibody (or mixtures of such antibodies), and the dishes are coated with immunoabsorbent-purified anti-Ig antibody of the appropriate specificity. Consequently those lymphocytes that bind the monoclonal antibody become bound to the plastic via a monoclonal antibody−anti-Ig bridge (indirect method). If highly purified subpopulation-specific antibody is available this may be adsorbed directly to the Petri dishes (direct method).

4.2 **Methods**

In this section examples of both negative and positive selection procedures for lymphocyte fractionation are given.

4.2.1 *B cell preparation by positive selection using the direct method*

Polystyrene bacteriological Petri dishes 100 × 15 mm (Sterilin) are preferred as tissue culture grade plastic increases the level of non-specific cell adherence.

(i)   Coat the dishes with affinity-purified anti-Ig to the appropriate species by adding 8 ml of PBS containing 10 μg/ml anti-Ig and leave at 4°C overnight.

(ii)   Decant the anti-Ig solution and wash twice with PBS.

(iii)   Add 5 ml of PBS/0.2% BSA and leave to stand at room temperature for 30 min; this saturates all protein-binding sites on the plastic surface and thereby reduces non-specific cell adherence.

(iv)   Wash once with PBS (5−10 ml), then add $2-4 \times 10^7$ cells per dish in 4 ml of PBS/0.2% BSA and incubate for 45 min at 4°C. Swirl the contents once at the mid point of the incubation period.

(v)   Resuspend the non-adherent cells by gently swirling the plate and decant them off. Discard the decanted fluid unless it is intended to recover the T cells contained in it (see Section 4.2.3).

(vi)   Wash the adherent cells three times with cold PBS/0.2% BSA by *very gently* swirling the washing fluid round the dish. Introduce the washing solution slowly down the side of the dish each time and remove it by decanting.

(vii)   Add 4 ml of pre-warmed 10% normal serum in PBS to the plates and incubate at 37°C for 30 min. This serum, which must be from the same species as that of the lymphocytes, reduces, by competition, the degree of anti-Ig binding to the cell surface Ig.

(viii)   Decant off the normal serum and mechanically disrupt the adherence of the cells to the plastic by forceful pipetting approximately parallel to the surface (to provide a shearing force), using cold PBS/0.2% BSA (~40 ml/plate).

(ix)   Wash the cells, count them and assay for purity as described in Section 2.1.

(x)   Note that the yield obtained by positive selection is markedly influenced by the strength of cell adhesion to the plastic and this depends upon the avidity of the anti-Ig preparation used. If low yields are obtained (i.e. <50% theoretical) try adding non-immune IgG to the anti-Ig solution used for coating the dishes. Ratios of 10:1 (normal:specific IgG) or above should be tried.

(xi)   A final incubation stage using xylocaine (4 mg/ml) for 15 min at room temperature has also been advocated to promote good recovery rates (9).

A typical example of positive selection for rat B cells is shown in *Table 2*.

4.2.2 *B cell preparation by negative selection using the indirect method*

In this procedure T cells are depleted from the mixed population by adherence to the anti-Ig-coated plates. To accomplish this the T cells must first be labelled with either polyclonal or monoclonal anti-T cell antibodies.

(i)   Prepare antibody-coated dishes as previously described (Section 4.2.1), using affinity purified anti-Ig to the species of origin of the anti-T cell antibody. This anti-Ig should be thoroughly absorbed to reduce cross-reactivity with B cell surface Ig (see Section 3.3).

(ii)   Add, to each dish, $2-4 \times 10^7$ cells, pre-labelled with anti-T cell antibodies (Section 3.4.1) in 4 ml of PBS containing 10% homologous normal serum. The serum blocks any final trace of remaining cross-reactivity.

(iii)   Incubate at 4°C for 45 min and swirl the plate gently once mid-way through the incubation period. Decant the non-adherent cells and retain.

(iv)   To increase the B cell recovery wash the plates with approximately 20 ml of cold PBS/0.2% BSA by gently swirling to recover the remaining non-adherent B cells. Pool all decanted washings.

(v)   Wash the cells in PBS/0.2% BSA, count and assay for purity as previously described. (See *Table 2*).

4.2.3 *Purification of T cells and T cell subpopulations — sequential panning*

The positive selection of B cells, as described in Section 4.2.1, is also a negative selection procedure for T cells if the non-adherent fraction is retained. This is a useful preliminary step to fractionation of the T cells into subpopulations, since the removal of most of the B cells contributes to the final level of purity achieved. Fractionation of the T cells into subsets may be carried out by incubating them with saturating quantities of the appropriate monoclonal antibodies, and separating the cells into bound and unbound fractions on plates coated with anti-Ig antibodies. Particular subsets may be recovered by either positive or negative selection. A typical example of a two-cycle

Table 2. Fractionation of lymphocyte suspensions by adsorption on plastic dishes ('panning')

Procedure	Sample	Total cell no. $\times$ 10^{-7}	% positive cells[c] Ig+	CD5+	CD4+	CD8+	Observed yield	Theoretical yield
A. B cell preparation by:								
1. Positive selection[a]	TDL pre-depletion	8	46.8	54.7	n.d.	n.d.		–
	post-depletion	1.9	96.9	3.3	n.d.	n.d.		50%
2. Negative selection[b]	post-depletion	2.9	94.5	5.6	n.d.	n.d.		69.4%
B. T cell subset preparation by two cycle negative selection:	TDL pre-depletion	40	53.1	n.d.	30.6	16.2		–
1. 1st cycle (B cell depletion)[d]	post-depletion	23	7.1	n.d.	58.6	34.8		108%
2. 2nd cycle (T subset depletion)[e]	T cells pre-depletion	10	7.1	n.d.	58.6	34.8		–
	post CD8 depletion	3.6	2.7	n.d.	94.1	3.2		58%
	post CD4 depletion	2.4	10.0	n.d.	9.1	80.8		61%

[a]Rat thoracic duct lymphocytes were depleted of T cells by decanting non-adherent cells following incubation on anti-rat Ig-coated Petri dishes. The adherent B lymphocytes were subsequently recovered by vigorous pipetting. Pre- and post-selection samples were examined on a Becton Dickinson FACS.

[b]B cells were negatively selected by removal of T cells labelled with anti-CD8 (MRC OX-8) monoclonal antibody and two non-competing anti-CD4 monoclonal antibodies (MRC OX-35 and W3/25), by panning on Petri dishes coated with rabbit anti-mouse IgG.

[c]Data are expressed as percentages of total T and B cells present in the respective preparations.

[d]First cycle B cell depletion was carried out by incubation on rabbit anti-rat Ig-coated Petri dishes as in A1. above.

[e]The T cell preparation above, B1., was incubated with either a combination of monoclonal antibodies, MRC OX-8, MRC OX-12 and MRC OX-6 (for depletion of CD8+ cells and remaining B cells), or W3/25, MRC OX-35, MRC OX-12 and MRC OX-6 (for depletion of CD4+ cells and remaining B cells) and subsequently incubated on anti-mouse Ig Petri dishes. This rabbit anti-mouse Ig reagent was immunoabsorbent-purified on a rat Ig column so that it was totally cross reactive. This facilitated the removal of rat B cells.

negative selection procedure for the preparation of rat T lymphocyte subsets is shown in *Table 2*.

4.3 General comments

The direct technique is less versatile than the indirect one since it requires purification of the subpopulation-specific antibodies used. These antibodies are frequently monoclonal and in the indirect method they can be used as hybridoma tissue culture supernatants without purification. Further, in the indirect method, mixtures of antibodies may be used to label the lymphocytes so that more than one subpopulation may be depleted in one step. In some cases, however, the direct method is useful, for example in the positive selection of B cells on dishes coated with anti-Ig.

Panning can be applied to the preparation of both major and minor populations of cells in a mixture, and purities of 95% or better have been reported using polyclonal antisera (8), but results with monoclonal antibodies may be less satisfactory (10). If the purified suspensions are subject to a second adsorption cycle, a further improvement in purity may be expected. Yields approaching the theoretical values can be obtained under optimal conditions but are more frequently in the range 50−70%.

5. SEPARATION OF LYMPHOCYTE SUBPOPULATIONS BY COMPLEMENT-MEDIATED LYSIS

This is a frequently used negative selection technique to obtain sub-populations of lymphocytes on the basis of their expression of unique surface molecules. This technique is of course limited to those antibodies which fix complement! Few of the currently available monoclonal antibodies specific for rat cell surface molecules for example, fix complement and thus alternative techniques must be employed for this species. Overall, however the technique is quick and simple to perform. However, like all of the techniques discussed in this chapter, certain limitations apply and these should be considered before the technique is employed (see Section 5.2 below).

5.1 Method

5.1.1 *Materials*

(i) Cell suspension prepared as described in Chapter 1.
(ii) Media. Balanced salt solutions or minimal essential medium are sufficient, while those such as PBS lacking Ca^{2+} and Mg^{2+} are not.
(iii) Specific antibodies (usually monoclonal).
(iv) Source of complement (fresh, or lyophilized normal rabbit or guinea-pig serum). Fresh serum should be stored at $-70°C$.
(v) Water bath at 37°C.

5.1.2 *One-step method*

(i) Resuspend the cells in warm medium containing the appropriate dilutions of antibody and complement. These dilutions must be determined by titration, but tissue culture supernatant diluted 1:4 and used at the rate of 1 ml/10^8 cells

should prove suitable for the antibody. Final complement concentrations between 1:4 and 1:10 should be tested.
(ii)   Incubate for 45−60 min at 37°C, shaking the mixture periodically.
(iii)   Pellet the cells and wash them twice with complete medium containing 5% heat-
inactivated fetal calf or homologous serum, or 0.2% BSA.
(iv)   Test for viability and purity by normal procedures.

5.1.3 *Two-step method*

(i)   Resuspend the cells at $5 \times 10^6 - 1 \times 10^7$ cells/ml in medium containing the appropriate dilution of antibody. Sodium azide may also be included here to prevent capping (see Section 5.2.ii), but is unnecessary if cells are maintained at 4°C.
(ii)   Incubate for 30 min at 4°C, shaking the mixture periodically.
(iii)   Pellet the cells, wash them once with cold medium, then resuspend the cells in
the original volume of warm medium, containing complement at the appropriate
dilution.
(iv)   Incubate for 45 min at 37°C, shaking the mixture periodically.
(v)   Pellet the cells and wash them twice with complete medium containing 5% serum,
or 0.2% BSA.
(vi)   Test for viability and purity by normal procedures.

5.2 Practical and theoretical considerations

(i)   Either a one- or two-step procedure may be employed, the latter of necessity
if the antibody has anti-complement activity (most unlikely with monoclonal antibodies). This will become apparent during preliminary titrations of reagents.
(ii)   Some surface markers 'cap' on exposure to antibody: this may be prevented by
employing a two-step procedure where antibody is first added at 4°C, with or
without 10 mM sodium azide. Excess antibody and azide are then washed off
before addition of complement at 37°C. This should not adversely affect the
viability of the remaining cells. Note that capping cannot occur with a monoclonal
antibody to a monomeric antigen, since multiple cross-linking is impossible.
(iii)   All reagents must be pre-tested to determine optimal but non-toxic working concentrations. Natural antibody in the complement may give high levels of
background toxicity. Absorption of the complement with agar (11), or the specific
tissue (e.g. spleen cells) may reduce this. These techniques however, particularly
the latter, may reduce the complement activity of the serum so are best avoided.
Preferably, a number of batches of complement should be pre-tested to obtain
one of low toxicity. Alternatively, low toxicity complement is available, from
Cedarlane Laboratories, for example. Fresh serum is generally preferable and
rabbit, rather than guinea-pig serum appears superior for lysis with most mouse
monoclonal antibodies to human leukocytes.
(iv)   Appropriate control tubes are essential and should consist of scaled-down versions of the 'preparative' batch. These controls are: cells incubated with antibody
but no complement, cells with no antibody but complement and cells with neither.
(v)   It is most important to understand the limits of this procedure. In particular, the
susceptibility of cells to lysis appears to be related, at least to some extent, to

the density of the target molecule on the cell surface: cells expressing low levels of a particular antigen may not be lysed (12,13). Thus, the cells which remain after this treatment, cannot be taken as lacking a particular surface molecule. This problem may be alleviated in some instances by using two, non-competing, antibodies to the same cell surface molecule (13). In this way pairs of IgG molecules may come into sufficiently close proximity to activate complement and cause cell lysis.

(vi)   The purity of the depleted population can be better than 95% under optimal conditions. For situations where purities must be 99% or better however, a combination of complement-mediated lysis and a positive selection procedure such as panning may be of value. This combined protocol (14) has been successfully employed to obtain very pure T cell populations. Assessment of purity by flow cytofluorography is recommended wherever possible.

6. COMPARISON OF THE DIFFERENT CELL FRACTIONATION TECHNIQUES

The four methods of separating cells described in this chapter all make use of antibodies. However, they are not otherwise strictly equivalent and each has advantages and limitations. Cell sorters are clearly the most discriminating. Not only do they allow the experimenter to choose just what he will regard as an antigen-positive cell, determined by its fluorescence brightness, but also because cells may be fractionated on the basis of several (usually four) criteria applied simultaneously. However, cell sorters are expensive and slow. It typically takes 10 h or more to obtain 50×10^6 sorted cells, when the cell preparation time is taken into account.

Rosetting and complement-mediated lysis are similar in that both are negative selection techniques. The latter method requires antibodies that fix complement, and this must result in cell death. Misleading results can be obtained — for example, based on complement-mediated lysis, the CD5 antigen (Lyt 1 in the mouse) was long considered to be a marker for murine T helper cells, whereas it is now known that the antigen is expressed on all T cells. Rosetting has the advantage that non-complement fixing antibodies may be used and it avoids the problem of selective resistance to complement-mediated lysis (12). Both techniques are superior to cell sorting with respect to cell numbers: up to 10^{10} rat lymphocytes can be subjected to rosette depletion in a few hours.

The separation of cells by panning in antibody-coated Petri dishes has the advantage, like cell sorting, of being both a positive and a negative separation technique. It is quicker than cell sorting, but slower than rosetting and complement-mediated lysis. As a negative selection method it suffers by comparison with rosetting, both with respect to purity of the depleted population and to the time required to process the cells. However, apart from cell sorting, it is the only positive selection method that we have described. While lacking the discriminatory capacity of cell sorters the method can handle relatively large numbers of cells. Yields and purities of positively selected fractions are comparable with those obtained from electronic devices, provided cells with moderately high levels of antigen expression are being selected.

Combinations of techniques are sometimes appropriate. For example, to maximize the recovery of subsets of T cells we sometimes rosette out the B cells, and then sort the depleted population using a monoclonal antibody that labels only a subset of the T cells isolated by rosetting. In other instances a combination of rosetting or complement-mediated lysis, for negative selection, and panning for positive selection may prove appropriate.

The powerful analytical capacity of cell sorters is invaluable for the assessment of cell purities after cell fractionation by whatever method. It is strongly recommended to all those that have access to such a machine.

7. REFERENCES

1. Loken,M.R. (1986) In *Monoclonal Antibodies*. Beverley,P.C.L. (ed.), Churchill Livingstone, Edinburgh, London, Melbourne and New York, p. 132.
2. Mason,D.W., Rackley,J.P. and Smith,D.T. (1985) In *Flow Cytometry: Instrumentation and Data Analysis*. Visser,J.W.M. and Tanke,H.J. (eds), Academic Press, London, p. 240.
3. Mason,D.W. and Williams,A.F. (1980) *Biochem. J.*, **187**, 1.
4. Parish,C. and Hayward,J. (1974) *Proc. R. Soc. Lond. (Biol).*, **187**, 47.
5. Mason,D.W. (1981) *Transplantation*, **32**, 222.
6. Catt,K. and Tregear,G.W. (1967) *Science*, **158**, 1570.
7. Mage,M.G., McHugh,L.L. and Rothstein,T.L. (1977) *J. Immunol. Methods*, **15**, 47.
8. Wysocki,L.J. and Sato,V.L. (1978) *Proc. Natl. Acad. Sci. USA*, **75**, 2844.
9. Lewis,G.K. and Kamin,R. (1980) In *Selected Methods in Cellular Immunology*. Mishell,B.B. and Shiigi,S.M. (eds), W.H.Freeman and Co., San Francisco, p. 227.
10. Rosenberg,J.S., Gilman,S.C. and Feldman,J.D. (1982) *J. Immunol.*, **129**, 996.
11. Cohen,A. and Schlesinger,M. (1970) *Transplantation*, **10**, 130.
12. Ledbetter,J.A., Rouse,R.V., Micklem,H.S. and Herzenberg,L.A. (1980) *J. Exp. Med.*, **152**, 280.
13. Howard,J.C., Butcher,G.W., Galfre,G., Milstein,C. and Milstein,C.P. (1979) *Immunol. Rev.*, **47**, 139.
14. Sprent,J. and Schaefer,M. (1985) *J. Exp. Med.*, **162**, 2068.

CHAPTER 3

Fractionation of lymphocytes by immunomagnetic beads

STEINAR FUNDERUD, KJELL NUSTAD, TOR LEA, FRODE VARTDAL, GUSTAV GAUDERNACK, PER STENSTAD and JOHN UGELSTAD

1. INTRODUCTION

1.1 Introduction to monosized magnetic polymer beads

A widespread use of magnetic particles for cell separation has only recently been initiated as a new generation of magnetic particles have been prepared by Ugelstad *et al.* (1–3). These particles have all the features needed for cell separation purposes.

A major problem for efficient application of magnetic beads in cell separation is due to differences in the preparation of beads which are well characterized regarding size and content of magnetizable material. The beads should be easily dispersible in water, they should allow a strong 'irreversible' binding of the antibodies applied in the selective cell separation, and they should not show any non-specific binding to cells.

Another requirement which turns out to be of great importance for the performance of the beads, is that they do not show any magnetic remanence after having been exposed to a magnetic field. In practice this means that they should be superparamagnetic. In the process of attaching antibodies to the bead surface the beads are repeatedly isolated from the dispersion by the use of a magnet, washed and thereafter redispersed. Any remaining magnetism would severely reduce the ease of re-dispersion.

Magnetic polymer beads which fulfil the above requirements have been obtained by a process which involves the continuous *in situ* formation of magnetic iron oxides and hydroxides inside the pores of highly porous polymer beads with an extremely narrow size distribution (2). After the final heat treatment all the beads not only have the same size, but they also contain the same amount of maghemite, γFe_2O_3. Because the maghemite exists as very small grains evenly distributed throughout the whole bead volume the beads show the desired superparamagnetic behaviour.

After introduction of the γFe_2O_3 the beads are still highly porous, with a surface of approximately 100 m^2/g. Originally the beads were applied in this form (4). In further development of the magnetic beads for cell separation (5–7) the pores are filled with a polymeric material which is bound chemically to the particles and leads to a dramatic reduction in the surface of the beads (3–5 m^2). A scanning electron micrograph of the beads is shown in *Figure 1*.

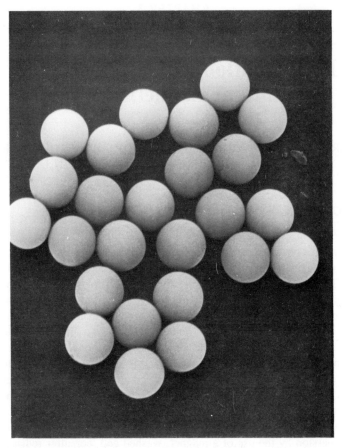

Figure 1. Scanning electron micrograph of magnetic M-450 beads. Magnification 2800×.

1.2 General considerations in lymphocyte separations

Over the last 10 years several methods for selection of lymphocytes in general and lymphocyte subsets have been developed, of which some are discussed elsewhere in this volume. Two main separation principles have been used:

(i)   separation based on physical properties of the cell such as size and density.
(ii) various techniques utilizing differences in receptors or antigens on the cell surface (see Chapter 2).

Methods based on the latter principle are the only satisfactory ones for purification of cell subsets. Due to the availability of monoclonal antibodies with a variety of defined specificities, it is possible to isolate pure cell populations if an appropriate separation system is applied. To achieve a sufficiently pure cell population with a satisfactory yield, several factors have to be considered. For instance, one has to choose between a negative and a positive selection principle. This is especially important if the cells are to be used in functional studies. To be able to decide which is the optimal in each case, knowledge about the functional properties of the receptor or antigen(s) used for selection is required. This chapter presents the versatility of positive selection via the CD8 and CD25 antigens on T cells and CD19 and CD37 antigens on B cells and demonstrates that the methods envisaged are not an obstacle to further studies of cell functions. Furthermore, procedures for negative selection of lymphocyte subsets are presented.

In the methods presented, antibodies (polyclonal or monoclonal) are adsorbed or coupled to a monosized super paramagnetic polymer particle (Dynabeads M-450). Such particles will be referred to as immunomagnetic beads in the following text.

Immunomagnetic beads make it easy to perform positive or negative selection whether the source of cells is peripheral blood leukocytes or whole blood. For both positive and negative selection the immunomagnetic separation may be carried out in two different ways:

(i)   indirect method — cells are first incubated with mouse monoclonal antibody and are subsequently rosetted with anti-mouse IgG-coated beads

(ii)   direct method — monoclonal antibody-charged immunomagnetic beads are bound directly to cells.

The system to choose for a particular purpose is discussed in Sections 3.1 and 3.2.

The morphology of the interaction between a cell and a bead is not dealt with here, but can be found in ref. (7).

In this chapter we describe techniques for separation of human lymphocytes. However, Dynabeads M-450 are equally well suited for separation of other cell types.

2. MATERIALS

2.1 Media and equipment for cell culture

Regular culture medium, balanced salt solutions, fetal calf serum (FCS) and plastic ware of any well known brand may be used.

2.1.1 *Equipment*

(i) *Magnets and devices.* Permanent magnets made from cobalt and samarium are available from many sources. Suitable sizes are squares of 10×10 mm which are 3 mm thick, or rectangles of 10×30 mm with 6 mm thickness, depending on the diameter of the tube/flask to be used. The magnet should be placed on a plate of soft iron which increases the magnetic field and makes it easier to handle.

Specially developed equipment which can hold one or six tubes with built-in magnets is available from Dynal A.S.

(ii) *Rock-N-Roller (Labinko).*

2.1.2 *Dynabeads M-450*

The particles described in the introduction above (Section 1.1) are now available commercially as Dynabeads M-450 from Dynal A.S. Uncoated Dynabeads M-450 are sold

Fractionation by immunomagnetic beads

Table 1. Properties of uncoated Dynabeads M-450.

Particle diameter	4.5 μm
Density	1.5 g/cm^3
Surface area	3 $-$ 5 m^2/g
Iron content	22% (w/w)
Particle/weight ratio	1.4 $\times$ 10^{10} particles/g

as sterile particles (30 mg/ml) in water in 2 and 10 ml bottles. The properties of these beads are given in *Table 1*. These particles are also available with sheep or goat antibodies to mouse IgG which binds all subclasses. The particles contain about 3.0 μg of antibody per mg. Coated Dynabeads M-450 are sold as sterile particles (30 mg/ml) in phosphate-buffered saline (PBS) supplemented with 0.1% bovine serum albumin (BSA) and 0.01% NaN$_3$ in 2 and 10 ml bottles. The particles are activated by *p*-toluene sulphonylchloride before binding of the antibodies.

2.2 **Preparation of antibodies**

2.2.1 *Polyclonal anti-mouse IgG antibodies*

High avidity polyclonal anti-mouse IgG antibodies which react equally well with all mouse IgG subclasses should be used. It is an advantage if the antibodies are Fc specific. The antibodies must be affinity purified and adsorbed for cross-reactivity on a solid phase. We usually adsorb against human IgG by passage of the antiserum through a column with human IgG coupled to CNBr-activated Sepharose 4B. The antiserum is then affinity purified on a Sepharose column coupled with mouse IgG and the bound fraction eluted with 4 M guanidine in PBS pH 6.2. Guanidine is removed by dialysis against PBS (0.15 M NaCl, 0.01 M sodium phosphate buffer pH 7.4). The antiserum is then sterile filtered and stored at 4°C before adsorption to the particles.

Commercial antisera might be used. However, we recommend that a comparison is performed with Dynabeads M-450 coated with sheep or goat anti-mouse IgG.

2.2.2 *Monoclonal IgM antibodies*

Monoclonal mouse IgM is purified from ascites by precipitation with polyethylene glycol as described by Neoh and co-workers (8). Other methods for purification of IgM antibodies can be equally satisfactory, although the polyethylene glycol method is superior in speed and simplicity. The precipitated IgM antibody is dissolved in PBS, sterile filtered and stored at 4°C.

The monoclonal IgM antibodies used in this presentation are the anti-CD8, ITI-5C2 clone (9) and the anti-CD19, AB1 clone (10).

2.2.3 *Monoclonal IgG antibodies*

The monoclonal IgG antibodies are used as culture supernatants, ascitic fluid or purified IgG. The monoclonal antibodies are either adsorbed onto the particles via anti-mouse Ig antibodies as described in Section 2.3.3, or used to sensitize the cells as described in Sections 3.1.2 and 3.2.2. The following antibodies have been used.

(i)   HH1, anti-CD37 (11)
(ii)   anti-IL-2 receptor, anti-CD25 (Becton Dickinson).

58

2.3 Coating of antibodies on Dynabeads M-450

Dynabeads M-450 have a mixed hydrophobic/hydrophilic surface. The polymers applied in preparation of the beads result in a hydrophobic surface mainly due to aromatic rings present in the polymers, whereas available hydroxyl groups can be used for chemical coupling to the beads. The strong adsorptive properties of the beads give a firm binding of antibodies. It should be noted that protein adsorption in general represents multiple protein/particle interactions and these interactions are very dependent on the structure of the protein to be adsorbed on a hydrophobic surface (12). We find that affinity purified antibodies adsorb much more readily than native IgG probably due to a partial denaturation during the isolation procedure affecting the Fc region. This results in a favourable antibody orientation on the particle surface as discussed by Nustad *et al.* (5).

The following conditions will usually be optimal:

Particle concentration:	20−50 mg/ml
Antibody concentration:	100−400 μg/ml
Antibody/particle ratio:	2−10 μg antibody/mg particle
Coating solution:	0.05−0.1 M Tris-HCl pH 9.5
Temperature:	2−8°C
Time:	2−24 h

Published data suggest a variety of coupling conditions, which indicate that a particular antibody might profit from experimenting around with the conditions for protein adsorption. Buffer, pH and ionic strength might be important variables.

Coating of antibodies to sulphonylchloride-activated particles follows the same rules as discussed above, since this activation procedure results in an increased hydrophobicity of the particles. The binding of antibodies is in this instance a two-step procedure, that is protein adsorption followed by chemical attachment (5).

It should be noted that we recently have found that some monoclonal IgM antibodies have a better antigen-binding capacity when only adsorbed to particles, compared with covalent binding to sulphonylchloride-activated particles. This is in contrast to polyclonal IgG antibodies which function equally well after chemical coupling and adsorption. The chemical coupling of polyclonal IgG antibodies gives about 30% better binding of soluble antigens, mainly due to an increased amount of antibody bound to the particles.

Table 2. Coating of polyclonal IgG antibodies to Dynabeads M-450.

1.	Place one bottle of uncoated Dynabeads M-450 (60 mg in 2 ml of water) on a magnet and aseptically remove water above the particles using a syringe.
2.	Add 2 ml of polyclonal anti-mouse IgG antibody (Section 2.2.1), 150 μg/ml in 0.05 M Tris-HCl pH 9.0, and mix well on a Vortex mixer.
3.	Rotate end-over-end overnight at 4°C.
4.	Place the bottle on a magnet and remove the supernatant aseptically with a syringe.
5.	Add 2 ml of PBS supplemented with 0.5% (w/v) BSA and mix. Place the bottle on the magnet after 5 min and remove the buffer as above.
6.	Repeat step 5 four times.
7.	Repeat step 5, but rotate end-over-end overnight.
8.	Remove the last washing buffer and add 2 ml of PBS supplemented with 0.1% BSA and 0.01% NaN$_3$. Store the final product at 4°C.

Table 3. Immunoadsorption of monoclonal mouse IgG.

1.	Place one bottle of Dynabeads M-450 coated with anti-mouse IgG antibodies (60 mg of particles in 2 ml of PBS supplemented with 0.1% BSA and 0.01% NaN_3) on a magnet. Remove the buffer aseptically with a syringe and add 2 ml of PBS.
2.	Wash twice in PBS and make up the particles in 2 ml of PBS.
3.	Add 120 μl of monoclonal mouse IgG, 1.0 mg/ml in PBS to the beads.
4.	Incubate by end-over-end rotation overnight at 4°C.
5.	Place the bottle on a magnet and remove the supernatant using a syringe.
6.	Add 2 ml of PBS, mix, place the bottle on a magnet and remove the supernatant.
7.	Repeat step 4 three times.
8.	Resuspend the particles in 2 ml of PBS and store at 4°C.

Monoclonal mouse IgG antibodies can be adsorbed directly to the surface of the particles. However, in most cases, we find that particles coated as presented in Section 2.3.3 are preferable.

2.3.1 *Coating of polyclonal IgG antibodies on Dynabeads M-450*

The procedure for adsorption of polyclonal anti-mouse IgG antibodies to the particles is given in *Table 2*. However, such particles should be compared with Dynabeads M-450 coated with sheep or goat anti-mouse IgG from Dynal A.S. as suggested above.

2.3.2 *Coating of Dynabeads M-450 with monoclonal mouse IgM antibodies*

Monoclonal mouse IgM antibodies should be purified and adsorbed directly onto the particle surface. We have not found polyclonal anti-mouse IgM antibodies which give a satisfactory binding to monoclonal IgM on a cellular surface. However, IgM monoclonals work perfectly when coated directly to the particle surface provided that the antibody avidity is sufficiently high. The coating procedure should be performed as described for polyclonal IgG in *Table 2*.

2.3.3 *Immunoadsorption of monoclonal mouse IgG antibodies on Dynabeads M-450 with sheep or goat anti-mouse IgG antibodies*

The procedures for immunoadsorption of monoclonal mouse IgG antibodies to anti-mouse IgG-coated particles is given in *Table 3*. The monoclonal antibody can be used as cell culture supernatant, ascitic fluid or as purified antibody.

The amount of antibody per milligram of particles should be optimized for each application, but will usually range between 0.2 and 3 μg monoclonal IgG per mg beads. The time needed for binding can be reduced to 1 h at room temperature. The final product is stable for months when refrigerated. Minute amounts of monoclonal antibody might leak off, and can easily be removed by simple washing. If smaller amounts of beads are to be used, it might be more convenient to transfer the amount needed to a sterile tube and to carry out the adsorption procedure in the tube.

3. LYMPHOCYTE SEPARATION

Isolation of cell subsets, especially for functional studies, should usually be carried out by depletion procedures. This ensures that the cells under study are neither influenced

Table 4. Direct method for positive selection of lymphocytes from blood.

1.	Collect blood in a 10 ml ACD-Vacutainer.
2.	Cool blood to $2-8°C$.
3.	Add Dynabeads M-450 coated with IgM antibodies ITI-5C2 or AB1 (see Section 2.2.2) (0.2 mg of beads per ml ACD blood) directly to the blood.
4.	Incubate the vacutainer for $5-10$ min at $2-8°C$ on a Rock-N-Roller.
5.	Place a cobalt−samarium magnet along the Vacutainer for 2 min to collect rosetted cells.
6.	Remove the blood from the Vacutainer while the rosetted cells are kept in the tube by the magnet.
7.	Wash the isolated cells four times in PBS. Use PBS with 0.6% sodium citrate in the first washing step. Each washing cycle is carried out as follows:
	(i) Add $5-10$ ml of PBS to the Vacutainer to suspend rosetted cells
	(ii) Place a cobalt−samarium magnet on the outside wall of the Vacutainer for 30 sec.
	(iii) Remove the PBS from the tube while the magnet is kept on the outside wall.
8.	Resuspend the rosetted cells and free particles in RPMI 1640 containing 10% FCS or 10% normal human serum.

by the monoclonal antibodies used for separation, nor by the separation procedure itself. Our experience with cell populations purified by negative selection have never demonstrated functional aberrations in the resulting cells (11). However, for certain purposes, even the most thorough depletion of cells with immunomagnetic beads cannot provide cell populations of sufficient homogeneity. For instance, negative selection procedures have never produced B cell populations of sufficiently high purity to accomplish a reliable assay for B cell growth factor (for further comments, see Section 3.1.2). In other situations, a particular monoclonal antibody has been developed against a specific cell population to be studied, and accordingly, positive selection procedures are the only alternative.

Examples of positive selections and negative selection (cell depletion) are given in Sections 3.1 and 3.2.

3.1 Procedures for positive selection of lymphocytes

In principle, any cell population defined by a monoclonal antibody can be isolated by positive selection with Dynabeads M-450, provided the following conditions are met:

(i)   the antibody does not bind non-specifically to other cell populations;
(ii)   the affinity/avidity of the antibody is sufficiently high;
(iii)   the density of the corresponding epitope on the target cell is not too low.

Given the speed with which such isolations can be performed, immunomagnetic separation by positive selection is the method of choice in many experimental systems. The possible applications of the method are, however, not only limited by the availability of suitable monoclonal antibodies. Considerations as to the involvement of the epitope in question in the regulation of distinct target cell functions must be taken into account before selection of a suitable monoclonal antibody. Thus, even with our present knowledge of the many cell surface components that might be involved in lymphocyte activation, it is still possible to use positive immunomagnetic selection for many purposes. Several examples of such applications are given in the sections below.

3.1.1 *Selection of lymphocytes by direct methods*

(i) *Selection of lymphocytes from blood.* In this technique, lymphocytes are positively isolated directly from blood by means of Dynabeads M-450 coated with monoclonal antibodies specific for T or B cells (*Table 4*). This technique permits fast and specific isolation of lymphocytes without gradient centrifugation and washing prior to specific cell isolation.

This technique achieves isolation of greater than 99% pure and functional intact lymphocytes from blood in approximately 15 min. Lymphocytes immunomagnetically isolated directly from blood may be recovered free of Dynabeads M-450 by using the procedure given in *Table 6* (steps 7−9). This procedure may be used to isolate various lymphocyte subsets, provided specific and high affinity monoclonal antibodies are available. The incubation time required for rosetting of lymphocytes will depend on the affinity of the monoclonal antibody coated onto the beads. The amount of Dynabeads M-450 required for isolation of the differet subsets will depend on the number of target cells expected in the blood sample. Thus, isolation of total T cells will require more Dynabeads M-450 than isolation of T cell subsets and B cells.

(ii) *From mononuclear cell suspensions.* A protocol for positive selection of lymphocytes from mononuclear cell suspensions by a direct method is outlined in *Table 5*.

An example using the procedure given in *Table 5*, for the purpose of positive selection of antigen-specific cytotoxic human T lymphocytes of the CD8-positive subset is given below.

As described in refs. 9 and 13, we have used Dynabeads M-450 directly coated with the monoclonal antibody ITI-5C2 (IgM anti-CD8) to isolate HLA class I-specific CD8-positive cytotoxic lymphocytes from mixed lymphocyte cultures. Typically, the above procedure yields 95−97% CD8-positive cells and 2−4% CD4-positive cells. With the low particle/cell ratio employed, the isolated cells retain their functional activity in the presence of the antibody-coated particles. Thus, functional tests can be performed immediately after isolation of cells, without an incubation step to remove the particles attached to the cells. Using the same procedure, CD8-positive cells having lymphokine-activated killer (LAK) activity can be isolated from human T cells cultured in the presence of high concentrations of interleukin-2 (IL-2). Also in this case, the presence of low numbers of particles does not seem to interfere with the cytotoxic effector mechanism of these cells.

Table 5. Direct method for positive selection of lymphocytes from mononuclear cell suspensions.

1.	Resuspend cells isolated by Isopaque−Ficoll centrifugation in Hanks' balanced salt solution (HBSS) with 1% FCS to a concentration of 20−40 × 10^6/ml.
2.	Add the desired amount of Dynabeads M-450 pre-coated with monoclonal antibody, in a small volume, resulting in 1−2 particles per cells carrying the membrane marker in question.
3.	Incubate the mixture for 20 min at 4°C on a Rock-N-Roller.
4.	Dilute the particle/cell suspension at least five times with cold HBSS/1% FCS.
5.	Place the culture tube or flask on an iron plate covered with cobalt−samarium magnets and pipette off the unrosetted cells.
6.	Wash the remaining rosettes/free particles thoroughly, at least five times, in HBSS/1% FCS by repeating steps 4−5 to get rid of contaminating cells before employing in functional assays.

Table 6. Indirect method for positive selection of lymphocytes from mononuclear cell suspensions.

1.	Isolate mononuclear cells from blood or other tissues by Isopaque-Ficoll gradient centrifugation.
2.	Wash the cells twice in HBSS with 2% FCS.
3.	Cool the cell suspension on ice.
4.	Add monoclonal antibodies to the cell suspension and incubate in an ice bath for 30 min.
5.	Wash the cells twice in ice-cold HBSS with 2% FCS.
6.	Resuspend the cells in ice-cold HBSS/2% FCS at a cell concentration of $20-40 \times 10^6$/ml.
7.	Add the desired amount of Dynabeads in a small volume, resulting in approximately two particles per cell expressing the membrane marker in question.
8.	Follow steps $3-6$ in *Table 5*.
9.	If cells free of particles are wanted; resuspend the rosettes in culture medium to approximately 10^6/ml, and incubate the cells overnight in a CO_2 incubator.
10.	Following the overnight incubation, stir the culture tube or flask gently and place it on the magnet. Pour off particle-free cells. If the cell yield is low, it can often be increased by either vortexing the rosettes or by pipetting through a narrow-bore Pasteur pipette before placing on the magnet.
11.	Wash the cells once in culture medium before employing in functional assays.

Table 7. Direct immunomagnetic depletion of cells.

1.	Isolate the cells from blood (or other tissues) by Isopaque−Ficoll gradient centrifugation.
2.	Wash the cells twice in HBSS supplemented with 2% FCS.
3.	Add Dynabeads M-450 coated with the monoclonal antibody specific for the cell subsets to be depleted.
4.	Incubate at 4°C for 30 min on a Rock-N-Roller.
5.	Increase the volume of the mixture by adding an appropriate volume of HBSS with 2% FCS.
6.	Place a cobalt−samarium magnet on the outside wall of the test tube or tissue culture flask for approximately 30 sec to collect rosetted cells and free Dynabeads on the inside wall of the vessel.
7.	Decant the supernatant containing non-rosetted cells into another tube or tissue culture flask.

Table 8. Indirect immunomagnetic depletion of cells.

1.	Follow steps $1-6$ in *Table 6*.
2.	Add Dynabeads coated with anti-mouse IgG (e.g. sheep anti-mouse IgG).
3.	The rest of the depletion procedure is carried out as shown in *Table 7*, steps $4-7$.

3.1.2 *Selection of cells by an indirect method*

In some situations, for instance when antibody avidity is low, the cells should first be sensitized with monoclonal antibody. *Table 6* gives parameters for an indirect positive selection procedure. It is crucial for the success of this procedure to reduce the amount of particles to the lowest possible, that is to a particle/cell ratio of approximately 2:1.

We have used anti-mouse Ig-coated Dynabeads M-450, with HH1 monoclonal antibodies (anti-CD37), to isolate resting human peripheral blood B lymphocytes in acceptable to good yield (11). For unknown reasons the recovery varies from separation to separation, but is usually between 40 and 70%. These cells are by most criteria resting B cells and not influenced by the separation procedure. Thus, we have used such cells in the study of early B lymphocyte activation parameters (11).

In the establishment of continuously growing, antigen- or mitogen-induced T cell lines or clones, a fractionation step on a density gradient like Percoll is generally included to isolate the activated blast cells. In our experience both the yield and purity of the cells varies considerably using this procedure. As an alternative, we have successfully used positive immunomagnetic selection of IL-2 receptor-bearing T lymphocytes. After 2 days in culture, IL-2 receptor-expressing cells can be isolated quantitatively. Following overnight incubation of the rosetted cells, more than 80% of the cells can be recovered free of particles for propagation in IL-2-conditioned medium.

3.2 Procedure for depletion of cells

This technique is used to deplete certain cell subsets from blood or other body fluids containing heterogeneous cell populations. The technique may be used to study how removal of these subsets may influence various functional parameters in cell culture experiments (14). It may also be used to deplete T cells from bone marrow grafts in order to avoid graft-versus-host disease in allogeneic bone marrow transplantation (14), or to carry out tumour cell purging in autologous bone marrow transplantation in treatment of neuroblastoma (4). The cell depletion technique may either be carried out directly (*Table 7*), or indirectly (*Table 8*).

Both direct and indirect methods accomplish very efficient depletion of T cells both when assayed for phenotypic markers (erythrocyte rosetting, immunofluorescence), and for T cell functions (abrogation of phytohaemagglutinin, pokeweed mitogen and PPD-induced responses as well as IL-2 production) (5,6).

The amount of beads required for depletion of a cell subset will depend on the concentration of that particular subset in the cell suspension. Note that depletion of cells requires higher particle/cell ratios than those employed in positive selection. To deplete T cells from a suspension of peripheral blood mononuclear cells (containing 50−70% T cells), 10−20 beads per cell are recommended. Depletion of many different cell subsets may be carried out simultaneously by sensitizing the cells with a cocktail of monoclonal antibodies (indirect technique), or by using beads coated with monoclonal antibodies specific for different cell subsets (direct method). In the depletion of T cells the direct method is at least as efficient as the indirect method. Additionally, the direct method is faster and less cumbersome than the indirect method. However, in depletion of, for example a tumour cell population having heterogeneous distribution of surface target antigens, sensitization of the cells with a cocktail of tumour-specific monoclonal antibodies may be preferable.

4. REFERENCES

1. Ugelstad,J., Mørk,P.C., Kaggerud,K.H., Ellingsen,T. and Berge,A. (1980) *Adv. Colloid Interface Sci.*, **13**, 101.
2. Ugelstad,J., Mfutakamba,H., Mørk,P.C., Ellingsen,T., Berge,A., Schmid,R., Holm,L., Jørgedal,A., Hansen,F.K. and Nustad,K. (1985) *J. Polym. Sci.*, **72**, 225.
3. Ugelstad,J., Berge,A., Schmid,R., Ellingsen,T., Stenstad,P. and Skjeltorp,A. (1986) In *Polymer Reaction Engineering*. Reichert,K.H. and Geiseler,W. (eds), Hüthig & Wepf, Basel, p. 77.
4. Treleaven,J.B., Gibson,F.M., Ugelstad,J., Rembaum,A., Philip,T., Caine,G.D. and Kemshead,J.T. (1984) *Lancet*, **1**, 70.
5. Nustad,K., Danielsen,H., Reith,A., Funderud,S., Lea,T., Vartdal,F. and Ugelstad,J. In *Microspheres: Medical and Biological Applications*. Rembaum,A. (ed.), CRD Press Inc., Cat. No. 6571, in press.
6. Lea,T., Vartdal,F., Davies,C. and Ugelstad,J. (1985) *Scand. J. Immunol.*, **22**, 207.

7. Danielsen,H., Funderud,S., Nustad,K., Reith,A. and Ugelstad,J. (1986) *Scand. J. Immunol.*, **24**, 179.
8. Neoh,S.H., Gordon,C., Potter,A. and Zola,H. (1986) *J. Immunol. Methods*, **91**, 231.
9. Gaudernack,G., Leivestad,T., Ugelstad,J. and Thorsby,E. (1986) *J. Immunol. Methods*, **90**, 179.
10. Melsom,H., Funderud,S., Lie,S.O. and Godal,T. (1984) *Scand. J. Haematol.*, **33**, 27.
11. Lea,T., Smeland,E., Funderud,S., Vartdal,F., Davies,C., Beiske,K. and Ugelstad,J. (1986) *Scand. J. Immunol.*, **23**, 509.
12. Norde,W. (1986) *Adv. Colloid Interface Sci.*, **25**, 267.
13. Leivestad,T., Gaudernack,G., Ugelstad,J. and Thorsby,E. (1986) *Tissue Antigens*, **28**, 46.
14. Vartdal,F., Kvalheim,G., Lea,T., Bosnes,V., Gaudernack,G., Ugelstad,J. and Albrechtsen,D. (1987) *Transplantation*, in press.

1.
2.
3.
4.
5.
6.
7.
8.

CHAPTER 4

Immunofluorescence and immunohistochemistry

GEORGE JANOSSY and PETER AMLOT

1. INTRODUCTION

The aim of this chapter is to summarize immunofluorescence (IF) and immunohisto-chemical (IHC) methods. To illustrate such methods examples are drawn from human clinical studies of:

(i)   lymphocyte subpopulations in immunoregulatory and infectious diseases such as acquired immune deficiency (AIDS) and related syndromes (ARC); and
(ii)   leukaemia/lymphoma diagnosis.

The methods are introduced in a step-wise manner, whereas each technique described opens up possibilities for tackling further questions about cellular phenotype and leads on to a further technique. Certain concepts, such as the correlation between immuno phenotype and function, or the correspondence between lympho/haemopoietic malignancies and stages in developments of 'normal-equivalent' cells are broached as the introduced techniques allow the investigation of these questions.

Modern IF techniques use incident light illumination with selective filters for fluorescein isothiocyanate (FITC, green elicitation) and tetramethylrhodamine isothiocyanate (TRITC, red elicitation). A more recently introduced fluorochrome, phycoerythrin (PE, orange elicitation) can be viewed together with FITC using the same FITC filter set (1). Membrane marker studies using fluorescence methods are combined with morphological analysis using phase contrast. Distinct populations such as granulocytes, monocytes and large granular lymphocytes can be distinguished from cells of classical lymphocyte morphology (2). These morphological observations are valuable for diagnostic work and the analysis of FITC and TRITC labelled cells by microscope represents the forerunner of the quantitative analysis recorded by flow cytometers.

IHC is also frequently used in both diagnosis and experimental work (3,4). IF and IHC are complementary techniques with unique advantages and disadvantages. Although IF is more frequently employed by immunologists and IHC by pathologists, in many laboratories such methods are used interchangeably depending upon the questions which need to be answered.

The advantages of the IF methods are as follows.

(i)   The speed of the technique. Staining of cells in suspension with directly labelled antibodies takes $10-15$ min, and with indirect IF assay $20-30$ min. Large numbers of samples can be assessed rapidly in a microplate assay.

(ii)   Its analytical precision when studying the expression of two different antigens by antibodies labelled with different fluorochromes. Only two-colour IF, viewed by separate filters, is capable of revealing the weak expression of a differentiation antigen in the presence of a strong reaction obtained with another molecule abundantly displayed on the same cell.

(iii)   The possibility of concomitant morphological assessment with phase contrast. It is also possible to stain the IF-labelled slides with haematoxylin without quenching the fluorescent label (5).

(iv)   The extension of the technique to flow cytometry for quantitative analysis.

The advantages of IHC methods are as follows.

(i)   The simultaneous examination of classical morphological features together with the phenotypic features of cells detected by antibodies.

(ii)   The investigation of antibody activity without filter changes or switching from dark field to light microscopy.

(iii)   The enhanced sensitivity which follows repeated layers of labelled antibody, for example during the alkaline phosphatase − anti-alkaline phosphatase (APAAP) method (3).

In the 1970s conventional antisera were established for the analysis of lymphocyte and monocyte subsets and also for the differential diagnosis of leukaemia (6). Careful absorptions against leukocytes from blood and bone marrow were necessary to eliminate unwanted reactivities and render these reagents specific and diagnostically useful. Examples of six specific heteroantisera used in clinical studies were: anti-immunoglobulin reagents made in various species (anti-human Ig), rabbit anti-T cell (anti-HuTLA; ref. 7) and, more recently, rat anti-T3 cell antisera (made against purified T3 antigens and capable of identifying T cells in formalin-fixed paraffin-embedded tissues (8), horse antiserum to suppressor/cytotoxic T cells (anti-TH$_2$; ref. 9), rabbit antiserum to common acute lymphoblastic leukaemia (anti-cALL; ref. 6) and a rabbit antiserum to a nuclear enzyme, terminal deoxynucleotidyl transferase which is detectable in immature cells of both the T and B lymphoid lineages (anti-TdT) (10). Some of these antisera, such as anti-human Ig and rabbit anti-TdT, are still in clinical use.

Diagnostic precision has now been refined by the development of new technologies which include the development of flow cytometry, linked to the use of FITC and PE in the two-colour investigations with a single laser. The most powerful impact on research and diagnosis has been made by monoclonal antibodies (MAbs), which liberated the scientist from the burden of extensive absorption during the preparation of antisera. The conferences on Leucocyte Differentiation Antigens have standardized the 'clusters' of MAbs (CD) reacting with the same differentiation antigens (12 − 14). Most CD include reagents of different Ig classes or subclasses. With specific goat antisera to murine IgM and IgG labelled with FITC and TRITC, these MAbs can be readily applied in various novel combinations.

Another important development has been the gradual simplification of diagnostic panels for leukaemia diagnosis. Over the last decade hundreds of reagents have been studied with two separate questions in mind: (i) which are the most useful antibodies? and (ii) what is the correct immunological diagnosis? There is now a widely accepted answer to the first question, and the leukaemia analysis now concentrates on the diagnostic enquiry using only a few crucial reagents with clearly established reactivity patterns on leukaemias (15) and these antibodies are now available from commercial sources.

The final introductory comment is about reagent control. Aggregated immunoglobulins bind to Fc receptors on many cell types including lymphocytic, monocytic and myeloid elements. When blood is taken from patients with circulating immune complexes, cells with Fc receptors may carry passively absorbed Ig. Most of these complexes can be eluted from the cells by a wash in acetate buffer (16). Aggregates can also bind to cells during the IF test: rabbit Ig has a particularly high affinity for human Fc receptors and should be avoided or used as $F(ab')_2$. Goat Ig does not bind efficiently to human Fc receptors and gives cleaner results. Reagents are centrifuged (100 000 g for 30 min) for removing aggregates, and stored frozen at $-30°C$ in small aliquots. These small aliquots are then spun again at 1000 g for 5 min before use. MAbs may also contain aggregates, particularly when stored in lyophilized form and reconstituted. The formation of aggregates in the culture supernatants of MAbs containing 10% fetal calf serum (FCS) is less noticeable, and these MAbs can be stored at $-30°C$. Finally, when particularly strong non-specific binding is observed on a subset of monocytes and on blast cells in acute monocytic leukaemias, the cell suspensions can be pre-incubated with rabbit serum in order to block Fc binding (Section 6).

2. SEPARATION OF MONONUCLEAR CELLS FROM BLOOD AND BONE MARROW

2.1 **Principle**

There are two convenient and efficient methods, and both of these have a rapid 'version'. In the first, anti-coagulated blood or bone marrow is layered onto Ficoll−Isopaque (also referred to as Ficoll−Hypaque, Lymphoprep, Ficoll−Triosil, see also Chapter 1). After centrifugation at 20°C, erythrocytes and polymorphs sediment to the bottom, while lymphocytes, monocytes, platelets and mononuclear bone marrow cells remain at the interface (17). The other separation fluid, Sepracell-MN is a silica colloid which is completely admixed with blood and after centrifugation the mononuclear cells are recovered from the upper layer (18).

2.2 **Materials**

(i)   Separation fluid mix: 10 parts of Isopaque (33% density 1.20 g/ml Triosil, Vestric Ltd) mixed with 24 parts of Ficoll (9%, Pharmacia) which gives a final density of 1.077 g/ml, or use proprietary brands such as Lymphoprep (Nyegaard Ltd).

(ii)   Alternatively, Sepracell-MN (Sepratech Corp.).

(iii)   Collect blood into lithium−heparin vials (10 ml), or use 10 IU of preservative-free heparin for each 1 ml of blood. Bone marrow is collected into lithium−heparin vials containing 2−4 ml of tissue culture medium.

(iv)   Sterile phosphate-buffered saline (PBS) containing 0.2% bovine serum albumin (PBSA) and tubes of 15 ml capacity.

2.3 **Method**

(i)   If the white blood concentration is less than $20 \times 10^9/l$ dilute blood twice with PBS; if it is greater than $20 \times 10^9/l$ dilute 4-fold.

(ii)   Place 4 ml of Ficoll−Isopaque into a tube and carefully layer on 8 ml of diluted blood. Spin at 400 *g* for 25 min. Alternatively, take a tube containing 6.7 ml of Sepracell−MN, add up to 6 ml of blood and mix gently. The length of centrifugation at 2000 *g* depends upon whether fixed angle rotor (10 min), or swinging bucket rotor (20 min) is used.

(iii) Transfer the cells at the interface of Ficoll−Isopaque and blood or in the upper layer of Sepracell−MN into another tube, and dilute the suspension five times in PBSA. Spin the cells at 40 *g* for 10 min; at lower speeds cell losses may occur. However, low-speed centrifugation allows further separation of platelets from mononuclear cells.

(iv)   Wash the cells again and then adjust the cell concentration to $1-2 \times 10^7$/ml PBSA after counting in a haemocytometer (Chapter 1).

(v)   Count viable cells using trypan blue (Chapter 1).

2.4 Comments

Variations in the Ficoll−Isopaque technique are described elsewhere (17, and Chapter 1). The Ficoll−Isopaque and Sepracell−MN methods give identical T and B cell yields, as well as stimulation values with T and B cell mitogens (18). A modification of these methods for a very rapid isolation of mononuclear cells from smaller samples is as follows.

(i)   Use polythene tubes with caps (volume 1.5 ml, e.g. Sarstedt) and a micro-centrifuge with fixed angle rotor (e.g. Eppendorf).

(ii)   Layer 1 ml of cell suspension onto 0.5 ml of Ficoll−Isopaque, alternatively, mix equal volumes of Sepracell−MN and undiluted blood.

(iii) Centrifuge for 1 min (600 *g* fixed speed).

(iv)   Collect the cells at the interphase of Ficoll−Isopaque or in the upper layer (on Sepracell−MN). This rapidly obtained sample is sufficient for a microplate assay allowing testing with 12 MAbs (see below).

3. MEMBRANE IMMUNOFLUORESCENCE STAINING (MICROPLATE METHOD)

3.1 Principle

Antibodies react with membrane antigens on viable cells in suspension. In order to prevent capping and shedding of antigens, 0.2% sodium azide is added to the cell suspension (19). In the *direct* method the antigen-specific antibody is labelled and used as a single-step procedure, while in the *indirect* method a labelled anti-Ig antibody is used as the second layer in a two-step procedure to identify the initial antigen-specific antibody. The indirect test is more sensitive than the direct test.

The microplate method allows processing of multiple samples and staining with multiple MAbs. Four elements contribute to the economy of the method (15).

(i)   Microplates with U-wells are used for simultaneous staining and washing of 96 samples.

(ii)   Antibody panels are constructed as multiples of six tests, and multipipettes are employed to handle six reagents and six samples simultaneously. These samples are transferred onto slides, for viewing, in a pre-arranged pattern of 2×6.

(iii)   Twelve-well multitest slides receive the 12 droplets of cells and are fixed in formalin and viewed on a standard microscope under coverslip. Bright $63 \times$ Phaco objectives with numerical apertures 1.4 are used without compromising optical quality.

(iv)   Depending on the results, it is possible

   (a)   to re-stain the residual cells left in the microplate wells using directly labelled second antibody (Section 6);

   (b)   to prepare cytospins from selected microwells and stain these for cytoplasmic or nuclear antigens (Section 7); or

   (c)   to analyse cells from selected microwells on the cell sorter (Section 5).

Although this method is specifically designed for lymphocyte membrane marker studies and leukaemia diagnosis, the economy of the technique in terms of reagents, cells and time readily allows its adaptation to other experimental situations in which a large number of tests need to be performed simultaneously and where the number of cells available is limited.

3.2 Reagents and materials

(i)   MAbs for investigating immune disorders and chronic leukaemias (*Table 1*) and those for diagnosing acute leukaemia (*Table 2*) together with normal control serum (from the same species). Goat anti-mouse Ig labelled with FITC (e.g. Sigma, or Seralab).

(ii)   PBS containing 0.2% BSA and 0.2% NaN_3 (PBSAA).

(iii)   Microplates with U-bottom wells (Sterilin).

(iv)   Adhesive microplate cover (Flow Labs).

(v)   Plastic stoppers for individual wells (e.g. Pierce and Warriner Ltd).

(vi)   Microplates with V-bottomed wells (in order to keep the panel of reagents in a standard order).

(vii)   Teflon-coated multispot slides with 12 wells (Hendley Engineering Ltd) and large coverslips.

(viii) Formalin vapour (40% formaldehyde in a moist chamber).

(ix)   Semipermanent mountant: 20 g of poly-vinylalcohol in 80 ml of PBS + 40 ml of glycerol containing 3 g of diazo-bicyclooctane (DABCO), pH 8.6 (ref. 20). Temporary mountant: PBS and glycerol in 1:1 (v/v) ratio.

3.3 Equipment

(i)   Centrifuge, for example Beckman TJ-6, or MSE Centaur 2 with plate carriers.

(ii)   Microscope with epi-illumination, filter sets for FITC and TRITC, phase contrast condenser and objective 63 Phaco $N.A = 1.3 - 1.4$

(iii)   Plate shaker (Dynatech).

(iv)   Titertek 8-fold multi-pipettes: $5 - 50$ μl; $50 - 200$ μl (Flow Labs), together with trays for solutions; also tips in unlimited quantity, changed after each operation.

(v)   Repette repeating dispensers, 2 ml total volume with Teflon piston (Jencons Scientific) for rapid repeated delivery of 50 μl cell suspensions.

3.4 **Microplate method**

(i)   Pipette $1-2 \times 10^5$ cells in 50 μl aliquots into each U-bottomed well of a 12-well row using a repeating dispenser.

(ii)   Transfer 50 μl aliquots of twelve (2×10^6) MAbs (*Tables 1* or *2*), (kept in an adjacent plate as a row of concentrated stock solutions and diluted with PBSA prior to use) in 50 μl volumes onto the cells with a multipipette (using six of the eight available channels).

(iii)   Cover the whole plate with an adhesive sheet and occasionally agitate while incubating for 10 min at 20°C.

(iv)   Top up the wells with 150 μl of PBSAA, spin in a centrifuge at maximum acceleration till it reaches to 2000 r.p.m. and then brake to a standstill. Flick the supernatants out.

(v)   Suspend the cells on a plate shaker, add 150 μl of PBSAA and repeat steps (iv) and (v) four times.

(vi)   Incubate the cells for 10 min with diluted goat anti-mouse Ig—FITC (30 μl), and wash as in steps (iv) and (v).

(vii)   After the last wash, add $5-6$ μl of PBSAA to each of the small cell pellets using a multipipette, and transfer 2 μl of resuspended cells, as two rows of six samples, onto a Teflon-coated multispot slide.

(viii) Place one slide (12 samples) for each patient into formalin vapour for 10 min, air dry at 20°C and cover with glycerol:PBS (1:1) and a coverslip.

3.5 **Comments**

Sodium azide under acid conditions yields toxic hydrazoic acid. Azide compounds should be diluted with running water before being discarded to avoid explosive deposits in copper piping.

It is important to adhere to the washing procedure (resuspension and number of washes). Residual traces of the first antibody in the supernatant can form soluble complexes with the second antibody and bind to Fc receptors on irrelevant cells.

3.6 **Interpretation**

The fine morphology of membrane staining is informative. Cap formation and shedding of antigens is prevented by azide but membrane movement (patch formation) does occur and helps to identify genuine membrane staining. The staining pattern of patch formation differs from the 'granular' appearance seen when Ig complexes bind to Fc receptors. Unfixed dead cells in the suspension may stain homogeneously with labelled antibodies.

Many laboratories use a fairly uniform primary panel of MAbs in the microplate assay for immunoregulatory disorders and chronic lymphoid leukaemias (see 'lymphocyte panel' in *Table 1*). These antibodies are referred to as (a) T cell-associated, (b) primarily reactive with large granular lymphocytes (LGL) and (c) B cell-associated. The T cell-associated markers are CD2, CD3 and CD7, together with the subset markers for T cells of predominantly helper function (CD4) and suppressor/cytotoxic function (CD8) (21). The LGL marker is MAb of the CD16 group, detecting Fc receptors of low affinity (22). The B cell-associated group includes anti-Class II reagents (which

Table 1. Diagnostic reagents in lymphoid disorders ('lymphocyte panel').

Antibody	Function and role	Mol. wt (kd)	Frequently used examples	Ref.
(i) T cell-associated				
1. CD2	E receptor	50	(OK)T11, 9-2, Leu5, RFT11	31
2. CD3	T cell receptor- associated	19,22,28	(OK)T3, UCHT1, Leu4	21
3. CD7	Receptor for Fcμ	40	3A1, WT1, Leu9, RFT2	30
4. CD5[a]	Pan T + CLL	67	T101, (OK)T1, RFT1	21,37,55
5. CD4	Helper type T	55	(OK)T4, Leu3	21
6. CD8	Suppr./cytotox. type T	32	(OK)T8, Leu2, RFT8	21
(ii) Large granular-lymphocyte associated				
7. CD16	Low affinity Fc receptor		Leu 11	22
(iii) B cell-associated				
8. Class II	B cells + activated T and monocyte	28,32	(OK)Ia, etc. RFDR2	7
9. CD19	Pre-B + B	95	B4, Leu12, SB4, RFB9	27
10. CD20	B cells	35	B1, Leu16, RFB7	29
11. + anti-ϰ and λ[b]	Direct anti-Ig double label combination			52,53
(iv) Control				
12. Normal mouse serum				

[a]CD5 is used in double label combination with anti-IgM.
[b]Monoclonality testing.

73

Table 2. Diagnostic reagents in leukaemia ('acute leukaemia' panel[a]).

Antibody	Function or role	Mol. wt (kd)	Frequently used examples	Ref.
(i) Stem cell-associated				
1. CD34	Lymphoid + myeloid precursors[b]		BI-3C5, My10	23
2. HLA-DR	Lymphoid + myeloid precursors + B cells[b]	28,32	anti-HLA-DR, RFDR2	7
(ii) Myeloid-associated				
3. CD13	Myeloblasts, granulocytes and monocytes[b]	150	My7, MCS2	24,25
4. CD14	Monocytes[b]	55	UCHM1	26
(iii) Common ALL and B lymphoid-associated				
5. CD19[c]	Pre-B + B	95	B4, Leu12, SB4, RFB9	27
6. CD10	Pre-pre-B and cALL	100	J5, VILA1, RFAL1, -3	28
7. CD20	B cells	35	B1, Leu16, RFB7	29,68
8. IgM	B cells	75	IgM goat anti-Hu IgM	6
(iv) Thymocyte and T lymphoid-associated				
9. CD7	Thymocyte + T cell	40	3A1, WT1, Leu9, RFT2	30
10. CD2	Thymocytes, T cells + NK	50	(OK)T11, Leu5, RFT11	31
11. CD3[d]	T cells	19,22,28	(OK)T3, UCHT1	57,62,63
12. Normal mouse serum				

[a]Leukaemic cells reflect many of the phenotypic features of lympho/haemopoietic precursor cells. An additional marker frequently used for ALL diagnosis is anti-terminal deoxynucleotidyl transferase (TdT) (ref. 10,61).

[b]See *Figure 8*.

[c]Weak antibody in sections and cytospins. CD22 (p135; including To15, RFB4) is another pan-B reagent when used for detecting cytoplasmic antigens (*Figure 6*) (see refs. 58,59).

[d]In cytospin preparations and tissue sections cytoplasmic CD3 is already present in early thymocytes (*Figure 7*) (see refs. 62,63).

under normal conditions bind strongly to B cells and weakly to monocytes) and antibodies of the CD19 and CD20 groups (*Table 1*).

The antibodies for the acute leukaemia panel (*Table 2*) are (a) stem cell-associated, (b) myeloid, (c) common ALL and B lineage-associated, and (d) T lineage-related; these descriptions are only convenient approximations for the predominant reactivity of these MAbs. Examples of leukaemic reactivity with these MAbs are shown in *Figure 2*.

As the pattern of reactivity with the first round of antibodies emerges, further tests might be required. These are largely dependent upon the location of the laboratory (i.e. leukaemia centre, general hospital or pediatric oncology group, etc.). An immediate task is double staining for TdT (Section 9). The 'second round' reagents include additional myeloid (CD33; e.g. My9), erythroid anti-glycophorin and megakaryocytic (CDw42; e.g. AN51 or CDw41, e.g. J15) reagents as well as anti-light chain (anti-κ and anti-λ) and anti-heavy chain antibodies (anti-IgM, -IgG, -IgA; heavy chain-specific) for monoclonality testing in B cell malignancies.

The microplate assay can be assessed by microscope or measured quantitatively by flow cytometer (fluorescence activated cell sorters). As illustrative examples, the findings seen in peripheral blood, AIDS and in chronic lymphocytic leukaemia (B-CLL) will be discussed together with this quantitative assay (see below).

4. STUDY OF LYMPH NODE CELLS IN SUSPENSION

4.1 Principle

Mechanical dissociation of lymphoid tissues is effective in releasing lymphocytes but is often damaging towards larger, blastic cells and invariably leaves histiocytic, dendritic and stromal elements in the debris. Gentle enzymatic digestion of tissues allows a more representative cellular population to be examined, particularly where sclerosis or epithelioid macrophages and giant cells are prominent (e.g. malignant lymphomas, sarcoidosis, etc.) (see also Chapter 1).

4.2 Materials

(i)   Enzymes: collagenase (Hoechst Type I); neutral protease (*B. polymyxa* – Hoechst, Grade II); and deoxyribonuclease (Sigma, Type IV).
(ii)   Tissue culture medium (e.g. RPMI 1640) containing 10% FCS.
(iii)   Carousel rotator.

4.3 Method

(i)   Place fresh, unfixed tissue in medium containing 10% FCS. Dice the tissue into 2–3 mm pieces using a sharp razor blade or skin graft blade (Weiss & Co). During this phase no further processing is necessary.
(ii)   The tissue to be digested should not exceed 15% of the total volume of digesting solution. Add collagenase (0.5 U/ml) and neutral protease (0.5–1.0 U/ml) to the solution and incubate at 37°C for 1 h, while being gently rotated on a carousel.
(iii)   Add DNase (1 μg/ml) to the digest after 1 h and disperse by aspirating up and down a syringe through a filler tube (internal diameter 2–3 mm) with sufficient force to draw tissue chunks up and down the filler tube.

(iv)   Allow the tissue digest to stand at 20°C for 5–10 min so that debris and aggregates of cells settle. Transfer the supernatant to a new container, spin the cells and wash them three times with medium containing 10% FCS.

4.4 Comments

(i)   The lymphocyte antigens regularly affected by the enzyme digestion with neutral protease are CD4 (OKT4, Leu3) and CD21 (C3dR).

(ii)   The panel of MAbs used for assessing markers on lymphoid tissues is similar to those shown in *Table 1* but differs in that RFD9, a newly standardized MAb reactive with lymphomata of centroblastic type (and also with early erythroid cells and some macrophages (32) and RFB5, a particularly strong 'unclustered' anti-B cell reagent (33), are used instead of RFT12 and RFT11.

(iii) The enzyme digestion removes erythrocytes so that further purification is only necessary if granulocytes or other cells (hepatocytes) heavily contaminate the lymphoid mononuclear cells.

5. QUANTITATIVE ASSESSMENT OF FITC STAINING INTENSITY

5.1 Principle

The advantages of flow cytometers over microscopy are the speed of analysis (>500 cells/sec) and the accurate quantitative assessment of independent parameters of the same cell: the light scatter and the fluorescent intensity (see Chapter 2). Modern flow cytometers routinely analyse two types of light scatter: (i) forward angle light scatter which is roughly proportional to cell size and (ii) '90° light scatter' (S), which is proportional to the cells' granularity. When information from these two types of light scatter are combined the analytical separation of red cells, lymphoid cells, monocytes, granulocytes and dead cells is excellent (34). Chronic lymphocytic leukaemic cells segregate into the lymphoid peak, and acute leukaemias are positioned amongst larger lymphocytes and monocytes. It is common practice to gate the flow cytometer so as to count IF-labelled cells exclusively within a defined population; the mature monocytic and granulocytic forms are commonly excluded from routine analysis.

5.2 Reagents

Same as Sections 3 and 4. In addition:

(i)   8% formalin or 4% paraformaldehyde in 0.85% saline (adjusted to pH 7.4 with 0.1 M NaOH or 0.1 M HCl).

(ii)   CaliBRITE beads, green (FITC) (Becton-Dickinson).

5.3 Equipment

(i)   Several instruments are used in flow cytometry. The most popular models are manufactured by Becton Dickinson (FACS Systems), Coulter Electronics (EPICS Systems) and Ortho Diagnostics (Cytofluorographs).

(ii)   Computer-controlled programs for quantitative analysis. In our laboratory we are familiar with the EASY.88 computer system which works on the EPICS analysers.

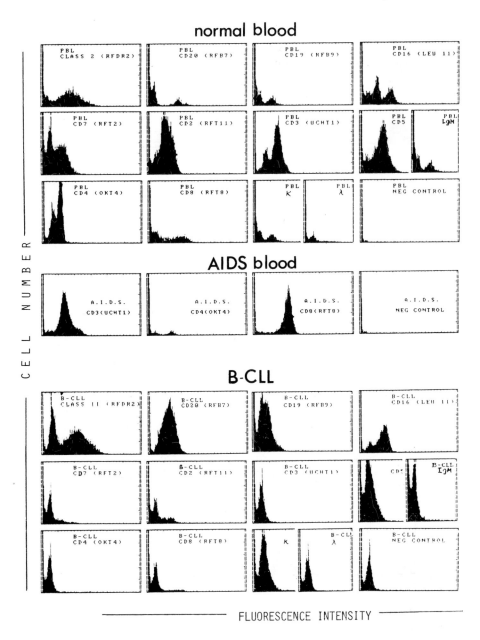

Figure 1. The typical reactivity of MAb panel used in the microplate assay on blood lymphocytes and in chronic lymphoid leukaemia as demonstrated by COMPOS plot on the EPICS V. Normal blood contains 10−15% B cells (Class II$^+$, CD20$^+$, CD22$^+$, CD21$^+$, IgM$^+$), some of which are $\varkappa^+$ and others are λ^+ in a normal 2:1 ratio. T cells are the majority (CD7$^+$, CD2$^+$, CD3$^+$, CD5$^+$). Most T cells are CD4$^+$, and others are CD8$^+$ in a 2:1 ratio. In acquired immune deficiency CD4$^+$ cells are absent. In B-CLL malignant B cells dominate which co-express CD5 and IgM. In this particular sample the B-CLL population is $\varkappa^+$ but λ^- (monoclonal).

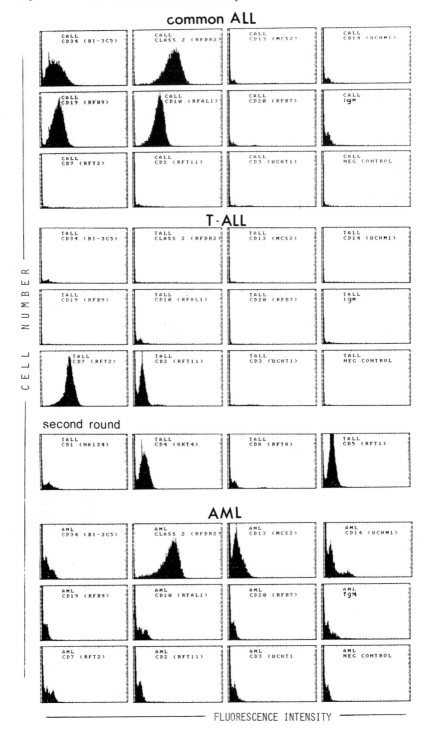

5.4 **Method**

(i)   Calibrate the flow cytometer according to manufacturers' instruction with caliBRITE (FITC) beads.

(ii)   Stain and wash the cell suspensions (Sections 3 and 4); add 100 μl of 8% formalin or paraformaldehyde solution to the cell pellets. Immediately, but gently, mix the cell suspension with a vortex mixer. These fixed cells can be stored for months in the dark at 4°C, allowing the operator to proceed with the study at convenience (35).

(iii)   FITC is routinely excited by monochromatic laser light at 488 nm wavelength. The required population is gated on forward angle and/or 90° light scatter. FITC fluorescence above 515 nm is collected, reflected 488 nm laser light being blocked out with filters; 10 000 cells are studied and the results are displayed in a histogram form.

(iv)   Most analysers have computer programs to calculate the percentages of fluorescence positivity, mean fluorescence of the studied population. Four graphic programs are available for the EPICS V with the EASY.88 computer system to produce comparative displays of results, such as the results obtained with a range of MAbs in a microplate assay. The first one is referred to as 'COMPOS' and lists histograms of the same set of analytical data in horizontal rows (*Figures 1 and 2*).

(v)   The second graphic program, 'COPLOT' is set up to graph a chosen number of histograms in vertical rows, while the third program 'NUCOPLOT' graphs at a diagonal. In all these displays, the graphs can be presented in boxes (*Figures 1 and 2*) or alone. The colours on the monitor are easy to change, and the graphs can be either lines or solid colours. Lines are preferred with IMMUNO and COPLOT, and solid colours alone without boxes are preferred with the NUCOPLOT.

(vi)   The fourth graphic program, OVERLAY, plots one or more histograms simultaneously and uses the full screen (*Figure 3*). This display helps compare these histograms visually, but it does not itself have analytical facility. Nevertheless, the percentages based on prior INTGRA and IMMUNO analysis (see below) can be displayed. The OVERLAY is particularly effective graphically in colour with 15 available different shades but does not print in box too well.

(vii)   The comparative analysis of observations is facilitated by two statistical programs: the 'INTGRA' and 'IMMUNO'. It is relevant here that the EPICS MDADs, the computer operating system of EPICS, already runs an integration program on histograms in order to obtain percentage results over selected channels. Here

Figure 2. The typical reactivity of MAb panels used in the microplate assay on malignant cells in acute leukaemia as demonstrated by the COMPOS programme on the EPICS V. cALL: common acute lymphoid leukaemia (Class II$^+$, CD19$^+$, CD10$^+$). T-ALL: thymic ALL (Class II$^-$· CD7$^+$, CD2$^+$). The study with additional markers confirms the thymic phenotype (CD1$^+$, CD4$^+$, CD8$^+$) although some of these Abs show weak or variable staining on T-ALL. AML: acute myeloid leukaemia (Class II mostly positive, MCS2$^+$). This particular case of AML shows some monocytic (UCHM1$^+$) differentiation.

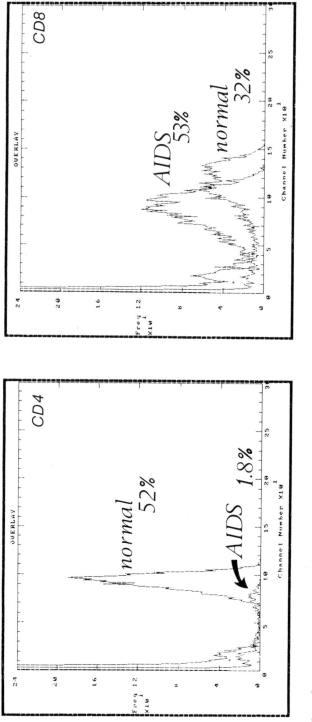

Figure 3. Investigation of peripheral blood taken from a normal individual (control) and from a patient with HIV infection. The overlay programme demonstrates the direct comparison between T cells of helper type (CD4) in the normal person and in AIDS, and a similar comparison with T cells of suppressor/cytotoxic type (CD8).

the cursors are simply set and the program calculates the percentage within the area chosen as compared with the whole histogram. This MDADS program allows only one area at a time to be examined, and further analysis involves repeated cursor setting. The EASY INTGRA program works on the same principle of integrating under chosen proportions of the histogram. Here up to eight ranges can be set by moving the mouse; these are referred to as 'cursor ranges'. Up to four % values can be displayed on the screen, and printed out. As the cursor ranges can be set in the memory, sequential samples can be studied and printed, and the percentages within fixed cursor ranges compared. Nevertheless, the INTGRA program does not allow for subtraction of control population: this is the role of the IMMUNO program.

(viii) Subtraction of control from test histograms is facilitated by programs such as IMMUNO (*Figure 4*). The IMMUNO program is useful for analysing samples where the positive cell distribution overlaps with the negative (or control) distribution. The program provides statistics for both the positive and negative (control) populations. For the limitations of the program see 'Immuno Program Notes' from Coulter Ltd.

5.5 Comments

In *Figures 1* and *2* the reactivity of the range of MAbs used in the microplate method is shown. In *Figure 1* the 'lymphocyte' microplate is demonstrated as it is applied to the analysis of AIDS and chronic B-CLL. In normal blood T lymphocytes dominate (CD3-, CD2- and CD7-positive, all showing varying fluorescent intensities) and represent a mixture of CD4- and CD8-positive cells. The $10-20\%$ B cells are CD19-, CD20- and IgM-positive, expressing $\varkappa$ or λ light chains in a normal 2:1 ratio. In the blood of a patient with AIDS the CD3-positive T cells are almost exclusively CD8-positive with a severe depletion of the CD4-positive population (see also *Figure 3*).

When normal blood is compared with CLL of B cell type, it is apparent that the numbers of B cells are high (Class II, CD19, CD20, IgM) and T cell number is virtually nil (CD7, CD2, CD3). The fluorescent intensity of B cell markers is lower than on normal B cells. The weak positivity of malignant B-CLL with CD5, otherwise a T cell marker, is a well-known phenomenon. The CD5/IgM double expression and the monoclonality assay with $\varkappa/\lambda$ labelling will be discussed in Section 7.

In *Figure 2* the diagnosis of common acute lymphocytic leukaemia (ALL) an early pre-B cell malignancy, is established by the strong reactivity with anti-Class II and CD10 (cALL antigen) and the weaker but still clear reactivity with CD19. This patient's leukaemic cells are reactive with CD34, a stem cell marker, and negative with CD20, a mature B cell marker (29).

The selected case of T-ALL, an early thymocyte malignancy, shows typically strong reactivity with CD7, whose staining intensity on T-ALL blast cells is frequently higher than observed on the majority of normal peripheral T lymphocytes (e.g. in *Figure 1*). Note the CD2 positivity of T-ALL and the lack of Class II expression. A small proportion of these T-ALL blasts also express CD10 (cALL) antigen weakly (36). The thymic features of T-ALL became evident upon the second round of additional reagents used in this case: these are the co-expression of CD1, CD4 and CD8 (ref. 37) together with

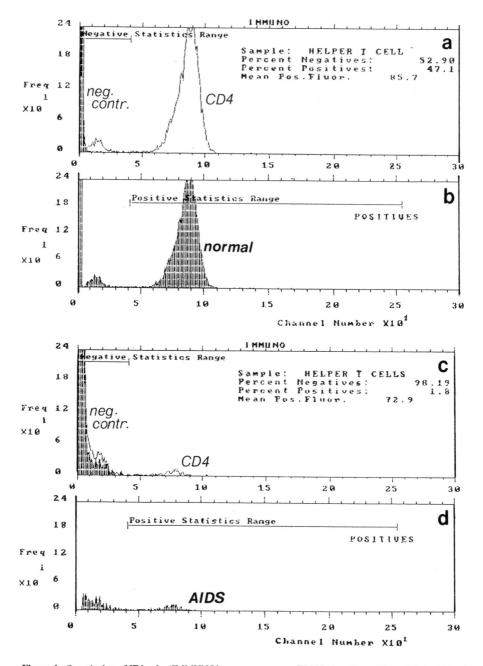

Figure 4. Quantitation of IF by the 'IMMUNO' programme on an EPICS V analyser. The staining of CD4+ cells is compared with irrelevant mouse antibody plus goat anti-mouse Ig−FITC [negative control in (**a**) and (**c**)]. The positive results are expressed following the subtraction of negative controls (**b,d**). Panels (**a**) and (**b**) are from normal blood; (**c**) and (**d**) are CD4-deficient samples from a case of AIDS with very low numbers (1.8%) of residual T4+ cells.

a lack of membrane CD3. The cytoplasmic expression of CD3 antigen by T-ALL will be re-investigated in cytospin smears (Section 9).

In the case of acute myeloid leukaemia (AML) shown, the weak background labelling with goat anti-mouse Ig (negative control) is higher than the negative controls seen in ALL and T-ALL. Labelling with a wide range of anti-lymphoid MAbs shows the same weak (negative) staining. Positive labelling is, however, seen with the anti-Class II, CD13 reagents, while the anti-monocytic CD14 MAbs 'marks' a subset of blast cells.

From the data presented in *Figure 1* the reactivity of lymphocytes with CD4 (T4) antibodies against T cells of helper phenotype were selected for statistical analysis using the IMMUNO program on the EPICS flow cytometer (*Figure 4*). Two samples, in this case CD4 antibody and its negative control are compared in *Figures 4a* and *c*. Then the control values are subtracted in order to show genuine positivity with CD4 (*Figures 4b* and *d*). The results demonstrate that 47% of mononuclear cells are strongly positive. These are normal T lymphocytes representing the 'positive range' (channels $40-250$). Cells in the other peak express CD4 very weakly (channels $2-40$). In the blood of a patient with HIV infection only 1.8% $CD4^+$ cells are present, indicating severe depletion. The low number of $CD4^+$ lymphocytes together with the clinical symptoms of opportunistic infections indicate that this HIV antibody-positive patient has AIDS.

With the sensitivity of programs such as the IMMUNO appropriate controls become crucial. For example, it is advisable to use, instead of murine serum (negative control, first layer), myeloma proteins having the same isotype and applied in the same concentration as the MAbs used in the parallel test.

5.6 Interpretation

The microplate assays above include the most informative reagents for the diagnosis of leukaemias. For reliable phenotyping multiple MAbs are necessary to identify cell lineages and the level of differentiation at which maturation 'arrest' has taken place. In addition, some breadth in the test system is required to detect 'lineage infidelity', that is deviations from the patterns seen during normal differentiation. The occasional cases of lineage infidelity found to have idiosyncratic phenotypes are often found to have multiple chromosomal aberrations in addition. For these reasons, the application of a rapid method using a panel of MAbs, as in the microplate assay, helps avoid misinterpretation of phenotypic data and allows additional investigations using further combinations of reagents. Examples of this process were seen in the cases of T-ALL and AML in *Figure 2*).

6. BLOCKING OF THE BINDING OF MONOCLONAL ANTIBODIES TO Fc RECEPTORS

6.1 Principle

Subpopulations of monocytes and leukaemias of monocytic origin often express $Fc\gamma$ receptors in high density. In these cases mouse MAbs of IgG type may give disturbingly high levels of binding even when used with $F(ab')_2$ second layers. This phenomenon is identified by the high background in the 'normal mouse serum' negative control, and can be proven by the efficient blocking of Fc binding using normal rabbit serum. Aggregated rabbit Ig has particularly high affinity for human Fc receptors, and incubation with rabbit serum saturates Fc receptors without affecting the specific binding of MAbs to their target antigens.

6.2 **Materials**

(i)   See Section 3. In addition:
(ii)   Normal rabbit serum stored for more than 1 month or freeze-thawed three times to facilitate the formation of Ig aggregates. Use at 1:10 dilution without previous centrifugation.
(iii)   Goat anti-mouse Ig−FITC, free of anti-rabbit Ig activity (negative on cells incubated with rabbit serum alone).

6.3 **Method**

(i)   Add 50 μl of rabbit serum diluted 1:10 to cells in microplate wells, and incubate for 10 min at 20°C, followed by two washes.
(ii)   Compare the results with the previous observations.

6.4 **Interpretation and comments**

The incubation of monocytes or leukaemic cells with rabbit serum can lead to a dramatic decrease in the binding of MAbs of IgG class and in the negative control (normal mouse serum). The staining intensity of both the anti-Class II and CD14 (anti-monocyte Ab) remains high. The conclusion is that this cell population expresses Fc receptors. The diagnosis of this type of leukaemia is acute (myelo)monocytic (AMoL or AMML).

7. TWO-COLOUR IF METHOD

7.1 **Principle**

This simple method is essential for immunobiologists who wish to investigate more closely the correlation between lymphocyte function and phenotype. The basic principle of double labelling for functional analysis is as follows. The major subset-specific antibodies used for subdividing lymphocytes into four major categories (*Table 3*) are relatively specific reagents but encompass cells with a wide range of functional capabilities. Major subset MAbs combined with antibodies detecting functionally related molecules (but which often are not lineage-specific on their own) allow distinctions of cells with much more restricted functional capabilities. Thus combinations of membrane molecules appear to subdivide the major categories of lymphocytes into functionally divergent populations (*Table 3*). The CD4$^+$ population can be further divided into helper-inducer and suppressor-inducer subsets by the Leu8 (38,39), CD45R (2H4; ref. 40) and CDw29 (4B4; ref. 41) MAbs. Both Leu 8 and CD45R react strongly with different B lymphoid populations (42) as well as with T lymphocytes. Similarly, CDw29 (4B4) is strongly reactive with monocytes, macrophages, polymorphs and, in tissue sections, with extracellular matrix. More recently a similar, though not identical, reagent with more restricted specificity for leucocytes (UCHL1) is being investigated for functional associations (43). Furthermore, there are also indications that a

Table 3. Correlations between lymphocyte phenotype and function.

	T helper type[a]		T suppressor/cytotoxic type[a]	Large granular lymphocytes (LGL)	B lymphocytes	Extra non-lymphoid activity
Major subset-specific antibodies[b]						
CD3	+		+	−	−	c
CD4	+		−	−	−	d
CD8	−		+	−/+	−	e
CD16[f]	−		−	+	−	
CD19	−		−	−	+	g
Secondary antibodies detecting secondary categories[b]						
	Helper inducer	Suppr. inducer				
Within CD4+	Leu8− CDw29+ (4B4+) CD45R−	Leu8+ CDw29− CD45R+ (2H4+)	Suppr.[i] Cytotox.	Cells of NK function[j]		h
Within CD8			? CD28+			
Within CD16[f]				HNK1(Leu7)+/− non MHC restricted cytotoxicity NKHI+ (Leu19)		

[a] Only these cells have T cell receptor (TCR) rearrangements; LGLs do not rearrange TCR.
[b] See *Table 2.*
[c] Occasional antibodies react with Purkinje cells or cytoplasmic filaments in all cells; otherwise a very specific reagent group.
[d] Weak reactivity on monocytes and Kupffer cells, weak to strong heterogeneous reactivity on subsets of macrophages.
[e] Sinus littoral cells in the spleen; and some large granular lymphocytes; otherwise very specific reagent group.
[f] Detecting Fc receptor of low affinity (e.g. Leu11).
[g] Specific antibody with uniformly weak expression on B cells.
[h] None of these antibodies are lineage specific and many react very strongly with non-lymphoid cells: these extra activities are too numerous to list. See ref. 14 for review.
[i] The phenotype of suppressor T cells is still elusive. Cytotoxic T cells are CD28+ (9.3+).
[j] Leu-7+,CD8− cells show strong NK activity but include only 50−60% of NK cells. Leu-7+,CD8+ cells or Leu-7+,CD4+ cells are less efficient NK cells. Most NK activity resides in the CD16+ population (Leu-11+); these cells are CD8−,CD4−. Another excellent marker for NK cells is HNK1 (Leu19). Positive population includes some CD3+ T cells which probably have TCR γ chain expression and show non-MHC restricted cytotoxicity.

subpopulation of CD8 cells reacting with the CD28 (9.3 and KOLT-2) MAbs (44) is involved in antigen-specific cytotoxicity. The phenotype of T suppressor cells is still elusive.

The subset structure of large granular lymphocytes (LGL) and the relationship of these cells to natural killer (NK) activity is equally intriguing. Only 50−60% of LGL and a similar proportion of functional NK activity in a given cell suspension is attributable to a population identified by the MAb Leu7 (HNK1). $HNK1^+$, $CD8^-$, $CD4^-$ cells have strong NK activity. Unfortunately, HNK1 is also found on some $CD8^+$ cells and on a population of $CD4^+$ lymphocytes with virtually no NK activity. It appears that CD16 antigen (low affinity Fc receptors) is a better 'marker' for the LGL and NK cell population than HNK1 antigen (*Table 3*). More recently a new set of reagents (NKH1; ref. 46, see also Leu-19) appears to be an interesting marker for NK cells but some of the positive cells express CD3 and may represent a subset of T cells with non-MHC restricted cytotoxic function. It is clear from this summary that only double and, in some cases, even triple marker techniques will accurately identify the lymphocyte phenotype with the cells' functional capacity.

The technical principles of two-colour IF are as follows. The double staining can be performed simultaneously with non-cross-reacting reagents directly labelled with different fluorochromes. The direct method is highly recommended when one wishes to investigate the absolute amounts of antigens expressed on the cells. The single layer antibodies are used at saturating conditions in such experiments. Commercial companies supply such labelled antibodies of high quality (47). One antibody in each pair is FITC labelled, the other can either be conjugated with TRITC or PE. The disadvantage of this system is that relatively large amounts of reagents are required in the absence of second layer amplification.

Although the *indirect* method is inappropriate for assessment of cell membrane antigen density, it can be used for other purposes. The advantages of indirect IF are 3-fold:

(i)   the second layer amplifies the intensity of labelling, and gives good results even if the given antigen is expressed in low density;

(ii)   it is economical with the first layer antibody, and

(iii) the same fluorochrome-labelled second antibody can be used with a wide variety of first layers.

When the first layer MAbs are of different classes, such as IgM and IgG, they can be identified separately using specific goat anti-mouse IgM and IgG conjugated with different fluorochromes. With the standardization of CD clusters it is relatively easy to find MAbs of the same specificity but belonging to different classes of the same CD (*Table 4*). An equally successful method is to conjugate MAbs with haptens such as biotin (48) (Section 8), or arsanilic acid and use avidin (or streptavidin) and goat anti-arsanilic antibodies, respectively as fluorochrome-conjugated second layers (49; reviewed in ref. 50).

A final variation in two-colour IF analysis can be applied when both first layer antibodies are of IgG class. One of the two antibodies is conjugated with biotin, and the other (usually purchased commercially in small amounts) left unconjugated (see Section 8; ref. 51).

Table 4. Examples of antibodies recognizing the same CD clusters but showing different isotypes.

	IgM		*IgG$_2$*		*IgG$_1$*	
T cell antibodies						
CD2 (T11) pan-T	9−2	(1)[a]	OKT11a	(2)	RFT11	(3)
CD3 (T3) periph.T (mitogenic)	T10B9	(4)	OKT3	(2)	UCHT1	(5)
CD4 (T4) helper	66.1	(6)	OKT4	(2)	Leu 3a	(7)
CD8 (T8) suppressor/cytotoxic	RFT8μ	(3)	OKT8	(2)	RFT8γ	(3)
Precursor cell-associated						
CD10 common ALL antigen	RFAL3	(3)	RFAL2	(3)	RFAL1	(3)
Class II non-polymorphic	RFDR1	(3)	RFDR2	(3)		
B cell antibodies						
CD19 pre-B + B	SB4	(8)			B4	(9)
CD20 pan-B	RFB7	(3)	B1	(9)		

[a]The numbers in brackets refer to the Laboratories where the reagents are made or distributed from. (1) Naito and Dupont, Sloan Kettering, New York; (2) ORTHO, Raritan, New Jersey; (3) Royal Free Hospital, London; (4) Thompson, Kentucky; (5) Beverley, University College Hospital, London; (6) Hansen, Seattle; (7) Becton-Dickinson, Mountain View, California; (8) Sanofi, Montpellier; (9) Coulter, Hialeah, Florida.

7.2 Reagents

(i)   For direct two-colour IF analysis use the following 'Simultest' kits:

     (a)   T and B cell test;

     (b)   CD4 and CD8 test;

     (c)   CD3 and anti-class II;

     (d)   the investigation of HNK-1 (Leu-7) and CD8$^+$ cells.

     These are available from Becton Dickinson. In these kits the first antibodies are FITC labelled and the second antibodies are PE labelled.

(ii)   For the simultaneous labelling of CD5 (T1; p67) antigen and surface immunoglobulin use CD5 + goat anti-mouse Ig−FITC or TRITC together with directly labelled goat anti-human IgM−TRITC (μ heavy chain-specific; Southern Biotechnology Associates) or rabbit anti-human IgM−FITC F(ab′)$_2$.

(iii) For establishing the monoclonality of B cell malignancies use goat anti-human $\varkappa$-TRITC together with goat anti-human λ−FITC, available from different companies including Southern Biotechnology Associates.

(iv) For examples of performing indirect two-colour IF with MAbs of different class see *Table 4*. The goat anti-mouse IgM−TRITC and anti-mouse IgG−FITC class specific column-purified second layers are available from Southern Biotechnology Associates, as is the alternative colour combination (IgM−FITC with IgG−TRITC).

(v)   Avidin and streptavidin are available in FITC, TRITC and PE conjugated form from a number of companies such as Becton Dickinson, Serotec and Amersham International.

(vi)   Directly conjugated secondary antibodies (see *Table 3*) are available from Coulter Ltd or from Becton Dickinson.

(vii)   TRITC-conjugated MAbs to Class II antigen (RFDR2−TRITC, Royal Free Hospital) or anti-HLA-DR−PE, Becton Dickinson).

(viii) Mouse serum used at 1:10 dilution.

(ix)   For equipment see Section 3.

7.3 Direct method with FITC and PE

(i)   Incubate mononuclear cells with CD4−CD8 Simultest or similar mixtures of CD4−FITC and CD8−PE for 10 min as described in Section 3.

(ii)   Add 8% formalin or 4% paraformaldehyde to the cell pellet and mix.

(iii)   Count 100−200 lymphocytes on the microscope, ignoring platelets and monocytes. Monocytes may exhibit weak CD4 labelling. Calculate the percentage of CD4 (green) and CD8 (orange) positive cells within the total lymphoid population.

(iv)   Gate the flow cytometer on cells with the scatter characteristics of lymphocytes. Count 10 000 cells and express the results, on the basis of two-colour histograms as % CD4−FITC-positive cells (green; X) and % CD8−PE-positive cells (orange; Y) within the lymphoid population.

(v)   Calculate the absolute numbers of CD4- and CD8-positive cells in the blood sample on the basis of the absolute white blood cell count, differential lymphocyte count and the proportions of CD4/CD8 in the lymphoid population.

7.4 Comments

Cells labelled with FITC and PE can be observed simultaneously without changing filters. Only a standard FITC filter set is required but the FITC-specific narrow band barrier filter has to be removed in order to allow the orange to be viewed. Using this illumination the PE fluorochrome fades very slowly while viewed under TRITC filters it fades rapidly.

7.5 Extension of the microplate assay with FITC/TRITC doubles

(i)   When the 'lymphocyte' microplate is performed (*Table 1; Figure 1*) place a mixture of goat anti-Hu-$\varkappa$−TRITC and goat anti-Hu-λ−FITC into the 11th well. After washing four times, FITC- and TRITC-positive cells can be counted by microscope with separate filters.

(ii)   The 8th well of the same microplate has been incubated with MAb of CD5 (T1-type) and to this well, in addition to goat anti-M-Ig−FITC, also add goat anti-Hu-IgM−TRITC. After washing four times and mounting on slides, examine the cells to see if CD5$^+$ (T) cells and IgM$^+$ (B) cells represent separate populations, as observed in normal blood, or, alternatively, whether malignant B cells of IgM$^+$ type co-express CD5.

(iii) Often cell populations in leukaemic blood and bone marrow are heterogeneous, with variable proportions of leukaemic cells admixed with normal myelo-erythropoietic cells and T lymphocytes. The cells remaining in the microplate wells can still be used for further staining: first add 20 μl of mouse serum for 5 min to block G-anti-M-Ig activity and wash the plate once. Now the cells can be stained with anti-Class-II−TRITC by incubation for 10 min, washed four times and the heterogeneity of leukaemia assessed by HLA-DR positivity (TRITC filter) in addition to other selected markers (CD10, anti-T or anti-myeloid in separate wells: FITC filter).

7.6 Comments and interpretation

In samples labelled for x and λ, the microscopic analysis of normal blood shows that 10−15% of lymphocytes form caps and patches on the membrane. These B cells have a 2:1 ratio of x/λ positivity on separate cells (*Figure 1*). Occasionally, some cells are doubly stained; this indicates the presence of Ig aggregates. In leukaemia/lymphoma the diagnosis of B cell malignancy can be made if the x/λ ratio is more than 10:1 or less than 1:5 (refs. 52,53). When the sample is not severely involved (e.g. when B lymphoma is studied in the bone marrow), a two-colour combination may be necessary for accurate diagnosis. It is important to emphasize that the percentage positivity with anti-Ig reagents has to be interpreted in the light of positivity with other B cell markers such as CD19, CD20 and anti-Class II, because some B cell malignancies express low or undetectable amounts of sIg, and still show the 'monoclonal' rearrangements of their Ig genes.

The CD5/IgM combination in normal blood is a convenient two-colour method to count T cells (CD5$^+$) and B cells (IgM) in the suspension, but in leukaemia this double staining is virtually a tumour-associated marker combination. These double cells are present in the primary nodules of fetal lymph nodes and spleen, and are also found in peritoneal wash-outs (54), but normally these B cells are rapidly diluted out with CD5-negative B cells and in adult lymphoid tissue, blood and bone marrow the CD5/IgM-positive cells are very rare (55).

The combination staining with anti-HLR-DR can also be very useful in leukaemia/lymphoma with low numbers of infiltrating cells. An example is provided by leukopenic common ALL where large numbers of Class II-negative T lymphocytes are present and the study has to be focused on sIg-negative, Class II$^+$ blast cells.

7.7 Standardization of indirect two-colour IF

(i) The standardization can be performed with any pair of MAbs of IgM and IgG class. Here we select a combination of Leu7 (HNK1, IgM) and RFT8 (CD8, IgG) reagents. Prepare cell suspensions (50 μl each into four tubes) from normal blood.

(ii) Add RFT8 (IgG) into tubes 1 and 2, and negative control (mouse serum) into tubes 3 and 4. Add Leu7 (IgM) into tubes 1 and 3, and negative control into tubes 2 and 4. Incubate for 10 min in the presence of 0.2% azide, and wash the tubes four times.

(iii) Add a mixture of appropriately diluted goat anti-mouse IgG−FITC and goat anti-mouse IgM−TRITC to all tubes, and incubate for 10 min and wash again three times.

(iv) Prepare slides and examine cells under sealed coverslips. The expected results are as follows. Both CD8 and HNK1 antibodies label subsets of lymphocytes (CD8$^+$: 25−30%; HNK1: 5−10%). There is some overlap: 3−6% of cells are double labelled in tube 1. Nevertheless, the antigens recognized by the two Abs are different, and the second layers do not cross-react with the irrelevant mouse Ig class or with each other. This is confirmed in tube 2 where only FITC-labelled cells can be detected, and in tube 3 where only TRITC-stained cells are seen. If the second layer reagents are well standardized, tube 4 is negative.

7.8 Comments

This standardization experiment for the two fluorochrome-labelled anti-mouse Ig class-specific reagents indicates that these particular second layers can be used with any of the dozens of IgG−IgM combinations for which MAbs are potentially available (*Table 4*). This assay is a powerful routine analytical tool in establishing the exact heterogeneity of lymphocyte populations in blood and other organs (Section 9) and in finding minute proportions of haemopoietic precursor cells.

8. IF STUDIES USING BIOTIN−AVIDIN

8.1 Principle

The conjugation of MAbs with biotin is a simple method, and antibody−biotin conjugates can be powerfully visualized by commercially available fluorochrome-labelled avidin or streptavidin. The principle of biotin conjugation is that biotin succinimide ester (BSE) dissolved in dimethyl sulphoxide (DMSO) binds to antibodies at pH 8.6 (48).

8.2 Materials

(i) MAb (purified antibody, 1 mg/ml) in 0.1 M NaHCO$_3$ (pH 8.6), without azide or preservative. Coupling is inhibited by extraneous amines, Tris or azide.

(ii) BSE (stored in desiccator), dissolved prior to use in DMSO: 1 mg/ml.

(iii) PBS (pH 7) with 0.2% NaN$_3$.

(iv) Avidin (Sigma) labelled with TRITC, FITC or PE in the laboratory. Alternatively: streptavidin−Texas Red or −FITC (both from Amersham International).

8.3 Method

(i) Take 3 × 1 ml samples of MAb solution and add 30, 60 and 120 μl of BSE in DMSO, respectively, mixing immediately they are added. Leave at 20°C for 4 h.

(ii) Dialyse against PBS overnight at 4°C.

(iii) Investigate which one of the three samples is the optimal conjugate with bright staining using (strept)avidin fluorochrome without non-specific IF or loss of anti-body activity.

(iv)   Incubate the cells with antibodies followed by washes in the following sequence: unconjugated MAb; goat anti-mouse Ig−FITC; mouse serum to saturate any excess activity of the previous layer; second biotin conjugated MAb, and finally avidin- or streptavidin−TRITC or −PE.

8.4 Comment

This technique is an alternative to the class-specific double combinations. It also gives a clean staining but takes much longer to perform (51). Most tissue culture media contain biotin which can lead to erratic results unless cells are washed first with PBS or other buffer not containing biotin.

9. INVESTIGATION OF CELLS IN CYTOCENTRIFUGE PREPARATIONS AND SMEARS

9.1 Principle

The analysis of IF of cytospins has led to the following observations.

(i)   Cells which have been labelled in suspension show superior morphology and can be stored, if necessary, in the dark at 4°C without loss of fluorescence for longer than 1 month and perhaps up to a year (56).

(ii)   Labelling of cytoplasmic and nuclear antigens dominates when *unstained* cells are labelled with antibodies *after fixation* (57). The reactivity of many MAbs may differ from those seen in suspension because of the appearance of intracellular staining. Strongly expressed membrane antigens are also stained. Instructive examples of this are encountered in the analysis of normal and malignant pre-B cells (58,59), and that of benign and malignant plasma cell disorders (60,61) with various anti-Ig reagents.

(iii)   Labelling of membrane antigens can be performed in suspension followed by staining the cytoplasmic antigens after cytospin preparation and fixation. Using different fluorochromes allows assessment of each antigen. This is illustrated by the investigation of cytoplasmic CD3, which first appears in the perinuclear space and then the cytoplasm of immature thymocytes before it is inserted into the membrane (57,62,63). Cytospins can also be re-stained for *nuclear antigens*. This allows the examination of membrane phenotype in relation to cells undergoing DNA synthesis and division by labelling with bromodeoxyuridine (BrdU, a thymidine analogue) followed by MAbs to BrdU (64), or alternatively by using the MAb Ki67 which detects a proliferation-associated nuclear protein (65).

(iv)   Finally, the detection of nuclear terminal deoxynucleotidyl transferase, a unique DNA synthetic enzyme in both immature B cells and thymocytes, has already been an established diagnostic test for some years in leukaemia, and a lymphoid stem cell marker in lymphocyte physiology (10,66).

        For cell suspensions there are three ways of preparing slides.

(i)   By the method used for routine haematological blood smears which requires a

50% packed cell volume in serum. In these spreads made from 'concentrated' suspensions the fluid rapidly evaporates and cells dry out without the damaging morphological effects shown by shrinking.

(ii)   By cytocentrifuge, optimally using $1-3$ drops of a 10^6 cells/ml in solution containing protein (0.2% BSA).

(iii)   By cell attachment to poly-L-lysine (PLL) coated slides onto which the cell suspension is layered and the cells allowed to settle and attach (~ 10 min). Excess fluid is shaken off. The second method is given here.

9.2 Materials

(i)   There is no single fixative suitable for all purposes: 5% acetic acid in 95% ethanol is optimal for demonstrating Ig in plasma cells (and disastrous for some other proteins); pure cold methanol is optimal for demonstrating most cytoplasmic antigens and nuclear TdT (10); NaOH solution (0.01 M: see below) is required for anti-BrdU staining, and acetone or formalin vapour can be tested for their efficacy with other antigens.

(ii)   Microscope slides, adsorbent cytospin paper, coverslips and mounting media for permanent storage as in Section 3.

(iii)   Glass micropipettes (2, 5 and 10 μl volume) for adding antibodies to smeared cells.

(iv)   Antibodies, for example for the demonstration of membrane, cytoplasmic and nuclear staining on human thymocytes: anti-CD3 MAb such as Leu4 (Becton Dickinson) or OKT3 (Ortho) with goat anti-mouse Ig $-$ TRITC (e.g. Southern Biotechnology Associates) as well as similar directly conjugated CD3 $-$ FITC; anti-BrdU $-$ FITC (Becton Dickinson), and BrdU (Sigma). Also required: 0.1 M NaOH solution and 0.1 M $Na_2B_4O_7$ solution.

(v)   Normal mouse serum (NMS) (1:20 dilution).

(vi)   Tissue culture medium with 10% FCS.

(vii)   Phytohaemagglutinin (PHA)-P (Wellcome) used at 2 μg/ml final concentration for lymphocyte activation.

9.3 Equipment

(i)   Bench centrifuge for Ficoll $-$ Hypaque separation (Section 3).

(ii)   Cytocentrifuge (Cytospin-2; Shandon).

(iii)   Moisture chamber, to prevent the evaporation of reagents from cytospins.

(iv)   Incubator, 37°C.

9.4 Method for double labelling of membrane and cytoplasmic antigens

(i)   Make cell suspensions ($5-10 \times 10^6$/ml), for example from normal blood or thymus and take PHA-stimulated cultures at day 4. Incubate cells with BrdU at a final concentration of 10 μM for 30 min in 5% CO_2 at 37°C.

(ii)   Following incubation, prepare two samples of cell suspension (4×10^5 cells/100 μl in PBSAA from blood (B), thymus (T) and PHA (P). PHA-stimulated clumps may have to be disrupted by pipetting and incubation with N-acetyl-galactosamine, 100 μg/ml for 2−3 min.

(iii) Wash the cells twice in PBSAA and incubate the test samples with CD3 antibody and negative control samples with NMS for 15 min at 20°C and wash three times. Add goat anti-mouse Ig−TRITC second layer and wash again three times.

(iv) Prepare three cytospins (S1−3) from each of the CD3-labelled B, T and P samples and from the three unlabelled negative controls. Draw rings with a diamond pencil around the cytospins. Fix two of these (S1, S2) in acetone at 20°C for 10 min. The first slide (S1) should be viewed to see membrane CD3 staining.

(v) Re-hydrate the second slide (S2) in PBS and add NMS (1:20−1:40 final dilution) for 10 min. Wash them in a Coplin jar with three changes of PBS for 1−3 min each change. Slides should not be allowed to dry out thus the procedure is carried out in a moist chamber.

(vi) Add CD3−FITC (1:10 diluted commercial antibody) for 20 min and wash in three changes.

(vii) Slides for BrdU labelling (S3) require special pre-treatment. These need to be fixed in cold methanol at 4°C for 30 min. Immerse these in 0.01 M NaOH for 10−15 sec and bring them rapidly to pH 5 by immersing into 0.1 M $Na_2B_4O_7$.

(viii) Incubate with NMS (1:20−1:40) for 10 min and wash as in (v).

(ix) Add pre-titrated anti-BrdU−FITC for 20 min, wash three times and mount. Observe the cells with membrane labelling (TRITC) and then investigate whether these are labelled in the nucleus for BrdU (DNA synthetic proliferating cells). In slide S2 look for cells with cytoplasmic CD3 (FITC) and membrane CD3 (TRITC). S1 is CD3 membrane staining alone (TRITC).

9.5 Comments

It is obvious from the description above that different antigens need different fixatives. The methods above demonstrate double labelling for membrane and cytoplasmic CD3 (slides S2) and for membrane CD3 and nuclear BrdU (slides S3) in normal blood, thymus and PHA-stimulated lymphocytes. A set of slides can be kept in reserve (S4) for nuclear TdT staining (see below).

The combined labelling of membrane or cytoplasmic antigens with BrdU needs particular attention. The practice recommended for BrdU staining in manuals destroys membrane and cytoplasmic antigens, because the concentration of NaOH is too high. Furthermore, the fixative recommended there (70% ethanol) allows the leakage of nuclear proteins into the cytoplasm and results in a rather homogeneous poor staining (e.g. with anti-TdT). For this reason the use of methanol fixative and the lower concentration of NaOH solution is critical to maintain the integrity of membrane, cytoplasmic and nuclear antigens and at the same time promotes the denaturation of DNA for BrdU staining (67).

9.6 Interpretation

The inspection of slides demonstrates that in blood only cells with membrane CD3

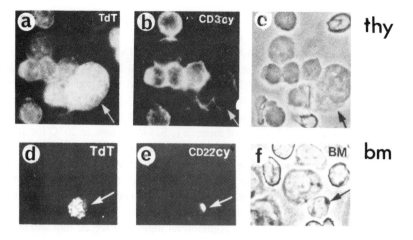

Figure 5. Double labelling for nuclear terminal transferase (TdT, **a,d**) and cytoplasmic antigens such as CD3 (**b**) and CD22 (**e**) in the normal thymus (**a,c**) and in the normal bone marrow (**d,f**). Large strongly TdT-positive blasts express perinuclear CD3 antigens. These thymic blasts are highly proliferative cells. In the bone marrow the TdT$^+$ cells have cytoplasmic CD22 being within the pre-B cell population.

positivity (TRITC) are co-labelled for CD3 when re-stained in smears (FITC in S2). When these cells are stimulated with PHA, surface CD3 might be down-regulated. Nevertheless, in suspensions made from the thymus, large blast cells (0.5−5% of total) and 20−40% of small thymocytes are membrane CD3-negative (TRITC) and distinctly positive for cytoplasmic CD3 (*Figure 5*).

When the BrdU staining is inspected, the lymphocytes from the blood contain few positive cells (<1%), but in PHA-stimulated cultures and in the thymus, larger proportions are recorded (10−40%). The large thymic blast cells are clearly included in the DNA synthetic population: these cells contain the highest proportion of cells (>90%) among thymocytes which incorporate BrdU. The large thymic blast cells also contain prominent, multiple nucleoli. When these cells are further studied for MAb reactivity, it is apparent that the cytoplasmic CD3 expressing thymic blast cells, unlike PHA blasts obtained from peripheral blood, are TdT-positive. The thymic blasts express CD7 antigens but hardly any other T-lineage associated antigens (CD1$^-$, CD2$^-$, CD5^{weak}, CD4$^-$, CD8$^-$; see *Figure 6*). Similar combinations of antigens which can be detected in the B cell system are summarized in *Figure 7*.

10. IMMUNOCYTOCHEMISTRY − PROCESSING OF TISSUES

10.1 **Principles**

Immunocytochemistry can be defined as a method of detecting molecular components within tissues or cells by microscopy using specific antigen−antibody reactions. Almost invariably antigen-specific antibody is used to detect cellular antigens and the antibody's site within tissues is demonstrated by labelling it either *directly* or *indirectly* with enzymes, fluorochromes or visible particles. As discussed previously, the indirect method is more sensitive than the direct, and further amplification can be achieved by using complexes of enzyme−anti-enzyme or other bridging methods (e.g. avidin−biotin−

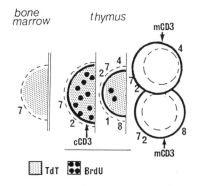

Figure 6. Thymocyte differentiation as defined by the expression of cytoplasmic CD3 (cCD3) and TdT together with BrdU uptake. The phenotypic features of the large thymic blasts (stage 1) correspond to those of T-ALL. These cells are absent in the bone marrow in which all TdT$^+$ cells are cCD3$^-$. The numbers refer to CD numbers of T cell-associated antigens, as established in the First Workshop on Leukocyte Differentiation Antigens in Paris, 1982. (Taken from ref. 63 with permission.)

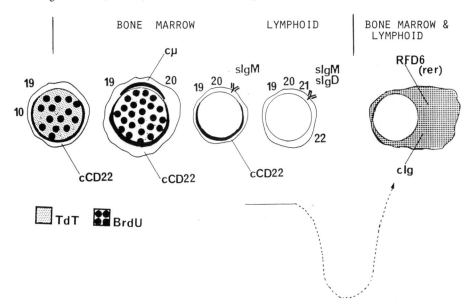

Figure 7. B lymphocyte differentiation as defined by double marker studies for nuclear (TdT) cytoplasmic (IgM heavy chain, CD22) and membrane antigens. The numbers refer to the CD groups as established in the Second Workshop on Leucocyte Differentiation Antigens in Boston, 1982.

enzyme complexes). A major practical consideration concerns the processing of tissue so as to preserve the antigens which are to be demonstrated. This is always counter-balanced by the need to keep adequate morphology of the tissues or cells to allow interpretation of the results.

10.2 Materials

(i)   Fixatives: refer to a Textbook of Histochemistry (72) for recipes of neutral buffered formol saline, Zenker's etc.

(ii)   PLL (Sigma), molecular weight 150 000 daltons.

(iii)   Protease VII (Sigma).

(iv)   Water repellent: mix iso-propanol (84 ml), concentrated sulphuric acid (1 ml) and dimethyl polysiloxane (15 ml) and allow to equilibrate before use. Use sparingly on glass slides.

10.3 Processing of tissue

(i)   Keep fresh samples for unfixed cryostat sections moist until freezing by immersion in physiological saline, tissue culture medium or in Michel's transport medium.

(ii)   Mount blocks of tissue 2−4 mm in size on cork blocks in tissue mountant (OCT, Tissue Tek) and snap freeze in isopentane at −70°C. This is achieved by suspending isopentane in a beaker in liquid nitrogen and waiting till the isopentane starts to freeze solid at the bottom of the beaker.

(iii)   After the block has thoroughly frozen (5 min), remove it, dry off liquid isopentane and store at −70°C until sections are cut. Freezing tissue directly in liquid nitrogen is more likely to produce cracking of the blocks when it comes to cutting cryostat sections; it is preferable to freeze first in isopentane. Storage can be for many years if the blocks are sealed in OCT and kept in liquid nitrogen, for about 1 year at −70°C and less at −20°C. Fluctuations in temperature are most damaging to stored samples and probably account for the shorter storage times at −20°C and −70°C.

(iv)   Fix blocks no larger than 0.5 × 1.5 cm in neutral buffered formol saline for 18−24 h at 20°C. Embed in paraffin according to conventional histological practice (72). These samples have well preserved morphology but the procedure, unfortunately, destroys most membrane antigens. Some cytoplasmic antigens are preserved or may be revealed by short treatment with proteolytic enzymes (trypsin or pronase). Other fixatives − formol sublimate (B5), formol acetic, Zenker's and Bouin's solutions − preserve many cytoplasmic antigens although they too destroy most membrane antigens. Proteases do not improve cytoplasmic antigens with these fixatives.

(v)   Fixation in periodate−lysine−paraformaldehyde (PLP) preserves glycoproteins and retains many but not all membrane and cytoplasmic antigens. This fixative allows the combination of good morphology with the preservation of certain membrane and cytoplasmic antigens (73).

(vi)   A recently described method is applicable to those who have restricted refrigeration space. Blocks of tissue 3−4 mm in size are freeze-dried overnight and then embedded in paraffin when they can be kept at room temperature (74).

10.4 Preparation of tissue sections from frozen tissue

(i)   Cut 5−8 μm cryostat sections from the frozen block once it has equilibrated with the cryostat temperature (optimum for lymphoid tissues is −20 to −28°C and for bone marrow −30 to −36°C). All the sections required from a block and any spares should be cut at one time. Blocks that are cut and re-frozen deteriorate rapidly and subsequent sections are often useless.

Table 5. Effects of fixation on detection of membrane and cytoplasmic antigens.

Fixative	Membrane	Cytoplasmic	IgG,A,M [a]	Morphology
FFS [b]				
Acetone−ethanol	+++	+++	+++	Poor
Acetone−chloroform	+++	+++	+++	Worse
Acetone-Methanol	+	++	+++	Good
Buffered formalin	−	+	++	Excellent
Periodate−lysine− paraformaldehyde	++	++	++	Excellent
Buffered formalin, formol saline, Zenker's or Bouin's	−	+	++	Excellent

[a]To detect membrane deposits of IgG or IgA in FFS post-fixed samples it is necessary to wash in saline for 24−48 h to remove serum IgG or IgA. Morphology of such samples is very poor.
[b]Fresh frozen section.

(ii)　Pick the cut sections up at 2−3 per glass slide and then allow to dry thoroughly at room temperature for 2−24 h. If the frozen blocks were in poor condition or had been pre-fixed then the sections should be placed upon glass slides pre-treated with PLL.

(iii)　The sections can then be fixed for 10 min in any of the following: acetone, equal volumes of acetone:chloroform, equal volumes of acetone:methanol, or for 10 min in acetone followed by 10 min in ethanol, and finally a brief wash in acetone. The choice depends on the antigens that one wants to detect and how important the preservation of morphology is (*Table 5*).

(iv)　Allow sections to dry again and store back to back wrapped in polythene cling film or aluminium at −20°C. Place the slides in a sealable plastic bag containing a desiccant (e.g. silica gel). At −20°C the slides will remain capable of being stained for at least 2 years. If the slides are not fixed then they should be processed and stained within a month.

(v)　Equilibrate slides taken from a freezer at −20°C to room temperature before unwrapping so as to avoid damage from the water of condensation. Draw rings around the sections with a diamond and paint the intervening areas with water repellent. This prevents mixing of primary antibodies if more than one section is placed on a slide. Sections are now ready for application of primary and secondary antibodies (Sections 11−13).

10.5 Processing of paraffin-embedded tissue

(i)　De-wax in xylene or other solvent.

(ii)　Hydrate the tissue through graded alcohol steps to the aqueous buffer used for applying the antibodies.

(iii)　With formalin-fixed tissue improved reaction with antibody may occur after protease treatment of the section. This has been attributed to the release of overfixed antigenic sites (75). Immerse the sections in 0.1% trypsin in Tris buffer at pH 7.8 for 10−30 min at 37°C. The time of digestion (or whether digestion helps) depends upon the antigenic sites being examined and this has to be determined by trial and error. In some situations, for example revealing immunoglobulin deposits, other proteolytic enzymes, such as protease VII, are preferable to trypsin. Sections are ready for staining as in Sections 10−12.

10.6 Poly-L-lysine treatment of slides

Prepare 0.1% (w/v) PLL in water and either dip in the solution or, more economically, spread a drop on the slide in the same way that blood smears are made. Drying occurs very rapidly (10−30 sec) so it is important to mark the side coated with PLL. Slides should be used within a week.

11. IMMUNOPEROXIDASE TECHNIQUES

11.1 Principle

Horseradish peroxidase (HRP) in the presence of a small amount of hydrogen peroxide catalyses a reaction with 3,3′-diaminobenzidine (DAB) to produce an insoluble golden brown product. When HRP is coupled either directly or indirectly to antibody then this reaction can be confined to the site of antibody binding. In this way a visible reaction product can be formed at sites of antigen−antibody reactions. This reaction product can be enhanced by metallic ions (72) or the colour reaction changed by using substrates other than DAB (76) but these carry the disadvantage that they are alcohol−xylene soluble and do not therefore make permanent preparations.

11.2 Materials and equipment

(i)   DAB: prepare solution consisting of either: (a) freshly made up 3,3′-diamino-benzidine tetrahydrochloride at 0.6 mg/ml in PBS containing 0.01% hydrogen peroxide (76) or, (b) 3,3′-diaminobenzidine free base at 40 mg/ml in ethylene glycol monomethyl ether, made up as a stock solution and stored at −20°C at which temperature it does not freeze. Just before use add 0.1 ml of this stock solution to 10 ml of 0.02 M phosphate buffer, pH 7.2 + 0.01% hydrogen peroxide. Working DAB solutions should be colourless. If there is a brown discolouration then filter the solution, otherwise background staining increases. Working solutions should be used within 2 h of preparation, kept cool and protected from the light. N.B. DAB may be carcinogenic so avoid inhaling or absorbing the product.

(ii)   Iron alum: 2% (w/v) dissolved in water.

(iii)   Meyer's haematoxylin. Haematoxylin 2 g, sodium iodate 0.2 g, aluminium persulphate 17.6 g, glacial acetic acid 20 ml all brought to 1 litre of water. Mix for several hours to dissolve completely and filter before use. This form of haematoxylin does not contain the stabilizer, polyethylene glycol, and should be used within a month. Its advantages are that it is not fluorescent (5) and following iron alum it gives a dark-brown/black coloured reaction product with peroxidase-precipitated DAB.

(iv)   PBS:phosphate buffered saline containing 0.01 M phosphate at pH 7.2 and 0.15 M sodium chloride.

(v) PBSAA: 0.01 M PBS + 0.2% BSA and 0.2% NaN_3.
(vi) Coplin staining jars, wet-boxes and staining racks.

11.3 Methods

Once sections have been rehydrated they should *never* be allowed to dry as this severely distorts the staining.

(i) Block endogenous peroxidase by treating the sections with buffer or methanol containing 1% H_2O_2 for 15–30 min, or nitroferricyanide (77) or 1% NaN_3 for 15–30 min. Another method is to use 2.5% periodic acid for 5 min. These methods can be applied to formalin-fixed material. Unfortunately, however, most of these methods damage membrane antigens in frozen sections. It is simpler to use the alkaline phosphatase method if intense endogenous peroxidase from cells such as eosinophils exist in the material for examination, and if the peroxidase blocking interferes with quality.
(ii) Add MAbs at appropriate dilutions in PBSAA directly to the sections without any prior hydration. MAbs from hybridoma supernatants are usually added neat, or up to a 1/50 dilution. Polyclonal antisera or ascites containing MAbs usually require careful titration and the use of antibodies in a high dilution ($1/500-1/10^6$). We prefer to use culture supernatants for immunohistology; 6 mm in diameter can be covered with 30–50 μl of antibody. Incubate at room temperature for 30–60 min in a wet-box to prevent drying out.
(iii) Wash the slides in Coplin jars with three changes of PBS for 1–3 min each change.
(iv) For mouse or rat MAbs add peroxidase-labelled rabbit or goat anti-mouse Ig at appropriate dilutions. Dilute peroxidase conjugates in PBS (azide-free) containing 20% of serum from the same species as the section to be stained. The serum cuts down non-specific binding of the rabbit antibody and absorbs out any reactivity against heterologous immunoglobulin. DAKO rabbit anti-mouse Ig can be used at a 1/50 dilution. Incubate for 30–60 min in the wet-box and wash as in (iii).
(v) Fix for 5 min in buffered formol saline and wash for 5 min in water.
(vi) Immerse for 2–10 min in DAB solution. The reaction can be enhanced by adding 10 mM imidazole in phosphate buffer pH 7.2. Wash for 5 min in tap water.
(vii) Immerse in iron alum for 1–2 min, dip in water to remove excess iron alum then stain with haematoxylin for 30 sec and differentiate in running tap water. Dehydrate through graded alcohols, clear in xylene and mount in DPX or Styrolite.

11.4 Comments

With immunocytochemical staining of any kind it is always important to run *positive* and *negative* controls at the same time as the test sample. *Negative* controls should consist of an irrelevant primary antibody which should not react with the tissue and a *positive* control should be performed on a tissue known to express the antigen being detected. Such controls are essential to allow accurate interpretation of the staining of an unknown test tissue. These precautions are necessary because non-specific staining of tissues can occur with any immunoenzyme technique and lead to general diffuse background staining or unexpected clear staining of certain parts of the tissues. Some of the causes are as follows.

(i)   Binding to Fc receptors. This occurs with polyclonal antisera or hybridoma ascites and can be counteracted by using $5-20\%$ of normal serum from the animal providing the secondary antibody, or using $F(ab')_2$ fragments.

(ii)   Binding by physical interaction. This can be counteracted by high dilution of the antisera, de-complementation at $56°C$ for 30 min (if due to complement binding) and the use of high salt buffers for washing, or as an antibody diluent (e.g. 2.5% sodium chloride or buffered EDTA).

(iii) Secondary antibody reacting with Ig of the species providing the section. This was dealt with in the method described by including 20% serum in the second layer.

(iv)   Reactive chemical groups present in the tissue. This may occur in formalin-fixed tissue which has been inadequately washed, leaving behind aldehyde groups. These can be neutralized by treating the section with sodium borohydride before staining.

11.5 Interpretation

The brown reaction product identifying the site of antigen—antibody reaction can be seen in relation to the conventional histological morphology. Apart from non-specific staining and a minority of cases in which endogenous peroxidase obscures the section, the main problem with immunoperoxidase and other immunoenzyme techniques concerns the balance between antigen and morphological preservation. For example, in a section containing 50% of malignant lymphocytes characterized by a distinctive nuclear or nucleolar pattern, interpretation becomes speculation if the nuclear morphology is so poor that the well preserved reaction product cannot with certainty be ascribed to the normal or malignant population of lymphocytes. On the other hand, it is useless to have perfect morphology and no antigens capable of detection.

Frustration with this dilemma has led to a vigorous search for MAbs capable of detecting lineage-specific antigens on formalin-fixed tissues. However, many of these MAbs lack the significance of functional antigens on living cells detected by MAbs.

We have found that much of the deterioration occurring in acetone or acetone:alcohol fixed sections occurs during the staining procedure and is caused by enzymic degradation. This can be diminished in susceptible tissues by adding a protease inhibitor to the diluent buffer (e.g. aprotinin), or by fixation with buffered formalin after the primary antibody has been applied. Immunoglobulin is relatively resistant to formalin fixation, and this extra step does not inhibit the binding of the second layer.

12. IMMUNO-ALKALINE PHOSPHATASE — ANTI-ALKALINE PHOSPHATASE (APAAP)

12.1 Principle

The principle is the same as for immunoperoxidase but immuno-AP has additional practical advantages and disadvantages. The advantages are that:

(i)   endogenous AP is easily inhibited by levamisole in all tissues except the intestine;
(ii)   its usual red reaction product gives a pleasing and more distinctive stain; and
(iii)   MAbs to AP are available which render alkaline phosphatase — anti-alkaline phosphatase complexes (APAAP) readily available for enhancing the detection of primary antibody.

The disadvantages of the method are:

(i)   most substrates give an alcohol- and xylene-soluble reaction product, and with these permanent preparations are difficult to make,
(ii)   APAAP is more time consuming than the immunoperoxidase method.

The easy inhibition of AP makes it particularly useful with blood and bone marrow preparations (69). Glucose oxidase and β-galactosidase are enzymes with no natural mammalian counterpart and which ought to make the ideal immunoenzymes but as yet lack appropriate substrates to give insoluble reaction products or those with a vivid stain.

12.2 **Materials**

(i)   AP substrate: there are two different types − (A) produces very delicate staining but a temporary preparation which needs an aqueous mountant, and (B) a permanent preparation.
(ii)   AP solution A: dissolve 2 mg of naphthol-AS-MX phosphate in 0.2 ml of dimethyl formamide in a glass vessel. Add 9.8 ml of 0.1 M Tris-HCl buffer, pH 8.2, and check the pH. This solution may be stored for several weeks at 4°C. Just before use add levamisole to make a 1 mM solution and Fast Red TR salt to make a 1 mg/ml solution; filter onto sections. The red reaction product can be changed, if required, to blue substituting Fast Blue BB for Fast Red at the same concentration.
(iii)   AP solution B: dissolve 12 mg of levamisole in 50 ml of propanediol buffer (see below), then add 2 ml of hexasotized new fuchsin and 0.5 ml of naphthol AS-BI phosphate at 5 mg/ml in ethylene glycol monomethyl ether. Mix well and filter onto sections. There are other methods described for new fuchsin-based permanent preparations (78).
(iv)   Aqueous mountant: dissolve 10 g of gelatin in 60 ml of hot distilled water, add 0.25 ml of phenol and 70 ml of glycerol and stir well to mix. This mountant solidifies on cooling and must be warmed in hot water before use.
(v)   Hexasotization: add freshly-made 4% sodium nitrite to an equal volume of new fuchsin solution. The solution becomes clear and straw coloured after 1 min.
(vi)   New fuchsin: dissolve 2 g of new fuchsin in 25 ml of concentrated HCl plus 200 ml of distilled water. Heat the mixture gently and add 2 g of activated charcoal for 1 h while mixing. Cool and filter.
(vii)   Propanediol buffer: prepare a stock solution 0.2 M (10.5 g/500 ml distilled water). For the working solution mix 25 ml of stock, 5 ml of 0.1 M HCl and 70 ml of distilled water.
(viii) TBS: prepare Tris-buffered saline from a stock Tris-HCl buffer at 0.5 M, pH 7.6.

Dilute this 1/10 in 0.15 M saline. A non-phosphate buffer is essential with the AP method.

12.3 Method

(i)   Carry out all dilutions in TBS *not* PBS.

(ii)   Add appropriately diluted primary antibodies to the sections for 30−60 min at 20°C. Wash with three changes of TBS for 1−3 min each time.

(iii)   Add unconjugated rabbit anti-mouse Ig in 20% serum from the same species as the section donor. The optimum titre for this step should be determined but DAKO RaMIg usually works between 1/20 and 1/50. As the antibody has to be in excess, veer on the generous side. Incubate at room temperature for 30 min, and wash as in (ii).

(iv)   Add APAAP complexes (e.g. DAKO, used at 1:50) and incubate for 30 min; wash again as in (ii).

(v)   To enhance staining repeat steps (iii)−(iv) again, and build up further layers of APAAP. If more than one round of APAAP stanining is envisaged then reduce the staining time to 15 min each time.

(vi)   Depending on the requirements add either AP solution A for 5−10 min or solution B for 30 min at 20°C with regular agitation. If solution A was used, wash in tap water, counter-stain and mount using an aqueous mountant. If solution B was used, wash in tap water, counter-stain with haematoxylin, differentiate, dehydrate rapidly through alcohols and mount using a permanent mountant.

12.4 Interpretation

This is the same as that encountered with immunoperoxidase apart from the advantages outlined above. The APAAP method of enhancing staining makes this a very sensitive technique, equal if not superior to immunofluorescence − particularly when the intensity is enhanced by more than one round of APAAP staining. It is interesting to observe that different cellular antigens can be optimally demonstrated by either APAAP or IF techniques, and the reason for the weak staining with one or the other of these

Table 6. Comparison of immunofluorescent, immunoperoxidase and alkaline phosphatase methods.

Qualities	Fluorescent	Peroxidase	Alkaline phosphatase
Microscope	U.v. light	Light	Light
Test time	75 min	120 min	180 min
Storage	2−4 weeks	Permanent	Semi-permanent
Colour	Vivid	Dull	Vivid
Counterstain	Possible	Integral	Integral
Cell suspension	Possible	Impossible[a]	Impossible[a]
Endogenous activity	Unavoidable	Poorly avoidable	Avoidable
Blood or BM	Good	Poor	Good

[a]Fluorescent labels can distinguish between surface and cytoplasmic staining while the other two cannot. Occasionally cells are incubated wtih MAbs in suspension, smeared and subsequently labelled with the corresponding substrate, which may allow some surface antigens to be detected.

techniques is not always clear. A comparison of the advantages and disadvantages of the various staining techniques is shown in *Table 6*.

13. THE AVIDIN−BIOTIN SYSTEM

13.1 **Principle**

There is an extremely high binding affinity between avidin and biotin ($K_a = 10^{-15}/M$) which is non-covalent and can only be dissociated under extreme conditions (e.g. pH 1.5). Avidin is a 60-kd glycoprotein obtained from egg white, consisting of four subunits providing four separate binding sites for biotin. It can be coupled to fluorochromes, enzymes and other tracers to act as a detector in immunochemical procedures. Avidin has two disadvantages which render it inappropriate for IHC. Firstly, its mannose and glucosamine residues can bind to lectin-like endogenous proteins. Secondly, its very high isoelectric point (pI 10.2) means that at the netural pH conditions used in IHC it will bind to negatively charged tissue components such as membranes and nuclei. These characteristics have led to high non-specific binding to tissues. They have largely been overcome by the use of streptavidin obtained from *Streptomyces avidinii* which is not a glycoprotein and has a neutral isoelectric point. Avidin or streptavidin can also be used to 'bridge' a biotinylated primary antibody with a biotinylated label or secondary antibody.

Biotin (vitamin H) is a small molecule (244 daltons). When in an activated state it can be coupled by a simple one-step procedure to a wide range of proteins.

13.2 **Materials**

(i)   Biotinylated antibody: made as in Section 7 or obtained commercially.
(ii)   Streptavidin label: can be obtained commercially or made as described below.
(iii) Avidin−biotin complex: obtained from Amersham International or made by mixing 1:25 w/w of avidin and biotinylated peroxidase (10).

13.3 **Method**

(i)−(iii) as in Section 11.
(iv)   Add biotinylated second layer at an appropriate dilution for 30−60 min at room temperature.
(v)   Wash three times in PBS.
(vi)   Add pre-formed avidin−biotin peroxidase complex for 30 min at room temperature. Optimal dilution should be determined but the Amersham complex can be used at 1:200.
(vii) Wash as in (v). Fix for 5 min in phosphate-buffered formalin. Wash again in water.
(iii) Add the DAB substrate for 2−10 min, wash and then stain as in step (vi) of Section 11.

13.4 **Interpretation**

Although avidin and biotin should provide good universal reagents, the staining obtained by *direct* or *indirect* methods does not give superior results to those obtained by using a good second layer antibody labelled with enzyme or fluorochrome. This

103

is because of unwanted binding by streptavidin to: (a) endogenous biotin present in tissues such as liver, breast, adipose tissue and kidney; and (b) to mast cells. Blocking of endogenous biotin can be partly achieved by incubating sections first with 1 mg/ml of avidin for 20 min and then 0.1 mg/ml of biotin for the same time followed by washes in PBS. However these steps are unnecessary when using the avidin−biotin complex method because this gives enhanced sensitivity without incurring an unacceptable increase in non-specific staining. It is not exactly clear why the avidin−biotin complex method should be free of some of the pitfalls found with the directer avidin−biotin methods but it is likely that the large aggregate of the complex can only bind efficiently to exposed biotin sites. Avidin binding to biotinylated antibody on tissue sections is considerably enhanced when the biotin has been linked to the antibody via a spacer arm. This significantly reduces any stereochemical interference in the binding of one to the other.

14. DOUBLE STAINING OF TISSUES

14.1 **Principle**

The purpose of double staining, as described in Section 7, is to determine the presence of different antigens on the same cell. In tissue sections there is also the possibility of demonstrating the relationship between cells of different phenotypes by using double or multiple staining. The localization of different cell types within lymphoid tissues and their relationship one to another, known as the microenvironment, has important functional implications.

Both immunoenzyme and immunofluorescent methods, described previously, can be used for double staining. Immunoenzyme techniques are very effective when demonstrating antigens on different cells (3,79) and have been adjusted to allow double staining of the same cell (3) but still lack the clarity with which IF techniques demonstrate two or more antigens on the same cell.

14.2 **Materials**

In addition to those materials described in Sections 10−13 use the following.

(i)   Rabbit anti-peroxidase anti-peroxidase. This can be obtained commercially (e.g. from Dakopatt).

(ii)   Antisera for the illustrative examples: CD21 (e.g. RFB6), anti-FDC (DAKO DRC, IgM), goat anti-human IgM and goat anti-human IgD (Southern Biotechnology Associates).

14.3 **Method**

Methods of double labelling using different fluorochromes have already been described in Sections 7−9. In summary, it can be achieved by: (i) using two *directly* labelled conjugates, for example a goat anti-$\varkappa$−FITC together with a goat anti-λ−TRITC; (ii) using two monoclonals of different mouse Ig classes or subclasses followed by mouse Ig class or subclass-specific antibodies.

Immunoenzyme methods of double labelling are more lengthy to perform and do not give such clear cut results, but allow cell morphology to be viewed simultaneously. A method is described below (see also 3, 50, 80).

(i) Process cryostat or formalin-fixed and paraffin-embedded tissue as in Section 10.
(ii) Add, for example a CD5 MAb and a rabbit anti-Hu IgM at appropriate dilutions. Incubate for 30−60 min at room temperature.
(iii) Wash three times in TBS for 1−3 min each wash.
(iv) Add sheep anti-mouse Ig and sheep anti-rabbit Ig at appropriate concentrations. Incubate for 30−60 min at room temperature and wash as in (ii).
(v) Incubate with monoclonal mouse APAAP and rabbit PAP for 30 min at room temperature and wash as in (ii).
(vi) Develop with DAB as described in Section 11.
(vii) Develop with AP solution A (Section 12) but use the Fast Blue BB salt at 1 mg/ml instead of Fast Red.
(viii) Wash as in (ii) and mount using an aqueous mountant.

14.4 Interpretation

With fluorochromes interpretation is straightforward. By switching from FITC to TRITC filters one can see whether a cell has been labelled with one or both antibodies. With immunoenzyme methods it is not so straightforward. Cells labelled with immunoperoxidase will give a golden-brown colour, cells labelled with alkaline phosphatase will be blue. Those labelled with both will be mauve. However, if the sections are too thick

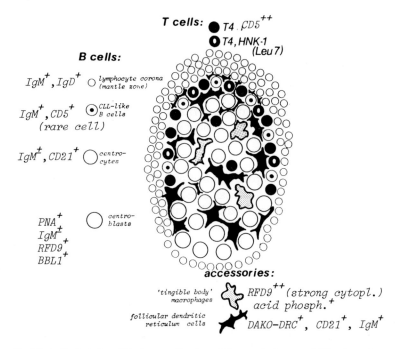

Figure 8. Schematic depiction of the immunohistology of the germinal centre. MAbs, heterologous antisera (to IgM and IgD) and other markers such as peanut agglutinin (PNA) and acid phosphatase staining help characterize the various T cell, B cell and accessory cell populations. In these studies double marker techniques, using either immunofluorescence or immunohistochemistry are particularly helpful, because virtually none of the individual markers are fully characteristic of the lineages.

then overlapping cells may falsely appear to be double stained and one cannot focus up and down in the plane of the section as one can with IF. Furthermore, cells may falsely appear to be positive with only one of the reagents used because one antigen is expressed much more densely than the other.

In the example used above in a normal tonsil the populations labelled with CD5 (T cells) and with rabbit anti-human IgM (B cells) are clearly separate. The CD5 staining is dominant in the paracortical region while the anti-IgM label is dominant in the germinal centres; $CD5^+$, IgM^+ cell are exceptionally rare (*Figure 8*). Nevertheless, in a lymph node taken from a patient with centrocytic lymphoma many cells may show an intermediate mauve colour; in this patient the malignant population is double labelled with CD5 and anti-IgM.

An illustrative example emphasizing points about double staining is given in *Figure 8*. Staining lymphoid tissues with anti-IgM and anti-IgD shows the recirculating B cells in the mantle zone to be IgM^+ and IgD^+ while B cells within the germinal centre lack IgD. Staining with an anti-FDC reagent (Dako-DRC) and CD21 (reacting with C3d receptor present on both follicular dendritic cells and B cells) reveals the characteristic FDC network within the germinal centre to be positive with both markers, while B cells are positive with only CD21. Anti-IgM also stains FDC due to the immune complexes deposited on these cells' surface. The T cell populations represent peculiar characteristics. Most of these cells are $CD4^+$ and about half of them are labelled by the HNK1 (Leu-7) MAb. This unusual T cell population is very rare in the circulating blood (1%). Finally the combination of MAbs reveal features of phagocytic, so-called tingible body, macrophages. These macrophages are strongly $RFD9^+$ in the cytoplasm but negative with panmacrophage reagents such as RFD7 (ref. 80). Similar macrophages can be detected in tissue granulomas. In conclusion, the double marker studies reveal unique features of cells which are peculiar to certain microenvironmental areas. These detailed observations can be used to separate the corresponding rare cells from the circulation or from the tissues, in order to perform functional studies *in vitro* in an attempt to understand the performance of these subsets in relation to their phenotypes.

15. ACKNOWLEDGEMENTS

We are indebted to Drs D.Campana and M.Bofill for advice and to Miss E.Coustan-Smith and Mr A.Timms for technical assistance. The investigation of leukaemia heterogeneity is supported by the Medical Research Council of Great Britain (UKALL trials: Grant No. SPG8417890) and by the Leukaemia Research Fund (Grant no. 84/15). The investigation of LAV/HTLV-III infections is supported by the Wellcome Trust (Grant No. 14386).

16. REFERENCES

1. Oi,V.T., Glazer,A.M. and Stryer,L. (1982) *J. Cell Biol.*, **93**, 981.
2. Schuitt,H.R.E. and Hijmans,W. (1980) *Clin. Exp. Immunol.*, **41**, 567.
3. Mason,D.Y., Naiem,M., Abdulaziz,Z., Nash,J.R.G., Gatter,K.C. and Stein,H. (1982) In *Monoclonal Antibodies in Clinical Medicine*. McMichael,A.J. and Fabre,J.W. (eds), Academic Press, London, p. 585.
4. De Mey,J. (1986) In *Immunocytochemistry. Modern Methods and Applications*. Polak,J.M. and Van Noorden,J. (eds), John Wright & Sons Ltd., Bristol, p. 115.
5. Chilosi,M., Pizzolo,G. and Vincenzi,C. (1983) *J. Clin. Pathol.*, **36**, 114.
6. Greaves,M.F. (1975) *Prog. Haematol.*, **9**, 255.

7. Janossy,G., Hoffbrand,A.V., Greaves,M.F., Ganeshaguru,K., Pain,C., Bradstock,K., Prentice,H.G. and Kay,H.E.M. (1980) *Br. J. Haematol.*, **44**, 221.
8. Christensen,K. and Mason,D.Y. (1987) Personal communication.
9. Evans,R.L., Lazarus,H., Penta,A.C. and Schlossman,S.F. (1978) *J. Immunol.*, **121**, 1423.
10. Bollum,F.J. (1979) *Blood*, **54**, 1203.
11. Loken,M.R. (1986) In *Monoclonal Antibodies*. Beverley,P.C.L. (ed.), Churchill Livingstone, Edinburgh, London, Melbourne, New York, p. 132.
12. Bernard,A., Boumsell,L., Dausset,J., Milstein,C. and Schlossman,S.F., eds (1984) *Leukocyte Typing I*. Springer Verlag, Berlin.
13. Reinherz,E.L., Haynes,B.F., Nadler,L.M. and Bernstein,I.D., eds (1986) *Leukocyte Typing II*. Springer Verlag, Berlin.
14. McMichael,A., Beverley,P.C.L., Hogg,N. and Horton,M., eds (1987) *Leukocyte Typing III*. Oxford University Press, Oxford.
15. Campana,D. and Janossy,G. (1986) *Blood*, **68**, 1264.
16. Habeshaw,J.A., Catley,P.F., Stansfield,A.G. and Brearley,R.L. (1979) *Br. J. Cancer*, **40**, 11.
17. Workshop,W.H.O. (1974) *Scand. J. Immunol.*, **3**, 521.
18. Dom,A.R., Moriarty,C.S., Osborne,J.P., Schultz,L.C., McCarthy,J.P., Lister,K.A. and Horne,L.A. (1986) *American Clinical Product Review*.
19. Taylor,R.B., Duffus,W.P.H., Raff,M.C. and De Petris,S. (1979) *Nature, New Biol.*, **233**, 225.
20. Johnson,G.D. and Holborow,E.J. (1986) In *Handbook of Experimental Immunology. Vol. 1. Immunochemistry*. Weir,D.M., Herzenberg,L.A., Blackwell,C. and Herzenberg,L.A. (eds), Blackwell Scientific Publications, Oxford, p. 2801.
21. Reinherz,E.L. and Schlossman,S.F. (1980) *Cell*, **19**, 821.
22. Lanier,L.L., Le,A.M., Phillips,J.H., Warner,N.L. and Herzenberg,L.A. (1983) *J. Immunol.*, **131**, 1789.
23. Tindle,R.W., Nichols,R.A.B., Chan,L., Campana,D., Catovsky,D. and Birnie,G.D. (1985) *Leukemia Res.*, **9**, 1.
24. Griffin,J.D., Linch,D., Sabbath,K., Larcom,P. and Schlossman,S.F. (1984) *Leukemia Res.*, **8**, 521.
25. Drexler,H.G., Sagawa,K., Menon,M. and Minowada,J. (1986) *Leukemia Res.*, **10**, 17.
26. Linch,D.C., Allen,C., Beverley,P.C.L., Bynoe,A.G., Scott,C.S. and Hogg,N. (1984) *Blood*, **63**, 566.
27. Nadler,L.M., Korsmeyer,S.J., Anderson,K.C., Boyd,A.W., Slaughenhoupt,B., Park,B., Jensen,J., Coral,F., Meyer,R.J., Sallan,S.E., Ritz,J. and Schlossman,S.F. (1984) *J. Clin. Invest.*, **74**, 332.
28. Greaves,M.F., Hariri,G., Newman,R.A., Sutherland,D.R., Ritter,M.A. and Ritz,J. (1983) *Blood*, **61**, 628.
29. Stashenko,P., Nadler,L.M., Hardy,R. and Schlossman,S.F. (1980) *J. Immunol.*, **125**, 1678.
30. Vodinelich,L., Tax,W., Bai,Y., Pegram,S., Capel,P. and Greaves,M. (1982) *Blood*, **60**, 742.
31. Verbi,W., Greaves,M.F., Koubek,K., Janossy,G., Stein,H., Kung,P.C. and Goldstein,G. (1982) *Eur. J. Immunol.*, **12**, 81.
32. Amlot,P. (1987) unpublished data.
33. Bofill,B. and Campana,D. (1987) unpublished data.
34. Loken,M.R. and Lanier,L.L. (1984) *Cytometry*, **5**, 151.
35. Lanier,L.L. and Warner,N.L. (1981) *J. Immunol. Methods*, **47**, 25.
36. Minowada,J., Janossy,G., Greaves,M.F., Tsubota,T., Sahai Srivastavia,B.I., Morkawa,S. and Tatsumi,E. (1978) *J. Natl. Cancer Inst.*, **60**, 1269.
37. Reinherz,E.L., Kung,P.C., Goldstein,G., Levy,R.H. and Schlossman,S.F. (1980) *Proc. Natl. Acad. Sci. USA*, **77**, 1588.
38. Gatenby,P.A., Kansas,G.S., Xian,C.Y., Evans,R.L. and Engelman,E.G. (1982) *J. Immunol.*, **129**, 1997.
39. Damle,N.K., Mohagheghpour,N., Kansas,G.S., Fishwild,D.M. and Engelman,E.G. (1985) *J. Immunol.*, **135**, 235.
40. Morimoto,C., Letvin,N.L., Boyd,A.W., Hagan,M., Brown,H., Kornacki,M.M. and Schlossman,S.F. (1985) *J. Immunol.*, **134**, 3762.
41. Morimoto,C., Letvin,N.L., Distaso,J.A., Aldrich,W.R. and Schlossman,S.F. (1985) *J. Immunol.*, **134**, 1508.
42. Kansas,G.S., Wood,G.S., Fishwild,D.M. and Engleman,E.G. (1985) *J. Immunol.*, **134**, 2995.
43. Beverley,P.C.L. (1987) unpublished data.
44. Ledbetter,J.A., Martin,P.C., Spooner,C.E., Wofsy,D., Tsu,T.T., Beatty,P.G. and Gladstone,P. (1985) *J. Immunol.*, **135**, 2331.
45. Abo,T. and Balch,C.M. (1981) *J. Immunol.*, **127**, 1024.
46. Hercend,T., Griffin,J.D., Bensussan,A., Schmidt,R.E., Edson,M.A., Brennan,A., Murray,C., Daley,J.F., Schlossman,S.F. and Ritz,J. (1985) *J. Clin. Invest.*, **75**, 932.
47. Becton-Dickinson, (1985) *Monoclonal Antibody Source Book*, Becton-Dickinson, Mountain View, CA.
48. Guesdon,J.L., Ternyuck,T. and Avrameas,S. (1979) *J. Histochem. Cytochem.*, **27**, 1131.

49. Simmonds,R.G., Smith,W. and Marsden,H. (1982) *J. Immunol. Methods,* **54**, 23.
50. Poulter,L.W., Chilosi,M., Seymour,G.J., Hobbs,S. and Janossy,G. (1983) In *Immunocytochemistry, Practical Applications in Pathology and Biology.* Polak,J.M. and Van Noorden,S. (eds), Wright PSG, Bristol, p. 233.
51. Janossy,G., Campana,D., Coustan-Smith,E. and Timms,A. (1987) In *Laboratory Haematology.* Cawley,J.C. (ed), Churchill Livingstone, Edinburgh, in press.
52. Galton,D.A.G. and MacLennan,I.C.M. (1982) *Clin. Haematol.,* **11**, 561.
53. Berliner,N., Ault,K.E., Martin,P. and Weinberg,D.S. (1986) *Blood,* **67**, 80.
54. Bofill,M., Janossy,G., Janossa,M., Burford,G.D., Seymour,G.J., Wernet,P. and Kelemen,E. (1985) *J. Immunol.,* **134**, 1531.
55. Caligaris-Cappio,F. and Janossy,G. (1985) *Sem. Haematol.,* **22**, 1.
56. Gathings,W.E. (1984) In *Monoclonal Antibody Source Book,* Becton-Dickinson, Mountain View, CA.
57. Moir,D.J., Ghosh,A.K., Abdulaziz,Z., Knight,P.M. and Mason,D.Y. (1983) *Br. J. Haematol.,* **55**, 395.
58. Gathings,W.E., Lawton,A.R. and Cooper,M.D. (1977) *Eur. J. Immunol.,* **7**, 804.
59. Campana,D., Janossy,G., Bofill,M., Trejdosiewicz,L.K., Ma,D., Hoffbrand,A.V., Mason,D.Y., Lebacq,A.M. and Forster,H. (1985) *J. Immunol.,* **114**, 1524.
60. Bast,E.J.E.G., Van Camp,B., Boom,S.E., Jaspers,F.C.A. and Ballieux,R.E. (1981) *Clin. Exp. Immunol.,* **44**, 375.
61. Caligaris-Cappio,F., Bergui,L.K., Tesio,L., Pizzolo,G., Malavasi,F., Chilosi,M., Campana,D., Van Camp,B. and Janossy,G. (1985) *J. Clin. Invest.,* **76**, 1243.
62. Furley,A.J., Mizutani,S., Weilbaecher,K., Dhaliwal,H.S., Ford,A.M., Chan,L.C., Molgaard,H.V., Toyonaga,B., Mak,T., Van den Elsen,P., Gold,D., Terhorst,C. and Greaves,M.F. (1986) *Cell,* **46**, 75.
63. Campana,D., Thompson,J.S., Amlot,P., Brown,S. and Janossy,G. (1987) *J. Immunol.,* **138**, 648.
64. Gratzner,H.G. (1982) *Science,* **218**, 474.
65. Gerdes,J., Lemke,H., Baisch,H., Wacker,H.H., Schwab,U. and Stein,H. (1984) *J. Immunol.,* **133**, 1710.
66. Janossy,G., Bollum,F.J., Bradstock,K.F. and Ashley,J. (1980) *Blood,* **56**, 430.
67. Bodger,M.P., Janossy,G., Bollum,F.J., Burford,G.D. and Hoffbrand,A.V. (1983) *Blood,* **61**, 1125.
68. Hokland,P., Rosenthal,P., Griffin,J., Nadler,L., Daley,J., Hokland,M., Schlossman,S.F. and Ritz,J. (1983) *J. Exp. Med.,* **157**, 114.
69. Falini,B., Martelli,M.F., Tarallo,F., Moir,D., Cordell,J.L., Gatter,K.C., Loreti,G., Stein,H. and Mason,D.Y. (1984) *Br. J. Haematol.,* **56**, 365.
70 Moldenhauer,G., Dorken,B., Schwartz,R., Pezutto,A. and Hammerling,G.J. (1986) In *Leukocyte Typing II.* Reinherz,E.L., Haynes,B.F., Nadler,L.M. and Bernstein,I.D. (eds), Springer Verlag, Berlin, p. 97.
71. Campana,D., Janossy,G., Bofill,M., Trejdosiewicz,L.K., Ma,D., Hoffbrand,A.V., Mason,D.Y., Lebacq,A.-M. and Forster,H.K. (1985) *J. Immunol.,* **134**, 1524.
72. Pearse,A.G.E. (1985) *Histochemistry, Theoretical and Applied.* Churchill Livingstone, Edinburgh.
73. Collings,L.A., Poulter,L.W. and Janossy,G. (1984) *J. Immunol. Methods,* **75**, 227.
74. Stein,H., Gatter,K., Asbahr,H. and Mason,D.Y. (1985) *J. Lab. Invest.,* **52**, 676.
75. Huang,S., Minassian,H. and More,J.D. (1976) *Lab. Invest.,* **35**, 383.
76. Nakane,P.K. (1968) *J. Histochem. Cytochem.,* **16**, 557.
77. Graham,R.C. and Karnovsky,M.J. (1966) *J. Histochem. Cytochem.,* **14**, 291.
78. Malik,D.Y. and Damon,M.E. (1978) *J. Clin. Pathol.,* **35**, 1092.
79. Lin,C.W., Fujime,M., Kirley,S.D. and Prout,G.J. (1984) *J. Histochem. Cytochem.,* **32**, 1339.
80. Janossy,G., Bofill,M. and Poulter,L.W. (1986) In *Immunocytochemistry. Modern Methods and Applications.* Polak,J.M. and Van Noorden,J. (eds), John Wright & Sons Ltd, Bristol, p. 438.

CHAPTER 5

The induction and enumeration of antibody-forming cells *in vitro*

KATHLEEN GILBERT and DAVID W.DRESSER

1. INTRODUCTION

Recent progress in cellular immunology owes much to the development of reliable *in vitro* techniques for culture and assay of antibody-forming cells. In this chapter we shall describe some simple methods for inducing specific antibody responses in cultures of unprimed lymphocytes from human and murine donors. The critical conditions required for *in vitro* immunization, including lymphokines and other essential ingredients for the tissue culture media, will be described and discussed. One of the more practical methods of demonstrating that successful induction of a response has occurred, is the haemolytic plaque assay. We shall therefore describe this assay in some detail together with variants such as the enzyme linked immunosorbent assay (ELISA) − plaque and the 'reverse' assay: the latter allows cells secreting substances other than antibody (i.e. antigens) to be enumerated with precision.

2. INDUCTION OF ANTIBODY PRODUCING CELLS IN VITRO

The analysis of the humoral immune response has been greatly assisted by the development of systems for *in vitro* immunization. These systems support the generation of antibody responses which supposedly mimic normal immune responses while allowing manipulations not possible *in vivo*. To recreate the *in vivo* environment of a B cell encountering and making antibody to an antigen, a culture system requires:

(i)   accessory cells;
(ii)   medium to provide nutrients for cell growth;
(ii)   serum proteins;
(v)   a stable pH.

A detailed description of these factors will be included in the delineation of systems which can be used to generate antigen-specific antibody responses by murine or human lymphocytes.

2.1 *In vitro* immunization of mouse spleen cells

The widely used culture system developed by Mishell and Dutton (1) allows the generation of an antigen-specific antibody response *in vitro* using dissociated spleen cells from non-immunized mice. We shall describe a protocol based on the Mishell − Dutton system, and discuss some of its variations.

2.1.1 *In vitro immunization of mouse spleen cells to sheep red blood cells (SRBC)*

(i)   Prepare dissociated spleen cells (as described in Section 3.3 or Chapter 1) and wash twice with RPMI 1640. Resuspend at a density of 5×10^6 cells/ml in supplemented Mishell−Dutton culture medium (*Table 1*) containing 5% (v/v) fetal calf serum (FCS).

(ii)   Pipette 1 ml aliquots of the cell suspension into 35 mm tissue culture Petri dishes.

(iii)   Add SRBC to a final concentration of 0.03% (5×10^6 SRBC/ml).

(iv)   Incubate the cultures at 37°C in an atmosphere of 7% O_2, 10% CO_2, 83% N_2 and 100% humidity. It has been observed that antibody production is augmented if the dishes are rocked at seven cycles/min through an angle of $\pm 11°$ for the duration of the culture. This necessitates incubating the cultures on trays in a hermetically sealed container, which can be filled with the special gas mixture and placed on a rocker platform. Specially made Perspex Mishell−Dutton boxes are often used for this purpose. As a cheap alternative, an air-tight plastic freezer storage container can be fitted with a gas inlet and outlet by cutting two holes and providing suitable bungs and a piece of tubing.

(v)   Add nutritional cocktail (*Table 1*) daily (0.05 ml/dish) to the cultures during the incubation period, to replace nutrients in the original medium used by the cells. The number of IgM anti-SRBC plaque forming cells (PFC), as determined using a direct haemolytic plaque assay (see Section 3.1.3) peaks between days 4 and 5 of culture. At this time, transfer the cells from the culture dishes to a centrifuge tube using a Pasteur pipette and wash once in balanced salt solution (BSS). Resuspend the cells from each culture in 1 ml of BSS (dilutions of the cell suspension may be necessary in highly active cultures) in readiness for the plaque assay.

2.1.2 *Additional medium components or lymphokines*

Accessory cells such as macrophages and helper T cells provide signals required for optimal B cell proliferation, differentiation, and eventual antibody production. The re-

Table 1. Media for Mishell−Dutton cultures.

Supplemented Mishell−Dutton culture medium:	
RPMI 1640 or MEM without L-glutamine	
2-Mercaptoethanol	5×10^{-5} M
Penicillin (10^4 U/ml)/Streptomycin (10 mg/ml)	1%
L-glutamine (200 mM)	1%
Sodium pyruvate (100 mM)	1%
Non-essential amino acids (100×)	1%
Nutritional feeding cocktail (ref. 1):	
Essential amino acids (50×)	5 ml
Non-essential amino acids (100×)	2.5 ml
Glutamine (200 mM)	2.5 ml
Dextrose	500 mg
MEM modified without $NaHCO_3$	35 ml
Adjust pH with 1 N NaOH to 7.2	
Add 7.5 ml of 7.5% $NaHCO_3$	
Sterilize by filtration (Millipore) and supplement with 33% FCS before addition to the cultures.	

quirement for these cells in culture can be met by the addition of the soluble factors (lymphokines) they produce. For example, macrophages can be replaced by interleukin-1 (IL-1) (2,3). Helper T cell activity is more complex and has been attributed to several factors including IL-2, B cell stimulating factor-1 (IL-4) and B cell growth factor-II/T cell replacing factor (IL-5). A detailed description of the role of lymphokines in antibody production is beyond the scope of this chapter (for reviews see 4,5 and Chapter 10). In practical terms, it is sufficient to note that the addition of lymphokines to culture:

(i) can augment antibody production by spleen cells and
(ii) is essential in order to stimulate antibody production by purified B cells.

Lymphokines may be purchased in purified or semi-purified form, or can be prepared from the supernatants of specific cell lines (see Chapter 10). Alternatively, the supernatant from Concanavalin A-stimulated spleen cells (Chapter 6) contains a variety of lymphokines and is still used to boost antibody production *in vitro* (6,7).

2.1.3 *Different immunogens*

When using erythrocytes from sheep, horse or donkey as the antigen in culture it is important to note that red blood cells (RBC) from different individuals within a species vary both with regard to their immunogenicity, and to their susceptibility to lysis by mouse anti-RBC antibody and complement. RBC obtained from several animals should be screened for suitability in the Mishell—Dutton culture system. For the sake of consistency a particular animal should then be designated as the source of RBC for all future experiments. The RBC can be stored in sterile Alsever solution at 4°C for several weeks.

Aside from RBC, a variety of other antigens have been used successfully to induce a primary antibody response *in vitro*. These include:

(i) microbial polysaccharides which are capable of inducing T cell-independent antibody responses;
(ii) naturally occurring or synthetic proteins, some of which are strongly immunogenic, and which are often used as carriers for less immunogenic molecules;
(iii) synthetic haptens, which are antigenic, but because of their small size are non-immunogenic unless attached to a carrier.

Table 2 lists these antigens and provided references concerning their use in *in vitro*. Most of these substances can be purchased but, when applicable, references concerning their preparation and/or conjugation have been included.

The murine antibody response to antigen is subject to Ir gene control. Thus, mouse strains may vary considerably in their responsiveness to a particular antigen. It is important to remember that low numbers of antigen-specific PFC may not signal a defect in the culture system, but may be due to the mouse strain used as the source of lymphocytes being a low responder to that antigen.

2.1.4 *Variation in the serum component*

Fetal calf serum is the source of serum components most commonly used in the Mishell—Dutton culture system. Batches of FCS differ considerably both in terms of their ability to support an antigen-specific antibody response and in terms of the induc-

Table 2. Antigens used for *in vitro* immunization.

Antigen	References	
	Preparation	Use in vitro
Polysaccharides:		
Dextran	8	8,9
Ficoll	10,11	10
Levan	12	9
SIII	16	9
S. pneumoniae R36A	17,18	17−20
Phosphorylcholine	21	22
Proteins:		
POL	13	14,15
Bovine serum albumin		22
Keyhole limpet haemocyanin		23
Ovalbumin		24,25
γ-Globulin	26	15,25,27
Insulins		28
PPD		29
β-Galactosidase	30	31
Synthetic polypeptides:		
GAT		32
TGAL		33
Haptens:		
2,4,6-Trinitrophenyl	34,35	23,36,37
2,6-Dinitrophenyl	10,11,34	9,38
Fluorescein	28	28
3,5-Dinitro,4-hydroxyphenyl	39	25

tion of their own non-specific polyclonal effects. It is therefore important to screen different batches of FCS to find one which effectively supports antibody production *in vitro*, but is not itself mitogenic.

Adult serum of several species is less effective than FCS in sustaining antibody production in murine culture systems. This may be due to the presence in adult, but not fetal serum, of a substance which inhibits the endogenous release of IL-1. The addition of IL-1 to cultures of murine spleen cells increased the antibody response to SRBC in the presence of adult mouse, human, or rabbit serum to the level observed in the presence of FCS (3).

The desire to avoid the non-specific stimulatory activity of FCS has led to the development of serum-free media, such as Iscove modified Dulbecco medium, which will support *in vitro* immunization. If supplemented with albumin, transferrin and soybean lipids, Iscove medium will support mitogen-induced antibody production, as well as secondary antigen-specific antibody responses in culture (40). Other media, including a serum-free modification of Mishell−Dutton medium containing fetuin and 2-mercaptoethanol, will support similar responses (41,42). These media are less successful in supporting a primary *in vitro* antibody response to a non-mitogenic antigen (43). However, it has recently been reported that if the supplements are altered to include insulin, progesterone, transferrin, 2-mercaptoethanol, BSA and certain trace elements (including linoleic acid) Iscove medium, alone or mixed with Ham F-12 medium, will support a primary anti-

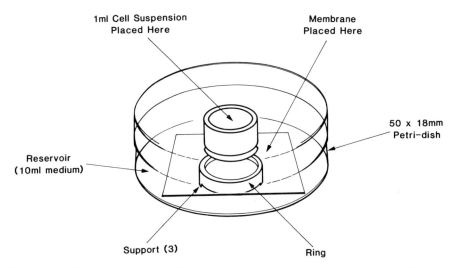

Figure 1. The Marbrook chamber (Hendley Engineering Ltd.). All the components are thoroughly washed and rinsed many times, with the final rinses in boiling double distilled water. The outer ring of the Marbrook chamber is placed over a disc of dialysis membrane and the bottom chamber. Assembled chambers are stored in Petri dishes kept humid with glass-distilled water and sterilized by autoclaving at 105°C. For special applications other membranes can be used. Sterilization of dialysis membranes by irradiation is not recommended since these membranes (cellulose) must be kept wet and irradiation of water leads to the formation of toxic peroxides. If irradiation is unavoidable it is essential to rinse the chambers three times in sterile medium for a period of at least 24 h.

body response to T cell-dependent and T cell-independent antigens by murine B cells (43,44). The media and supplements can be purchased, and a detailed recipe for modified Iscove/F12 medium has been published (43).

2.1.5 *Different culture vessels*

In vitro immunization of murine spleen cells by SRBC can be performed in both 96-well flat-bottomed microtitre plates and Terasaki plates. The concentrations of spleen cells and SRBC are similar to those described in Section 2.1.1, but cells are usually added to microtitre plates in volumes of 0.1 or 0.2 ml/well. It is important that all culture vessels and equipment which come into contact with the cells during the culture period or during the assay procedure should be scrupulously clean: even the minutest trace of detergent can be inhibitory.

2.1.6 *Use of Marbrook chambers*

A culture system which uses Marbrook chambers (*Figure 1*) may be useful to extend the culture period beyond 5 days (4−5 days is optimal for the Mishell−Dutton culture system). Marbrook chambers allow close cell−cell contact in the context of a large volume of medium, which provides a continuous source of nutrients, and prevents the by-products of cell growth from reaching toxic concentrations (45). Such a system can be useful, for example if one wishes to examine a murine primary IgG antibody response which usually peaks between day 7 and 9 of culture. The procedure is as follows.

(i)   To set up the cultures pipette 10 ml of complete Mishell−Dutton culture medium (see *Table 1*), containing 5% FCS into deep (50 × 18 mm) sterile polystyrene Petri dishes.

(ii)   Place the sterile assembled Marbrook chamber in the Petri dish, taking care to avoid air bubbles beneath the membrane.

(iii)   Pipette a 1-ml aliquot of spleen cell suspension ($8-16 \times 10^6$ cells/ml) in complete medium inside the Marbrook chamber.

(iv)   Add SRBC in aliquots of 50 μl of 0.1% to the chambers.

(v)   Incubate the cultures and assay as described above (feeding with nutritional cocktail is not necessary). Anti-SRBC IgM PFC peak on day 6, and IgG PFC peak on days $8-9$.

2.2 *In vitro* immunization of human lymphocytes

Lymphocytes from a variety of human tissues can be induced to form antibodies *in vitro*. Most culture systems use peripheral blood lymphocytes (PBL), since blood is the most easily attainable source of human immunocompetent cells. PBL will generate a secondary antibody response *in vitro* if stimulated with the priming antigen (e.g. Tetanus toxoid) (46,47), or an antigen-non-specific response if stimulated with polyclonal B cell activators [e.g. pokeweed mitogen (PWM)] (48−50). The development of a reproducible culture system with which to induce a primary antigen-specific antibody response by human PBL has proved more difficult. The results obtained using several different systems show that a small, variable but antigen-specific primary antibody response (e.g. $30-300$ PFC/10^6 cultured cells) can be generated by PBL in a modified Mishell−Dutton culture system (51−53). If, in addition to antigen, a small amount of a non-specific proliferative stimulus is added to the cultures of PBL, the number of antigen-specific PFC can be increased 10-fold (54). The addition of lymphokines to the cultures may further augment the response (55,56). We shall describe in detail a model culture system designed by Hoffmann [a modification of his previously published method (56)] for the generation of a primary antibody response to SRBC by human PBL. We shall then discuss some of the ways in which other systems vary from this one.

2.2.1 *In vitro immunization of human PBL to SRBC*

(i)   Isolate PBL from heparinized venous blood by the Ficoll−Hypaque density centrifugation method (described in Chapter 1).

(ii)   Wash the cells twice with RPMI 1640 medium and resuspend in supplemented Mishell−Dutton medium (see *Table 1*), containing 5% heat-inactivated human serum (incubated for 40 min at 56°C). This serum preparation consists of pooled allogeneic serum from normal donors, the blood type of whom seems to be irrelevant.

(iii)   Mix the cells with SRBC (0.03% final volume) and add 0.1-ml volumes to 96-well flat-bottomed microtitre plates at densities ranging from 1.25 to 5×10^6 PBL/ml.

(iv)   Add to the cultures 100 Units/ml of both IL-1 and IL-2 (used in commercially available recombinant form), and 0.003% heat-inactivated *Staphylococcus aureus* Cowan strain I [(American Type Culture Collection) which is cultured as described in ref. (57)] as a selective B cell mitogen. Alternatively use the supernatant fluid of lipopolysaccharide-stimulated adherent human mononuclear cells as a source of IL-1 (56).

(v)   Incubate cultures for $6-7$ days on a rocker platform at $37\,°C$ in an atmosphere of 7% O_2, 10% CO_2, 83% N_2 and 100% humidity, and feed every other day with nutritional cocktail (see *Table 1*).

(vi)   After incubation wash the cells twice in RPMI 1640 containing 5% FCS, resuspend in BSS and test for IgM anti-SRBC PFC in a direct haemolytic plaque assay (see Section 3.1.3).

2.2.2 *Different immunogens*

Antigen-specific antibody responses by human PBL have also been induced using as antigen DNP-KLH (53), ovalbumin (24,58), hapten conjugates of polyacrylamide beads (51), rabbit immunoglobulin (59), dog serum albumin (59), renal cell carcinoma extract (59) and Rh(d) on human erythrocytes (59).

2.2.3 *Different non-specific activators*

Apart from *S. aureus* (described in Section 2.2.1), non-specific stimulants which have been used to boost antigen-specific antibody responses of human PBL *in vitro* include Epstein–Barr virus (EBV) (54), polyethylene glycol (54), C8-guanine ribonucleosides (55) and PWM (60, 61).

Dosch and Gelfand (58, 62) have described an assay system in which relatively large numbers of antigen-specific PFC can be generated in the absence of polyclonal stimulators or exogenous lymphokines. This system is not however universally popular, due partly to the technical difficulty of the assay procedure (SRBC are centrifuged onto the bottom of poly-L-lysine-coated microtitre plates). In addition, the relatively rapid deterioration of the erythrocyte monolayer used in the assay procedure restricts the time available for the development and subsequent enumeration of plaques.

2.2.4 *Medium components or lymphokines*

The effect of lymphokines on the antigen-specific cell responses of B cells are less well defined for the human than the murine system. The addition of IL-1 to cultures of human PBL enhances the production of PFC (56,63,64). In addition, it has been shown that IL-2, a receptor for which (IL-2R) has been demonstrated on human B cells (65), is required to stimulate antibody production to SRBC by T cell-depleted human lymphocytes (55,66). The ability of BCGF, BSF-1 and BCDF to control polyclonal antibody production by human B cells has been demonstrated (67,68), but their effects on antigen-specific antibody synthesis are as yet unclear.

2.2.5 *Serum components*

Some investigators use horse serum (66), or autologous human serum (59) as the source of serum components. FCS seems less effective than human serum in promoting antibody synthesis by human PBL, and in some systems FCS may inhibit antibody production (52).

The use of human plasma is sometimes associated with the appearance of pseudoplaques during the assay procedure. Pseudoplaques are thought to result from the passive transfer of specific or cross-reactive antibody for the immunogen. The serum may be absorbed with the antigen (e.g. SRBC) to avoid this problem. However, Misiti and Waldmann have reported that, in comparison to unabsorbed serum, absorbed serum increases the number of PFC in culture: this is presumably because the serum contains unknown amounts of antigen eluted from intact erythrocytes during absorption (52). They recommend that it is better to risk a few pseudoplaques and use unabsorbed serum. Serum with unusually high haemolytic activity can be discarded.

Farrant *et al.* (69) have described a method in which human B cells grown in hanging drops in Terasaki plates under serum free conditions will generate a secondary antibody response to Tetanus toxoid. This system, though technically difficult, results in high antibody production by relatively few cells (see Chapter 9).

2.2.6 *Variation in the culture vessels*

Primary antibody responses by PBL have been successfully generated in 35 mm tissue culture dishes (52), 17 × 100 mm capped plastic tubes (58) and Terasaki plates (69).

2.2.7 *Additional points*

(i) The conditions required for the generation of a primary antibody response by human PBL are stringent. It is likely that optimum conditions of cell density, culture vessel geometry, antigen concentration and length of incubation will have to be determined by individual investigators for their particular experimental system.

(ii) When using unseparated PBL to induce antibody responses, care should be taken to avoid culture conditions which stimulate suppressor cells. Suppressor T cells are present in PBL and may be activated by histamine released during blood collection and plasma preparation (55,70), or stimulated by immune complexes, IL-2, or certain concentrations of polyclonal B cell activators (71,72). Adherent monocytes, while essential for antigen-specific antibody responses, can under certain conditions, inhibit B cell activation. Antibody production by PBL has been shown to increase following depletion of monocytes (64,73). The investigator may find that optimal antibody production occurs in lymphokine-supplemented culturs of PBL from which suppressor T cells and macrophages have been removed. Cell separation procedures are described in Chapter 2.

(iii) To induce an antigen-specific antibody response *in vitro* it is important to avoid conditions which favour a polyclonal response. These include round-bottomed culture vessels, low concentrations of cultured PBL, and high concentrations of antigen (47).

2.2.8 *In vitro immunization of human spleen or tonsil cells*

Cells from these organs give more reproducible responses than PBL. The protocols used to generate antibody responses with human spleen or tonsil cells are similar to these designed for PBL. Optimal antigen-specific antibody production seems to require the addition of a polyclonal B cell stimulant, and a source of lymphokines (particularly IL-2) (66,73−76). Again, removal of suppressor cells from the preparations of spleen or tonsil cells enhances antibody synthesis (73,76).

2.3 *In vitro* immunization of lymphocytes from other species

Systems similar to those using human PBL have been described for *in vitro* immunization of PBL from other large animals including calves (77), stump-tailed macaques (78),
and rabbits (79). Culture systems using rabbit (80), or guinea pig (81) spleen cells are
very similar to those used for mouse spleen cells described in Section 2.2.1.

3. ENUMERATION OF CELLS SECRETING ANTIBODY

3.1 Haemolytic plaque assay

3.1.1 *General description*

In this assay a plaque visible to the naked eye is formed in a lawn of indicator
erythrocytes, round an individual lymphoid cell secreting antibody. For example, a
suspension of spleen cells from a mouse immunized previously with SRBC, is mixed
in a culture medium with SRBC (indicator cells) and suitably diluted fresh guinea-pig
serum as a source of complement. During incubation at 37°C, anti-SRBC antibody
is secreted into the medium by some of the lymphocytes (plasma cells). The antibody
diffuses freely until it meets a vacant antigenic site on a target erythrocyte (SRBC),
to which it binds forming a complex which activates complement. The ensuing local
haemolysis round the antibody-secreting cell results in discrete, distinct and readily
countable plaques, clearly visible under dark ground illumination.

The assay outlined above is the simplest possible, detecting mostly cells secreting
IgM antibodies directed against antigenic determinants of the target SRBC. The IgM
antibodies produced by these cells are capable of fixing complement on their own, and
are consequently said to form *direct* plaques. Most other classes (isotypes) of mouse
antibody are either unable or inefficient at activating guinea pig complement, requir-
ing the formation of immunoglobulin complexes by (xeno- or allogeneic) anti-Ig-
developing (facilitating) sera for haemolysis to occur: the cells secreting these antibodies
are said to produce *indirect* plaques. An advantage of the indirect assay is that the use
of class-specific anti-Ig reagents allows the separate visualization of plaques of different
isotypes.

The range of possible target antigens is large, since SRBC can be passively coated
with a wide variety of protein or carbohydrate antigens and used as target cells in both
direct and indirect assays. The assays mentioned so far, in which target SRBC (or
antigen-coated SRBC) are used to detect cells secreting antibody are called *conventional* plaque assays. In contradistinction, SRBC coated with antibody can be used to
detect cells secreting antigen in a *reverse* assay. The reverse assay can therefore be
used to identify cells secreting Ig independently of the specificity for antigen of the
secreted molecules. The reverse plaque assay is a powerful means of identifying cells
secreting a wide range of proteins other than immunoglobulins, for example enzymes,
hormones and components of complement.

Haemolytic plaque assays can only be carried out satisfactorily if the medium containing the target and secretory cells is immobilized so that diffusion effects are para-
mount. This can be achieved with liquid media by the use of extremely thin planar
glass chambers or by the use of a suitable gel. An example of both these alternatives
will be given in the following sections. A microtechnique for assaying lymphocytes

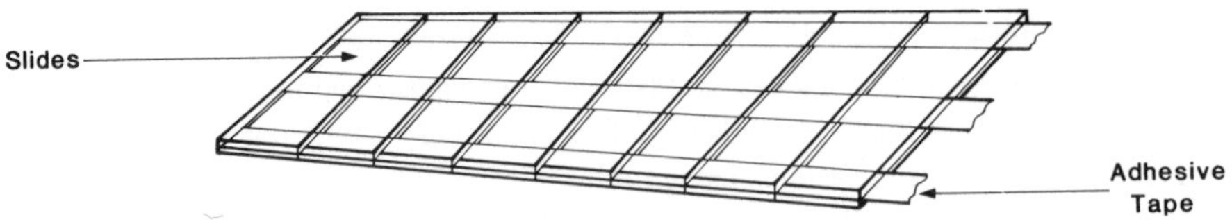

Figure 2. Preparation of 'Cunningham' chambers. The procedure is described in the text. Individual chambers can easily be broken off from the array, ready for loading with the mixture of medium, cells, developing reagents and complement.

in situ in 96-well tissue culture plates has been described by Kappler (80). The haemolytic plaque assay is a very sensitive technique. For example, 50 PFC in a lymph node draining a site of injection could be a highly significant result, although the antibody secreted by these cells into the circulation is probably undetectable. This high precision for looking at the individual compartments of the immune response system makes the assay unsuitable, on its own, as a method for measuring overall levels of immunity in the animal as a whole.

3.1.2 *Haemolytic plaque assays in liquid medium*

A mixture of target cells, cells secreting antibody, appropriately diluted complement and possibly also a developing reagent, in a suitably buffered BSS are loaded into a thin planar chamber, which is then placed horizontally on a level surface to allow the cells to settle and form a monolayer. After incubation at 37°C (>30 min) plaques become visible and can be counted under dark ground illumination and slight magnification.

(i)   Lay plain glass microscope slides (25 × 75 mm; pre-cleaned) flat in a row with their short edges aligned against a straight edge. Apply three strips of 6 mm wide double-sided self-adhesive tape (Scotch No. 410) in parallel strips as illustrated in *Figure 2*.

(ii) After the backing is peeled off place a layer of slides precisely on top of the first layer and press down firmly, using a rubber-faced roller. Individual chambers are separated and are then ready to be loaded.

(iii) The chamber has a volume of about 180 μl (90 μl for each part), so prepare 200 μl of plaquing medium. For example, pipette 150 μl containing a suitable number of spleen cells in Hepes Eagle gelatin medium (HEG: 0.02 M Hepes, 0.5% Difco Bactogelatin in Eagle MEM) into a small (~5 × 40 mm) tube, followed by 20 μl of an appropriately diluted developing (anti-Ig) serum, 20 μl of a 16% (packed cell volume) target erythrocyte (SRBC) suspension, and 10 μl of fresh, target cell absorbed guinea pig serum. For high precision 160 μl can be prepared and the residual space in the chamber filled with medium.

(iv) Air bubbles in the chamber lead to movement of the liquid with consequent loss of resolution of plaques: avoid this by ensuring that the slides are clean and grease free and allow the suspension to warm to ambient temperature before loading the chamber.

(v)   Seal the chamber after loading by dipping the long edge in molten wax-petroleum jelly at 70°C (see *Figure 3*).

118

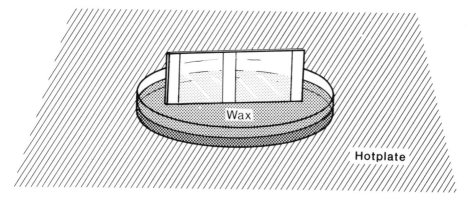

Figure 3. The open edges of a 'Cunningham' chamber are sealed after loading by dipping the long edges in a hot (70°C) wax mixture. The mixture consists of equal volumes of wax (pastillated paramat wax, m.p. 56−57°C, Gurr) and petroleum jelly BP.

3.1.3 *Further comments*

This assay was first described by Cunningham and Szenberg (83), who demonstrated the convenience and sensitivity of the method for detecting direct (IgM) plaques. There is some evidence (84) that the Cunningham (closed) assay is less sensitive for indirect plaques than the slide (open) method described in Section 3.1.4. In Cunningham's version of the assay secreting and target cells are mixed with developing reagent and complement at the start of incubation, whereas in the slide method complement is usually added towards the end of the incubation period. It may be this early contact with complement which leads to lower numbers of observable plaques. Further factors which may be disadvantageous in some circumstances, are (i) the closed nature of the culture which prevents any form of direct access to the PFC and (ii) Brownian movement and slight convection currents which can lead to the occlusion of small plaques in a few hours. It is therefore necessary to count the plaques soon after the end of the incubation period. The obvious advantages are speed, relative sensitivity and the lack of a need for special apparatus such as slide trays or gassed incubators.

3.1.4 *Haemolytic plaque assay in gel*

This procedure is a modification of the method originally described by Jerne *et al.* (85). The mixture of medium and cells used here is similar to that mentioned in Section 3.1.2, differing in being a gel at physiological temperatures, so that it is possible to form a thin stable layer on a standard microscope slide. Since the culture is open, in the sense that there is glass on one side only, it is possible (and the usual practice) to add complement towards the end of the incubation period.

(i)   Use pre-cleaned glass microscope slides (25 × 75 mm), frosted on one side at one end. Sub these by dipping briefly in hot (70−95°C) 0.5% w/v agarose (A37 or A45, Indubiose, L'Industrie Biologique Francaise), made up in distilled water and allow to dry. Metal or glass histology racks may be used to hold the slides for both subbing and drying. If dry, subbed slides may be kept indefinitely.

(ii)   Number the slides on the frosted end using a soft (B) graphite pencil.

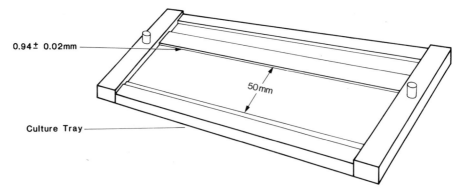

Figure 4. Perspex tray used for the slide method of the haemolytic plaque assay. Slides are placed on the tray gel-side down. When required, complement (5% fresh guinea pig serum) is flooded into the narrow space between the gel layer and surface of the tray.

(iii)   Prepare a 0.75% w/v solution of 'SeaPlaque' agarose (low gelling temperature, FMC Corp.) in Eagle medium buffered with bicarbonate (pH 7.2) as follows. Place the required weight of agarose in a conical flask, add distilled water (90% of the final volume) and bring the mixture to the boil with constant stirring (magnetic stirrer hotplate). When the agarose is completely 'dissolved', add 10% of the final volume of ×10 concentrated Eagle MEM (Wellcome), containing phenol red. Adjust the pH to 7.2−7.4 by the dropwise addition of a 5.6% w/v sodium bicarbonate solution. Keep the medium at 35−37°C until required: since it is not sterile, maintenance of the medium at this temperature should be as brief as practicable.

(iv)   In a typical assay, pipette 0.2 ml aliquots of the gel medium into small glass test tubes (~7 × 45 mm), held in a water bath at 35−37°C. Add aliquots (10 μl) of a suitable dilution of developing reagent (see Section 3.4) to appropriate tubes.

(v)   Meanwhile place warm subbed and numbered slides and Pasteur pipettes on a level warm plate at 30−35°C. Also prepare a level cooled palte, since the Sea-Plaque agarose remains liquid at temperatures down to 28°C. Place plaquing trays (*Figure 4*) within reach ready for the next stage of the process.

(vi)   Add aliquots (say 20 μl) of an appropriate dilution of lymphoid cells to selected tubes using an Eppendorf or Oxford pipette, immediately followed by 10 μl of a 7−9% suspension of target SRBC, which can conveniently be dispensed by a Hamilton repeater. Shake the tubes to mix the contents and then transfer to a warm slide using a warm Pasteur pipette.

(vii)   Spread the gel over the non-frosted portion of the slide using the thin part of the pipette and leave the slide on the warm plate for up to 10 sec to ensure that the gel layer is even. Then transfer the slide to the cold plate for solidification. After about 60 sec on the cold plate transfer the slides face down onto the plaquing trays.

(viii)   Place the loaded trays in a 37°C CO_2 (3% in air) gassed humid incubator for 2−3 h prior to the addition of complement.

(ix) Absorb guinea-pig serum (fresh; stored at −70°C; or freeze-dried stored at −20°C) at 4°C for 5 min with 5−10% packed cell volume of target erythrocytes (SRBC); dilute to 5% in Hanks' gelatin (HG: Hanks' BSS plus 0.5% w/v Difco gelatin) (or Dulbecco PBS) and flood into the space between slide and tray: about 1 ml of diluted complement will be required for each slide.

(x) Return the trays to the 37°C incubator for a further 30−35 min. Then load the slides into slide racks, which are put into a solution of 0.25% glutaraldehyde in 0.15 M NaCl for 3−5 min for fixation. Wash fixed slides in tap and distilled water for 20−30 min before laying them out face upwards on absorbent paper to dry.

The advantages of this method over the closed 'Cunningham' method, include:

(i) the possibility of using autoradiographic techniques;
(ii) the ability to use chemical manipulations, such as reduction and alkylation of secreted immunoglobins (86);
(iii) the possibility of studying the effect of early, late or sequential addition of developing reagents;
(iv) the opportunity to examine the stained secretory cells in the plaques histologically on fixed slides.

The description given in this section is for a simple assay for cells forming plaques against SRBC. It was pointed out in Section 3.1.2 that the haemolytic plaque assay is much more flexible and wide ranging than this. While other species of target erythrocyte can be used, for example donkey (burro) RBC which have an extremely low level of cross-reactivity with SRBC, it is possible to coat SRBC with haptens, proteins and carbohydrates to form target cells with a very wide range of antigenic specificities (see Section 3.1.5). The preparation of isotype- and allotype-specific developing reagents which permit detailed analysis of the structure of the immune response at the level of the constituent cells, is summarized in Section 3.4.

3.1.5 *Non-erythrocyte antigens*

Cellular humoral responses may be measured to a wide range of antigens by passively sensitizing target erythrocytes with proteins, glycolipids, carbohydrates or haptens.

(i) *Proteins.* Chromic chloride is probably the simplest and most reliable coupling reagent available and is thus the method of choice (87). There are two versions (88), one using a 'matured' solution and the other a freshly prepared solution. While the former gives excellent results for the preparation of indicator cells for agglutination or rosetting assays (see Chapter 2), the latter is recommended for assays relying on haemolysis.

(1) Wash SRBC (centrifugation, ~1500 g, 5 min, etc) four or five times in 0.15 M NaCl at 20°C: it is essential that phosphate ions are avoided at this stage. It is also important to note that the RBC of some sheep are not suitable, since they agglutinate spontaneously on contact with $CrCl_3$, so it may be necessary to select a suitable sheep. It has been found that SRBC suitable for Mishell−Dutton cultures (Section 2) can be successfully coated with protein using the chromic chloride method.

(2)   Dissolve chromic chloride (reagent grade) in 0.15 M NaCl at a concentration of 10 mg/100 ml ($\sim 4 \times 10^{-5}$ M) shortly before use. All glassware must be scrupulously clean.

(3)   Add one volume of 50% SRBC (packed cell volume) to 10 volumes of a solution of protein in 0.15 M NaCl at 20°C in a 15 ml graduated plastic centrifuge tube (Falcon 2095). The exact concentration of a particular protein has to be determined experimentally: 1−2 mg/ml is ideal for goat and bovine IgG being coated onto sheep, horse or goat RBC.

(4)   While the tube containing SRBC and protein is being briskly vortexed, quickly add 10 volumes of the chromic chloride solution.

(5)   Incubate the mixture at room temperature (20°C) for 15−20 min, then stop the reaction by the addition of a phosphate buffered BSS such as HG.

(6)   Wash the coated RBC three or four times in HG. They can be used at once or stored at 0°C for at least 2 days.

Economy of protein may be effected by reducing the volumes of chromic chloride and protein solutions used in the procedure outlined above, keeping the *concentration* of protein and the *absolute amount* of $CrCl_3$ the same. Proportions optimal for haemolysis may not be optimal for haemagglutination or rosetting. Some viral antigens can be coupled to SRBC using this method (89).

(ii) *Glycolipids and carbohydrates*. SRBC are quickly coated with lipopolysaccharide (LPS) simply by mixing a solution of LPS with washed SRBC. For example mix 1 ml of PBS containing 1 mg of LPS (*Escherichia coli* — phenol extract; Sigma) with 0.5 ml of washed packed SRBC in PBS, mix carefully and incubate at 37°C for 30 min. Then wash the SRBC thoroughly in HG before use in the plaque assay.

The polysaccharide of *Pneumococcus* type III (SIII) can be coupled to SRBC by mixing crude dialysed (0.15 M NaCl) culture broth with the washed erythrocytes. The exact proportions will need to be determined experimentally for each batch. Unfortunately purified SIII and other carbohydrates are difficult to couple successfully to erythrocytes. An alternative is to couple the carbohydrate to latex micro beads (1.0−1.5 μm diameter; Dow Diagnostics). Coated beads are then mixed with SRBC (50:1) in a plaquing medium. Complement fixation initiated on the beads, leads to lysis of closely adjacent SRBC in a 'by-stander effect' (90).

(iii) *Haptens*. Haptens can be coupled to SRBC to form functional target cells, in two ways; (i) by direct chemical coupling which is suitable for a limited number of haptens, and (ii) indirectly through the use of a protein carrier: the hapten/protein is then coupled to SRBC by the method for proteins outlined earlier. While being more complicated, this method, at least in principle, should be suitable for all haptens.

For method (i) SRBC are readily coated directly with picryl (TNP, trinitrophenyl) as follows.

(1)   Wash SRBC four times in PBS.

(2)   Dissolve 10−20 mg of trinitrobenzyl sulphonic acid (TNBS; Sigma) in 7 ml of PBS containing sufficient phenol red to allow the pH to be adjusted to 7.0−7.2 by the addition of 0.5 M NaOH (caution — TNBS is a skin sensitizing agent).

(3)   Add 1 ml of packed SRBC to the TNBS solution and stir gently for 20 min at 20°C.

(4)   Add triglycine (Sigma) (1.1 mg for each milligam of TNBS), dissolved in PBS to the reaction mixture to block all active groups.

(5)   Finally, wash the coated SRBC in PBS or HG until no free colour is detectable (4−5 times). After each centrifugation (1500 g, 5 min) resuspend the SRBC gently using a Pasteur pipette.

It is essential that the guinea pig complement used in assays with these TNP−SRBC, is absorbed by TNP(DNP)−Lys−Sepharose and SRBC immediately before use. Different levels of coupling can affect the sensitivity of the target cells to antibodies of different affinities (91): high coupling ratios (40−50 mg TNBS in recipe above) favour low affinity antibody, while low coupling ratios (5−10 mg TNBS) favour high affinity antibodies.

For method (ii) haptens may be coupled to proteins such as serum albumin, IgG or KLH (39,92), which may then be coupled to SRBC using one of the protein methods outlined earlier. DNP may be coupled to a polysaccharide such as SIII (93), although for haemolytic plaque assays this is of less usefulness than coupling to protein carriers.

An alternative is to use anti-SRBC as the vehicle for binding haptens to SRBC. IgG is prepared from a hyperimmune rabbit anti-SRBC serum (94), then Fab fragments are prepared from the IgG (95). Hapten is then coupled to the Fab, which forms a haptenated reagent with natural affinity for SRBC without an ability to cause spontaneous lysis in the presence of complement. Once the optimum proportion Fab/hapten to SRBC is known, aliquots can be frozen down ready for use. Preparation of target cells for each day's assay is both reliable and simple.

A quick way to prepare Fab_2 anti-SRBC for this assay is as follows.

(1)   Run the antiserum through a Sepharose−Protein A (Pharmacia) column which binds the IgG.

(2)   Wash the column free of unbound protein, elute the IgG using 0.2 M glycine/HCl pH 2.4 and concentrate by pressure dialysis against 0.2 M phosphate buffer (Sorensen), containing 0.008 M EDTA, pH 7.2.

(3)   To the concentrated IgG add Mercuripapain suspension (Worthington): 10 mg enzyme preparation for every gram of protein).

(4)   Make the mixture to 0.01 M with 2-mercaptoethanol and incubate for 8 h at 37°C.

(5)   Stop the reaction by the addition of 1/33 volume of 0.5 M iodoacetamide in Tris.

(6)   Dialyse against PBS pH 7.2 before passing down a Sepharose−Protein A column: undigested IgG and Fc fragments bind to the column and the Fab passes through. After concentration the Fab is ready for the coupling of haptens.

A 1.5 g (~5 ml) column of Sepharose−Protein A should bind about 18 mg of rabbit IgG and should stand at least 25 cycles of treatment with pH 2.4 buffer.

3.1.6 *Reverse assay*

Cells secreting 'antigen' can be detected in a haemolytic plaque assay using as indicator cells, RBC coated with antibody to the antigen (96). The method, commonly used to study cells secreting Ig, has also been used to detect cells secreting growth hormone

(97), thyroglobulin in an autoimmune situation (98) and also for general clinical studies (99). There are two commonly used procedures using either (i) Protein A (ex *Staph. aureus* Cowan I) coated erythrocytes (usually SRBC) or (ii) target cells coated directly with antibody using $CrCl_3$ (Section 3.1.5).

For method (i) SRBC are coated with Protein A (Sigma) by a slight modification of the procedure described in Section 3.1.5, to allow for economy of the Protein A which is expensive:

(i)   Mix 0.2 ml of 50% packed, washed (in 0.15 M NaCl) SRBC with 0.2 ml of 0.5 mg/ml Protein A in 0.15 M NaCl.

(ii)   To this add with vigorous vortex mixing 2 ml of a freshly prepared solution of $CrCl_3$ in saline (10 mg in 100 ml; $\sim 4 \times 10^{-5}$ M). Otherwise the procedure is as described earlier.

Protein A-coated SRBC are used in the standard plaque assay (liquid or gel medium), together with a (rabbit) developing antiserum specific for the secreted protein. Complexes of secreted protein and IgG of the developing reagent are bound by the Protein A which has a high affinity for the Fc of rabbit IgG. Local haemolysis occurs where bound complexes activate complement. The effectiveness of the developing serum has

a   **b**

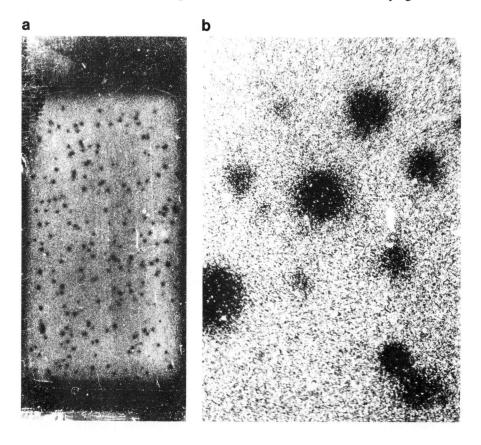

c

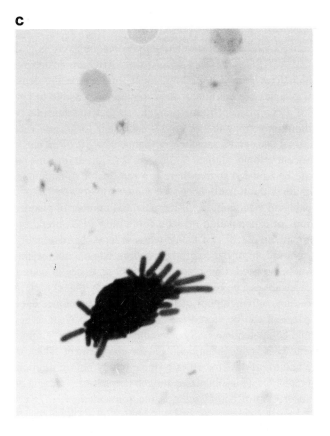

Figure 5. Haemolytic plaques. **(a)** A fixed and dried slide with plaques viewed with dark ground illumination; **(b)** a similar view under higher magnification. This illustrates the wide range of size and quality of plaques which may be obtained; **(c)** a germinating fungal spore at the centre of a pseudoplaque. Three unlysed (target) SRBC give the scale.

a pronounced maximum (prozone effect): it is therefore essential to titrate this carefully.

Where the secreted 'antigen' is Ig direct coupling of anti-Ig (by $CrCl_3$) to the target erythrocytes is preferable:

(i)   Prepare IgG from the serum of a goat hyperimmunized against (for example) mouse IgG, and dialyse against saline (see Section 3.4).

(ii)   Couple the goat IgG, usually at $1-2$ mg/ml, to SRBC by the standard chromic chloride method already described. Since the goat IgG in these circumstances is usually IgG_1 (which does not fix guinea pig complement), there is no spontaneous lysis of the target cells on addition of complement: local haemolysis to form plaques is ensured by the presence of a rabbit anti-mouse Ig developing serum.

(iii)   The developing serum used in the reverse plaque assay can be the same and at a similar concentration to that used in the indirect form of the conventional assay described earlier. As with method 1 above, there is a prozone effect with the developing sera, so careful titration to find the optimum concentration is essential.

3.1.7 *General comments*

One of the commonest problems in the haemolytic plaque assay is generalized lysis of all indicator cells (SRBC). This can arise if the SRBC are coated with an antigen such as IgG_2 which fixes guinea pig complement, or because the density of PFC is so high that their plaques are confluent. It is sometimes possible to coat SRBC with a lower density of a complement-fixing antigen, so that spontaneous lysis is greatly reduced, but without preventing the local lysis necessary for plaque visualization: the window between total lysis and a satisfactory plaque assay is often narrow, so careful titration of the concentration of antigen for coating is required for each batch. The density of PFC should be adjusted so that there is a reasonable minimum number of plaques and a maximum without confluence (see *Figure 5*). Between 20 and 150 plaques on a slide is probably an ideal number. If the potential number of plaques is unknown, a range of dilutions of a population of cells containing PFC should be assayed.

Sometimes there are no plaques on a slide when several can reasonably be expected. This can be due to a failure of the coating procedure when a non-erythrocyte antigen or reverse assay is being used. Phosphate in the BSS or traces of detergent on inadequately rinsed glassware can be responsible. It is unlikely that complement would be a cause of total failure, although poor quality plaques is sometimes due to this cause. Guinea pig complement can be stored freeze dried at $-20°C$ or as serum at below $-50°C$, and should be diluted in a BSS containing Ca^{2+} and Mg^{2+} immediately before use. Rarely, general lysis is due to antibodies in the complement. This can be corrected by absorbing the serum, at 4°C for 10 min immediately before dilution and addition to slides, with target RBC and insolubilized antigen (Sepharose—antigen or coated target cells). Routine absorption of complement is recommended.

Artefacts which look like plaques can be caused either by small bubbles in the medium, or by foreign bodies secreting or releasing haemolytic substances. Bubbles are usually fairly obvious, being large and very sharp edged. 'Plaques' round clumped cells, or germinating fungal spores (*Figure 5c*) are not so obvious, especially as these 'plaques' often increase in size in the presence of complement. If the slide (open) assay is being used, the fixed and dried slides may be stained and examined microscopically, under high power if necessary, to determine the source of the problem. Another source of artefacts can be a transient chilling of a gel medium to its setting temperature prior to the addition of target cells, which are excluded from the microfoci of gelling. On being spread these look superficially like plaques, but can be easily excluded if a test slide is examined before commencement of the assay procedure.

Plaques may be photographed using dark ground illumination and a single lens reflex camera fitted with an appropriate macro lens. Alternatively, fixed and dried slides may be mounted on the plate or film carrier of a standard photographic enlarger and the image printed directly onto a high contrast photographic paper. The latter method is suitable if the prints are to be used for the measurement of plaque size.

3.2 **Non-haemolytic plaque assays**

3.2.1 *Nucleated target cells*

Cells secreting antibody to antigens on nucleated cells can be enumerated in a manner analogous to that described for the haemolytic plaque assay (100,101). A monolayer of target cells is allowed to grow and form in appropriate conditions of culture. Antibody-forming cells are added and allowed to settle onto the monolayer where they secrete antibody for a time after which rabbit complement is added and local lysis occurs. The plaques are visualized by fixing and staining the unlysed cells. With target cells such as mastocytomas a prolonged period (24 h) of culture after complement addition is required for lysis to occur.

It is not necessary however, to depend on lysis of the nucleated target cells. Providing that a cytotoxic antibody is secreted, plaques can be visualized by the use of a vital dye such as Trypan blue: live cells exclude the dye and the dead cells are stained (102). Intact bacteria have also been used as targets for a plaque assay (103).

3.2.2 *ZIPP assay*

Cells secreting antibodies specific for viral antigens can in many cases be detected in a standard haemolytic plaque assay using SRBC coated with viral proteins by the chromic chloride technique (qv). In addition 'plaques' may be visualized as ZIPPs (zones of inhibited phage plaques) in a lawn of phage-infected bacteria surrounding cells secreting anti-phage antibody (104). Antibody-secreting cells are incubated at 37°C in a thin layer of agarose containing tissue culture medium and a target phage such as ϕX174 or Fd. This gel is then overlaid by a thin layer of an appropriate strain of bacteria in nutrient agar. After a short incubation at about 24°C, the active lysis of bacteria is stopped by the addition of a large excess of hyperimmune anti-phage antiserum.

3.2.3 *ELISA plaque (Elispot) assay*

Solid-phase immunoabsorption techniques for the localization of cells secreting antibody by means of a radioactive anti-globulin reagent and autoradiographic techniques, were first developed about two decades ago (105,106). The advent of ELISA technology (107,108) has led to the development of the ELISA-plaque (Elispot) assay (109,110). In these assays anti-globulin reagents coupled to an enzyme such as peroxidase or alkaline phosphatase are localized on antibody bound to antigen immobilized on a solid phase. The position of the localized enzyme is identified by the addition of a substrate which produces an insoluble coloured product. This technique is much simpler and quicker than the autoradiographic procedure and consequently is of much greater practical value. The procedure summarized here is basically that described by Sedgewick and Holt (111).

The substrate and plates for the assay may be prepared a day in advance.

(i)   Use 24-well tissue culture plates (Nunclon Linbro). Add 1 ml aliquots of antigen [e.g. human IgG at 10 μg/ml in PBS (or bicarbonate buffer (107))] to each well. Incubate for 1 h at 37°C and overnight at 4°C.

(ii)   Prepare the 2-amino-2 methyl-1-propanol (AMP) (substrate) buffer by dissolving 150 mg of $MgCl_2.6H_2O$, 0.2 ml of Triton X-405 and 1.0 g of sodium azide in a small amount of water, to which is added 95.8 ml of stock AMP solution (Sigma) with stirring. Make the solution up to about 900 ml with water and adjust the pH to 10.2−10.3 with concentrated HCl. Leave the buffer overnight at 20°C, and the next day re-adjust the pH and bring the volume to 1 litre prior to storage at 4°C until required.

(iii)   Wash lymphoid cells carefully to remove all traces of free antibody and suspend at 4°C in RPMI 1640 containing 5% FCS.

(iv)   Wash an antigen-coated plate several times in 0.05% Tween 20 in PBS (PBS/Tween) by adding about 1 ml to each well, allowing it to stand for 3 min before flicking the contents out in one swift movement.

(v)   Add about 0.5 ml of a 1 mg/ml solution of BSA in PBS/Tween to the plate 1 h before addition of cells, to block non-specific binding: some workers find that this step is unnecessary in their system.

(vi)   Remove the BSA and add 1 ml aliquots of cells at an appropriate concentration to each well.

(vii)   Incubate the plate at 37°C for 1−3 h, taking care to ensure that it is not shaken or moved during this time.

(viii) Wash the cells off the plate with at least three washes of PBS/Tween at 4°C: since cells tend to stick to the plates these washes should be vigorous.

(ix)   Add an enzyme-linked anti-Ig reagent in PBS/Tween (or PBS/Tween 1% BSA) (0.5 ml of a suitable concentration, e.g. 1/200−1/2000).

(x)   Leave the plate for 1 h at 20°C (or overnight at 4°C), then wash the wells in PBS/Tween ready for the addition of agarose/substrate.

(xi)   Prepare the substrate (for alkaline phosphatase) the previous day by dissolving 10 mg of 5-bromo-4-chloro-3-indolyl phosphate (BCIP) (Sigma) in 10 ml AMP buffer, for 1 h at 20°C before filtration and storage at 4°C overnight.

(xii)   Also prepare a 3% w/v stock solution of agarose in distilled water. On the day of assay melt a suitable volume in a boiling water bath. After cooling to 70°C, add 1 vol. of the agarose to 4 vols of BCIP/buffer (0.6% w/v agarose) and pipette quickly 0.75 ml aliquots of the molten substrate/agarose mixture into each well. The agarose should be allowed to set without moving the level plate.

(xiii) Incubate at 20°C for about 30 min when blue dots will appear which identify antibody (plaque) forming cells. The plates can be examined under a microscope to check that the plaques (spots) are not artefacts.

The ELISA-plaque technique has a very wide application providing that the antigen can be bound to the solid phase and that suitable enzyme-linked anti-globulin reagents can be prepared.

3.3 Preparation of lymphoid cells

Since this topic is dealt with in detail in Chapter 1, only the briefest mention will be made of a simple method suitable for use in plaque assays.

Spleens and individual lymph nodes of mice can be homogenized using a loose fitting Teflon (PTFE) pestle in a glass test tube. These homogenizers can be made from 15 ml round-bottomed centrifuge tubes with the pestles being turned on a lathe so that there is a 1−2 mm clearance.

(i)   Cut the pellicle of the lymphoid organ with a scalpel or pair of scissors as it is placed in a small amount of HG in the centrifuge tube. After homogenization rinse the pestle with HG and pass the cell suspension through a fine (30−35 holes/cm) stainless steel sieve.

(ii)   Centrifuge the cells (600 *g*, 5 min), resuspend in an appropriate volume of HG and transfer to an ice bath (0°C): until this point all procedures are carried out at ambient temperature (20°C).

(iii)   The cells are usually assayed at once, but may be kept for 1 or 2 days at 0°C, although the resulting plaques are somewhat less distinct and the plaque counts obtained are often reduced by as much as 25%. It is relatively easy to prepare several different suspensions and to keep these sterile since pestles, centrifuge tubes and sieves can all be autoclaved. Methods for preparing lymphoid cells from other organ systems including peripheral blood are described in Chapter 1.

3.4 **Anti-immunoglobulin sera**

Anti-Ig sera are used both for the development and inhibition of haemolytic plaques, and as specific reagents for linking enzymes for ELISA. Many of the sera required for these purposes are commercially available: those produced for ELISA are often particularly well prepared. IgM (direct) plaques can be specifically inhibited by anti-μ antibodies of the IgG_1 subclass, since these do not fix guinea pig complement. Specific inhibition does not interfere with the development of indirect (non-IgM) plaques by isotype specific developing antibodies of the IgG_2 subclass (112). Very low levels of indirect plaques can therefore be detected despite concurrent high levels of IgM plaques. It is of some practical importance that most goats immunized with antigen in Freund type adjuvants produce a largely IgG_1 response, while rabbits produce an IgG_2 type of response. Since the isotype, specificity and optimal working strength must be known accurately, it is sometimes necessary to carry out further absorptions and specificity testing if commercial sera are to be used as developing reagents for haemolytic assays. A summary of methods for raising antisera and absorbing them ready for use in haemolytic plaque assays has been included in two recent reviews (84,94).

4. ACKNOWLEDGEMENTS

We thank Paddy Hutchings (Department of Immunology, Middlesex Hospital Medical School, London) and Angela Popham for helpful discussion and practical advice related to the techniques described in this chapter.

5. REFERENCES

1. Mishell,R.I. and Dutton,R.W. (1967) *J. Exp. Med.*, **126**, 423.
2. Hoffmann,M.K. (1980) *J. Immunol.*, **125**, 2076.
3. Hoffmann,M.K., Mizel,S.B. and Hirst,J.A. (1984) *J. Immunol.*, **133**, 2566.
4. Hamaoka,T. and Ono,S. (1986) *Annu. Rev. Immunol.*, **4**, 167.
5. Marrack,P., Graham,S.D., Kushnir,E., Leibson,H.J., Roehm,N. and Kappler,J.W. (1982) *Immunol. Rev.*, **63**, 33.
6. Dutton,R., Falkoff,R., Hirst,J., Hoffmann,M., Kappler,J., Kettman,J., Lesley,J. and Vann,D. (1971) In *Progress in Immunology*, Amos,B. (ed.), Academic Press, Vol. I, p. 355.
7. Harwell,L., Kappler,J. and Marrack,P. (1976) *J. Immunol.*, **116**, 1379.
8. Coutinho,A., Moller,G. and Richter,W. (1974) *Scand. J. Immunol.*, **3**, 321.
9. Desaymard,C. and Feldmann,M. (1975) *Eur. J. Immunol.*, **5**, 537.
10. Inman,J.K. (1975) *J. Immunol.*, **114**, 704.
11. Sharon,R., McMaster,P.R.B., Kask,A.M., Owens,J.D. and Paul,W.B. (1975) *J. Immunol.*, **114**, 1585.
12. Hammerling,U. and Westphal,O. (1967) *Eur. J. Biochem.*, **1**, 46.

13. Ada,G.L., Nossal,G.J.V., Pye,J. and Abbot,A. (1964) *Austr. J. Exp. Biol. Med. Sci.*, **42**, 267.
14. Feldmann,M. and Basten,J.A. (1971) *J. Exp. Med.*, **134**, 103.
15. Schrader,J.W. (1974) *Eur. J. Immunol.*, **4**, 20.
16. Howard,J.G., Zola,H., Christie,G.H. and Courtenay,B.M. (1971) *Immunology*, **21**, 535.
17. Cosenza,H. and Kohler,H. (1972) *Proc. Natl. Acad. Sci. USA*, **69**, 2701.
18. Du Clos,T.W. and Kim,B.S. (1977) *J. Immunol.*, **119**, 1769.
19. Abruzzo,L.V., Mullen,C.A. and Rowley,D.A. (1986) *Cell. Immunol.*, **98**, 266.
20. Stout,J.T., Strickland,F.M. and Cerny,J. (1985) *J. Immunol.*, **134**, 1926.
21. Chesebro,B. and Metzger,H. (1972) *Biochemistry*, **11**, 766.
22. Imperiale,M.J., Faherty,D.A., Sproviero,J.F. and Zauderer,M. (1982) *J. Immunol.*, **129**, 1843.
23. Feldmann,M., Greaves,M.F., Parker,D.C. and Rittenberg,M.B. (1974) *Eur. J. Immunol.*, **4**, 591.
24. Ballieux,R.E., Hiejnen,C.J., Uytdehaag,F. and Zegers,B.J.M. (1979) *Immunol. Rev.*, **45**, 3.
25. Cheers,C., Breitner,J.C.S., Little,M. and Miller,J.F.A.P. (1971) *Nature, New Biol.*, **232**, 249.
26. Schimunkevitz,R., Kappler,J., Marrack,P. and Gray,H. (1981) *J. Exp. Med.*, **158**, 303.
27. Schrader,J.W. (1973) *J. Exp. Med.*, **138**, 1466.
28. Jensen,P.E. and Kapp,J.A. (1984) *Cell. Immunol.*, **87**, 73.
29. Coutinho,A., Moller,G., Andersson,J. and Bullock,W.W. (1973) *Eur. J. Immunol.*, **3**, 299.
30. Eardley,D.D. and Sercarz,E.E. (1976) *J. Immunol.*, **116**, 600.
31. Eardley,D.D. and Sercarz,E.E. (1977) *J. Immunol.*, **118**, 1306.
32. Kapp,J.A., Pierce,C.W. and Benacerraf,B. (1973) *J. Exp. Med.*, **138**, 1107.
33. Hodes,R.J. and Singer,A. (1977) *Eur. J. Immunol.*, **7**, 892.
34. Makela,O. and Seppala,I.J.T. (1986) In *Handbook of Experimental Immunology.* Weir,D.M., Herzenberg,L.A., Blackwell,C. and Herzenberg,L.A. (eds), 4th edition, Blackwell, Vol. 1, p. 31.
35. Rittenberg,M.B. and Amkraut,A.A. (1966) *J. Immunol.*, **97**, 421.
36. Jacobs,D.M. (1975) *J. Immunol.*, **114**, 365.
37. Slowe,A. and Waldmann,H. (1975) *Immunology*, **29**, 825.
38. Segal,S., Globerson,A., Feldmann,M., Haimovich,J. and Sela,M. (1970) *J. Exp. Med.*, **131**, 93.
39. Brownstone,A., Mitchison,N.A. and Pitt-Rivers,R. (1966) *Immunology*, **10**, 465.
40. Iscove,N.N. and Melchers,F. (1978) *J. Exp. Med.*, **147**, 923.
41. Burger,M. (1977) *J. Immunol.*, **117**, 906.
42. Tanno,Y., Arai,S. and Takishima,T. (1982) *J. Immunol. Methods*, **52**, 255.
43. Mosier,D.E. (1981) *J. Immunol.*, **127**, 1490.
44. Tittle,T.V., Mawle,A. and Cohn,M. (1985) *J. Immunol.*, **135**, 2587.
45. Marbrook,J. (1967) *Lancet*, **2**, 1279.
46. Geha,R.S. (1979) *Immunol. Rev.*, **45**, 275.
47. Lane,H.C., Volkman,D.J., Whalen,G. and Fauci,A.S. (1981) *J. Exp. Med.*, **154**, 1043.
48. Bird,A.G. and Britton,S. (1979) *Immunol. Rev.*, **41**, 67.
49. Fauci,A.S. (1979) *Immunol. Rev.*, **45**, 93.
50. Ringden,O., Rynnel-Dagoo,B., Kunori,T., Smith,C.I.E., Hammarstrom,L., Freijd,A. and Moller,E. (1979) *Immunol. Rev.*, **45**, 195.
51. Galanaud,P., Delfraissy,J.F. and Dormont,J. (1979) In *Antibody Production in Man.* Fauci,A.S. and Ballieux,R. (eds), Academic Press, p. 159.
52. Misiti,J. and Waldmann,T.A. (1981) *J. Exp. Med.*, **154**, 1069.
53. Morimoto,C., Reinherz,E.L. and Schlossmann,S.F. (1981) *J. Immunol*, **127**, 69.
54. Luzatti,A.L. (1981) In *Immunological Methods.* Lefkovits,I. and Pernis,B. (eds), Academic Press, Vol. II, p. 241.
55. Goodman,M.G. and Weigle,W.O. (1985) *J. Immunol.*, **135**, 3284.
56. Hoffmann,M.K. (1980) *Proc. Natl. Acad. Sci. USA*, **77**, 1139.
57. Kessler,S.W. (1975) *J. Immunol.*, **115**, 1617.
58. Dosch,H. and Gelfand,E.W. (1976) *J. Immunol. Methods*, **11**, 107.
59. Cavagnaro,J. and Osband,M.E. (1983) *Biotechniques*, **1983**, 31.
60. Olsson,L., Kronstrom,H., Cambon-de Mouzon,A., Honsik,C., Brodin,T. and Jakobsen,B. (1983) *J. Immunol. Methods*, **61**, 17.
61. Sjoberg,O. and Kurnick,J. (1980) *Scand. J. Immunol.*, **11**, 47.
62. Dosch,H. and Gelfand,E.W. (1977) *J. Immunol.*, **118**, 302.
63. Lipsky,P.E. (1985) *Contemp. Top. Mol. Immunol.*, **10**, 195.
64. Pollack,S., Reisner,Y., Koziner,B., Good,R.A. and Hoffmann,M.K. (1985) *Immunology*, **54**, 89.
65. Mittler,R., Rao,P., Olini,G., Westberg,E., Newman,W., Hoffmann,M.K. and Goldstein,G. (1985) *J. Immunol.*, **134**, 2393.
66. Tan,L.J., Booth,R.J., Prestidge,R.L., Watson,J.D., Dower,S.K. and Gillis,S. (1985) *J. Immunol.*, **135**, 2128.

67. Kehrl,J.H., Muraguchi,A., Buttler,J.L., Falkoff,R.J.M. and Fauci,A.S. (1984) *Immunol. Rev.*, **78**, 75.
68. Mayer,L., Fu,S.M. and Kunkel,H.G. (1984) *Immunol. Rev.*, **78**, 119.
69. Farrant,J., Newton,C.A., North,M.E., Weyman,C. and Brenner,M.K. (1984) *J. Immunol. Methods*, **68**, 25.
70. Wang,S.R. and Zweiman,B. (1978) *Cell. Immunol.*, **36**, 28.
71. Lipsky,P.E. (1980) *J. Immunol.*, **125**, 155.
72. Pryjma,J., Flad,H.D., Ernst,M., Brandt,E. and Ulmer,A.J. (1986) *Immunology*, **59**, 485.
73. Chiorazzi,N., Fu,S.M. and Kunkel,H.G. (1979) *Immunol. Rev.*, **45**, 219.
74. Booth,R.J., Pang,G.T.M. and Watson,J.D. (1984) *J. Biol. Resp. Modifiers*, **3**, 205.
75. Ho,M., Rand,N., Marray,J., Kato,K. and Rabin,H. (1985) *J. Immunol.*, **135**, 3831.
76. Lagace,J. and Bradeur,B.R. (1985) *J. Immunol. Methods*, **85**, 127.
77. Filion,L.G., Ohman,H.B., Owen,P.H. and Babiuk,L.A. (1984) *Vet. Immunol. Immunopathol.*, **7**, 19.
78. Reed,M.J., Borkow,I. and Staple,P.H. (1981) *J. Peridontol.*, **52**, 111.
79. Luzatti,A.L. and Ramoni,C. (1981) *J. Immunol. Methods*, **47**, 201.
80. Theis,G.A. and Thorbecke,G.J. (1970) *J. Exp. Med.*, **131**, 970.
81. Cohen,S.A. (1981) *Cell. Immunol.*, **60**, 354.
82. Kappler,J.W. (1974) *J. Immunol.*, **112**, 1271.
83. Cunningham,A.J. and Szenberg,A. (1986) *Immunology*, **14**, 599.
84. Dresser,D.W. (1986) In *Handbook of Experimental Immunology*. Weir,D.M., Herzenberg,L.A., Blackwell,C. and Herzenberg,L.A. (eds), 4th edition, Blackwell, Vol. 2, p. 64. 1.
85. Jerne,N.K., Nordin,A.A. and Henry,C. (1963) *Cell-bound Antibodies*. Amos,B. and Koprowski,H. (eds), Wistar Institute Press, p. 109.
86. Plotz,P.H., Talal,N. and Assovsky,R. (1968) *J. Immunol.*, **100**, 744.
87. Gold,E.R. and Fudenberg,H.H. (1967) *J. Immunol.*, **99**, 859.
88. Goding,J.W. (1976) *J. Immunol. Methods*, **10**, 61.
89. Steinmann,J. and Marzock,H.-J. (1983) *J. Immunol. Methods*, **59**, 221.
90. Bagasra,O. and Damjanov,I. (1982) *J. Immunol. Methods*, **49**, 283.
91. Passanen,V.J. and Makela,O. (1969) *Immunology*, **16**, 399.
92. Eisen,H. (1964) *Methods Med. Res.*, **10**, 94.
93. Mitchell,G.F., Humphrey,J.H. and Williamson,A.R. (1972) *Eur. J. Immunol.*, **2**, 460.
94. Dresser,D.W. (1986) *Handbook of Experimental Immunology*. Weir,D.M., Herzenberg,L.A., Blackwell,C. and Herzenberg,L.A. (eds), 4th edition, Blackwell, Vol. 1, p. 8.1.
95. Strausbauch,P., Sulica,A. and Givol,D. (1970) *Nature*, **227**, 68.
96. Molinaro,G.A. and Dray,S. (1974) *Nature*, **248**, 515.
97. Frawley,L.S. and Neill,J.D. (1984) *Neuroendocrinology*, **39**, 484.
98. Row,V.V. and Voloe,R. (1984) *J. Clin. Lab. Immunol.*, **15**, 219.
99. Tauris,P. (1983) *Scand. J. Immunol.*, **18**, 249.
100. Fuji,H., Zaleski,M. and Milgrom,F. (1971) *Transplant. Proc.*, **3**, 852.
101. Nordin,A.A., Cerottini,J.-C. and Brunner,K.T. (1971) *Eur. J. Immunol.*, **1**, 55.
102. Lake,P. (1976) *Nature*, **262**, 297.
103. Schwartz,S.A. and Braun,W. (1965) *Science*, **159**, 200.
104. Tao,T.-W. and Dresser,D.W. (1972) *Eur. J. Immunol.*, **2**, 262.
105. Pick,E. and Feldman,J.D. (1967) *Science*, **156**, 964.
106. Klinman,N.R. and Taylor,R.B. (1969) *Clin. Exp. Immunol.*, **4**, 473.
107. Engvall,E. and Perlmann,P. (1971) *Immunochemistry*, **8**, 871.
108. Van Weeman,B.K. and Schurs,A.H.W.M. (1971) *FEBS Lett.*, **15**, 232.
109. Sedgwick,J.D. and Holt,P.G. (1983) *J. Immunol. Methods*, **57**, 301.
110. Czerkinski,C.C., Nilsson,L-A., Nygren,H., Ouchterlony,O. and Tarkowski,A. (1983) *J. Immunol. Methods*, **65**, 109.
111. Sedgwick,J.D. and Holt,P.G. (1986) *J. Immunol. Methods*, **87**, 37.
112. Dresser,D.W. and Popham,A.M. (1980) *Immunology*, **41**, 569.

CHAPTER 6

In vitro culture of T cell lines and clones

PAT M.TAYLOR, D.BRIAN THOMAS and KINGSTON H.G.MILLS

1. INTRODUCTION

In recent years, advances in the methodology for propagating antigen-specific T cell clones *in vitro*, have had a major impact on molecular and cellular immunology (1). Structural analyses of T cell receptor genes have established the mechanisms responsible for generating repertoire diversity (2,3), and rapid progress is being made in our understanding of the role of immune-response gene products in antigen presentation (4). Moreover, T cell clones promise to be of enormous practical value for the future development of synthetic vaccines. For effective vaccine production by recombinant DNA technology, it is essential that B and T cell epitopes are included in the peptide/polypeptide construct. Ground rules for T cell recognition of proteins and synthetic peptides are now being established with cytotoxic T cell (Tc), and helper T cell (T_h) clones (5−9): armed with this information, it may be possible to produce synthetic vaccines that elicit either Class I or Class II restricted T-cell immunity. *In vitro*, the survival of T lymphocytes is critically dependent on interleukin 2 (IL-2), a tissue-specific growth factor produced by T_h cells activated with antigen, or polyclonal mitogens (10,11). Given an adequate source of exogenous IL-2, it is now a routine procedure to establish clonal populations of antigen-specific T_h and Tc cells from both mouse and man. Suppressor cells remain an *in vivo* activity resisting most attempts at their *in vitro* propagation, and will not be considered here. We will discuss methods for propagating murine T cells. For a discussion of human T cell culture see (1).

1.1 Different strategies for establishing Tc and T_h cell lines

The phenotypes of mouse Tc and T_h cell lines are summarized in *Table 1*. Here, we will contrast the requirements for their initial propagation. First, Tc lines can be established with resting populations of either virgin (alloreactive), or memory (virus or hapten-specific) T cells. However, T_h lines specific for soluble proteins can only be initiated with lymphoblasts, previously activated *in vivo*, since resting T_h cells do not proliferate *in vitro*. Conditions for priming T_h cells to soluble proteins are stringent and the most reliable procedure is that of Corradin *et al.* (12): draining lymph node cells are cultured 8−10 days after injection of antigen emulsified in Freund's complete adjuvant. Since Tc cell precursors are resting lymphocytes, spleen cells are commonly used, although lymph node cells are equally responsive to allo-stimulation.

Secondly, T_h lines produce autocrine IL-2 and do not require an exogenous source to maintain viability, apart from the cloning step, whereas Tc cells require exogenous IL-2 after the third or fourth round of antigenic stimulation. Apart from these differences

In vitro culture of T cell lines and clones

Table 1. Phenotypes of murine Tc and T_h cell lines.

	Major histocompatibility restriction	
	Cytotoxic T cells *Class I: K or D*	*Helper T cells* *Class II: I−A or I−E*
Surface phenotype	Lyt2$^+$; L3T4$^-$	Lyt2$^-$; L3T4$^+$
Lymphoid tissue of origin	Resting spleen cells	Activated lymph node cells
Antigen priming *in vivo*	Optional	Essential
IL-2 dependence	Yes	No

in activation requirements, conditions for culturing T_h and Tc cells are broadly similar: bulk cultures are initiated with spleen cells and irradiated stimulator cells (Tc), or with lymph node cells and soluble protein antigen (T_h), and are assayed for effector functions after 4−5 days. Thereafter, viable cells are stimulated repeatedly with antigen and antigen-presenting cells (APC) to establish T cell lines, and clones are selected after the third round of antigen stimulation. The time intervals between antigenic stimulations differ for T_h and Tc, although cloning procedures are identical.

2. PREPARATION OF LYMPHOID CELL SUSPENSIONS

The preparation of responder T cells and target or accessory cells (feeder cells or APC) for long-term tissue culture require rigid adherence to aseptic techniques. Filter sterilize all tissue culture reagents through 0.22 μm Millipore filters. Autoclave glassware and instruments at 121°C for 20 min.

2.1 Tissue culture medium and culture conditions

(i)   Carry out all cell preparation and culture in RPMI 1640 medium supplemented with 2 mM L-glutamine, 50 μM 2-mercaptoethanol, 100 units/ml penicillin, 100 μg/ml streptomycin, and 5−10% heat-inactivated fetal calf serum (FCS) (complete medium).

(ii)   Maintain cultures at 37°C in a humidified incubator and an atmosphere of 5% CO_2 in air.

2.2 Preparation of spleen and lymph node suspensions

(i)   Place the organ on a sterile stainless steel mesh in a Petri dish, with 10 ml of RPMI and press through the grid with the barrel of a 5 ml plastic syringe.

(ii)   Transfer the cell suspension to a 10 ml centrifuge tube and allow the debris to settle.

(iii) Transfer to a further centrifuge tube, and centrifuge at 400 g for 5 min.

(iv)   Resuspend the cell pellet in complete medium and count.

2.3 Viable cell counts

2.3.1 *Vital staining with acridine orange (AO) and ethidium bromide (EB)*

Caution: Reagents are **carcinogenic**, avoid contact with skin.

134

(i)   Prepare a stock solution containing 0.1 mg of both AO and EB (Sigma), in 100 ml of phosphate-buffered saline (PBS) containing 0.1 mg of sodium azide. Keep in the dark at 3°C.

(ii) Mix $50-100$ μl of the cell suspension at 10^5-10^6 cells/ml with an equal volume of AO/EB solution, and fill the haemocytometer.

(iii) Count the number of green (viable), and orange (non-viable) cells using a fluorescence microscope, and a combination of u.v. and visible light.

2.3.2 *Eosin (yellowish) vital stain*

The advantage of this procedure is that a light microscope is sufficient and reagents are non-carcinogenic. However, dye uptake is affected by the presence of serum, so cells must be resuspended in protein-free medium for counting.

(i)   Prepare a stock solution of 0.2 g eosin (yellowish) (Gurr) in 100 ml of PBS containing 0.1 mg of sodium azide. (There are several other eosin dyes that are not suitable as vital stains.)

(ii) Mix equal volumes of cells (10^5-10^6/ml) and eosin solution and, using a haemocytometer, count the numbers of viable (unstained) and non-viable (red) cells. Cell counts should be made within $5-10$ min of dye addition.

2.4 Removal of dead cells with metrizamide

(i)   Prepare a stock solution (35.3% w/v) of analytical grade metrizamide (Nyegaard) in distilled water. Filter sterilize and keep at 4°C for up to 3 months.

(ii)   Dilute to 18% (v/v), that is 1.02 ml of stock, 0.94 ml of PBS and 0.04 ml of FCS. (Refractive index of 1.3613.)

(iii) Dispense 1 ml of 18% metrizamide into 12×75 mm tubes.

(iv)   Carefully overlay 1×10^7 cells in 1 ml of medium.

(v)   Centrifuge for 15 min at 500 g.

(vi)   Recover the viable cells from the interface and wash twice with 1 ml of complete medium. Cell recovery is greater than 80%.

2.5 Target cells for Tc cells

2.5.1 *Thioglycollate-induced peritonal exudate cells (TG-PEC) (13)*

(i)   Prepare a stock solution of 3% (w/v) fluid TG (Difco) in distilled water; sterilize by autoclaving and store aliquots at 4°C.

(ii)   Inject mice i.p. with 1.5 ml of TG using a 23-gauge needle.

(iii) Kill the mice with ether $3-5$ days later (cervical dislocation may produce haemorrhage).

(iv)   Inject 5 ml of PBS i.p. (19-gauge needle) and withdraw the fluid. Repeat once. (Yield: $0.5-1 \times 10^7$ cells/mouse.)

2.5.2 *B or T cell lymphoblasts*

(i)   Prepare stock solution (1 mg/ml; Dulbecco's PBS-A) of Concanavalin A (Con A; Sigma), or lipopolysaccharide (LPS: *Escherichia coli* 055:B5W; Difco). Sterilize Con A by filtration and LPS by boiling for 30 min.

(ii)   Prepare spleen cells (Section 2.2) and dispense at 1×10^6/ml in 10 ml of complete medium in upright 50 ml culture flasks.

(iii) Add LPS (to 10 μg/ml) to generate B lymphoblasts, or Con A (to 2.5 μg/ml) for T lymphoblasts.

(iv)   Culture for 48–72 h. Cell recovery should be 80–100% with more than 50% blasts.

2.6 Irradiated spleen cells

Irradiated syngeneic spleen cells are the most convenient source of large numbers of feeders or APC for routine maintenance of T cell lines or clones.

(i)   Prepare spleen cells (Section 2.2), and suspend them in PBS with 10% FCS in a 10 ml plastic centrifuge tube.

(ii)   Place the cells on ice within irradiation chamber of a ^{60}Co source, or X-ray machine and irradiate to 1500–3000 rad. (The exact dose required to inhibit proliferation of lymphocytes must be established for each source of X- or γ-rays.)

(iii) Wash the cells and resuspend in complete medium.

3. IL-2 PRODUCTION

There are three principal sources of IL-2 for cloning and maintaining T cells *in vitro*.

(i)   Supernatants from Con A-stimulated rat spleen cell cultures (Con A-sup).

(ii)   Supernatants from cultures of the EL4 mouse thymoma stimulated with phorbol myristic acetate (PMA) (EL4 sup).

(iii) Auto-IL-2, produced by T_h cell lines after 48 h exposure to antigen and APC.

For the routine maintenance of T_h and Tc cell lines or clones, we recommend Con A-sup, while for 'one-off' expansion of Tc clones, EL4-sup. Auto-IL-2 is reserved for cloning autologous T_h lines.

3.1 Con A supernatant

(i)   Prepare rat spleen cell suspensions. Each spleen should yield $2-3 \times 10^8$ viable cells.

(ii)   Culture at 2×10^6/ml in complete medium, containing 2.5 μg/ml Con A for 48 h. Maintain the cultures horizontally as 250 ml volumes in 500-ml tissue culture flasks.

(iii) Transfer the cultures to 50-ml tubes and centrifuge at 400 *g* for 10 min.

(iv)   Aliquot the supernatants into 20-ml Universal containers containing 0.4 g of α-methyl mannoside (Sigma) and store at $-20°$C. (α-Methyl mannoside dissolves on thawing at 37°C.)

(v)   Filter sterilize before use.

(vi)   Screen each batch for IL-2 activity before use (Section 8.2).

3.2 EL4 thymoma supernatant

The EL4 thymoma (H-2^b) (14) may be obtained from the European Collection of Animal Cell Cultures, PHLS, Porton Down, UK. A reliable procedure for obtaining large numbers of EL4 cells is to grow directly from frozen stocks, as mouse ascites. Frequent *in vitro* passage may select for non-IL-2 producing variants.

(i) Rapidly thaw a vial of EL4 cells (1×10^7) at 37°C. Wash once with complete medium, once with PBS.

(ii) Inject 5×10^6 cells i.p. into two C57Bl mice, using a 25-gauge needle.

(iii) When mice are visibly swollen (10−14 days) harvest ascitic fluid aseptically as follows: inject 5 ml of PBS i.p. using 19-gauge needle, and withdraw fluid using the same needle and syringe. Repeat twice. (Yield/mouse ~5×10^8 cells.)

(iv) Freeze the cell stock at this point [1×10^7/vial in RPMI + 20% FCS + 10% dimethyl sulphoxide (DMSO)].

(v) Prepare stock solution of PMA (Sigma). (**Caution:** this is a known tumour promoter, so avoid contact with skin.) Dissolve 1 mg/ml in DMSO and store at −70°C.

(vi) Pellet EL4 cells. Resuspend (1×10^6/ml) in RPMI (1% FCS) containing 10 ng/ml PMA. Incubate at 37°C in 250 ml cultures/500 ml flask, horizontally for 48 h.

(vii) Centrifuge, collect the supernatant and filter sterilize. Store aliquots at −20°C. Use at 3−5% (v/v).

3.3 Auto-IL-2

T_h cell lines produce high levels of autocrine IL-2 after 2 days exposure to antigen. Auto-IL-2 is recommended for cloning T_h cells at high efficiency.

(i) Maintain T_h lines (e.g. ovalbumin-specific) by a repeat 'feed−starve−feed' cycle (Section 4.2), as upright 10-ml cultures in 50-ml flasks.

(ii) Feed T_h cells (2×10^5/ml) with ovalbumin (100 μg/ml) and 2×10^6/ml APC for 2 days.

(iii) Aspirate 50% of medium, (auto-IL-2) and replace it with fresh complete medium. Culture for a further 2 days before the starve cycle.

(iv) Aliquot auto-IL-2 and store it at −20°C. Use at 5−20% (v/v) as dictated by the IL-2 assay.

4. GENERATION OF T_h CELL LINES

4.1 *In vivo* priming of T_h cells to soluble proteins (12)

(i) Emulsify equal volumes (1−2 ml) of Freund's complete adjuvant (Difco) and the protein antigen (4 mg/ml in PBS) of choice (e.g. ovalbumin; Sigma).

(ii) Load a 1-ml syringe using a wide gauge needle and replace with a 27-gauge needle for injection.

(iii) Inject mice s.c. at the base of the tail with a volume of 50 μl. This requires some practice: it is best done by placing mice on a wire cage top and restraining them by the tip of the tail while injecting. Some leakage of fluid is inevitable.

(iv) After 8−9 days (time is crucial) kill the mice by cervical dislocation and remove the inguinal and periaortic lymph nodes aseptically.

(v)   Place these in a Petri dish containing cold RPMI. Dissect away any excess fat. (Successful priming is evident from the considerable increase in lymph node size.)

4.2 Initiation and maintenance of T_h cell lines

(i)   Prepare lymph node cell suspensions and establish cultures at 4×10^6/ml in 20 ml of complete medium in upright 50-ml culture flasks.

(ii)   Add 1 ml of antigen stock solution, for example ovalbumin (2 mg/ml in saline) and culture for 4 days.

(iii)   Harvest, count the viable cells and resuspend them at 2×10^5/ml in 20 ml of medium in upright 50-ml culture flasks.

(iv)   Prepare APC (Section 2.6) and add this to flasks at a final concentration of 2×10^6/ml.

(v)   Incubate for 4 days. Harvest and count the viable cells.

(vi)   Re-culture T_h cells (2×10^5/ml) and APC (2×10^6/ml) for $6-8$ days without antigen. This is the starve period.

(vii)   Thereafter, maintain T_h lines by a 'feed' ($3-4$ days, antigen and APC), 'starve' ($6-8$ days, APC alone), 'feed' cycle.

(viii) Freeze cell stocks 3 days after the second antigen stimulation.

(ix)   Assay for T_h cell proliferation, or IL-2 release (Section 8), 8 days after a 'starve' period.

(x)   Clone 3 days after third (or more) round of antigenic stimulation.

5. GENERATION OF Tc CELL LINES

5.1 Priming for Tc cells

There are two distinct methods of priming for Tc cells. Firstly, mice may be primed with antigen *in vivo*. This may involve immunization with tumour or allogeneic cells (1×10^7 i.v. or i.p.), or infection with live virus, for example influenza (13). Poor immunogens may require hapten coupling to be effective inducers of Tc cells, for example the male-specific transplantation antigen HY (15). In these examples the spleen, which now contains Tc memory cells, is removed $1-6$ months later. These memory cells must now be re-stimulated *in vitro* by antigen in bulk cultures.

Alternatively, Tc cells to MHC antigens can be primed *in vitro*. Here, normal spleen cells are cultured with either allogeneic spleen cells, or hapten-modified syngeneic spleen cells (16).

5.2 Initiation of cytotoxic T cell lines

(i)   Prepare a sterile suspension of responder spleen cell suspensions (Section 2.2).

(ii)   Establish at $1-2 \times 10^6$/ml in 40 ml of complete medium in upright 250-ml culture flasks.

(iii)   Prepare irradiated stimulator cells, for example allogeneic cells, virus-infected or hapten-modified syngeneic cells (Section 2.6). These are usually spleen cells, but other cell types may be used (*Table 2*).

(iv)   Add stimulator cells to responder cell cultures (at a ratio of 1:5 to 1:10).

Table 2. Cell types commonly used as stimulators for Tc cells.

Cell type	Source	Use to stimulate
Spleen	Normal mouse	Bulk cultures Lines Clones
TG-PEC	Normal mouse	Bulk cultures
B or T lymphoblasts	Spleen cells cultured with either LPS, or Con A (Section 2.5.2)	Bulk cultures Lines

(v) Incubate for 5 days at 37°C and then test for cytotoxic activity against appropriate target cells (Section 9).

(vi) After 10−12 days *in vitro* stimulation, harvest the cultures. Cell recovery is usually 30−60% of the initial responder cell number.

(vii) Resuspend the viable cells in complete medium at $1-2 \times 10^6$/ml.

(viii) Repeat the stimulation cycle (10−12 days with irradiated stimulator cells) twice.

(ix) At this stage cell viability will be low ($<10\%$) and dead cells may be removed (Section 2.4).

(x) Re-stimulate the Tc cell line every 10−12 days. After the fourth stimulation, add IL-2 to the cultures to maintain viability. Also, the stimulator cell number may be increased to equal that of responder cells, and thereafter to a 5- to 10-fold excess.

6. CLONING T CELLS

Conditions for cloning, and expanding T_h and Tc cells are identical: the optimal time is 3−4 days after the third or subsequent antigenic stimulation. If attempts are made to obtain clones earlier the efficiency of cloning will be extremely low, although a wider sample of the repertoire may be obtained (9). The efficiency of cloning varies greatly between individual T cell lines. To ensure absolute clonality, it is essential to re-clone *at least* once at 0.3 cells/well.

6.1 Cloning by limiting dilution

(i) Prepare irradiated spleen cell suspensions (3000 rad; $4-6 \times 10^6$/ml), in complete medium supplemented with 20% IL-2 (Con A-sup or auto-IL-2), and soluble antigen (200 μg/ml) in the case of T_h cells.

(ii) Plate out 100 μl/well in flat-bottomed, 96-well microtitre plates. A minimum of four plates is recommended.

(iii) Count the T_h or Tc lines. Prepare a range of cell concentrations in complete medium plus 20% IL-2, (e.g. 10, 50, 150, 500 cells/ml).

(iv) Plate out 100 μl/well and allow one plate each for the lowest cell numbers.

(v) Add 25 μl of IL-2 (100%) to all wells on day 7.

(vi) Score the plates after 10−12 days for wells containing growing cells.

Due to the large number of background feeder cells in the wells, T cell clones are often difficult to identify by a novice. Scoring is best done by examination of the wells

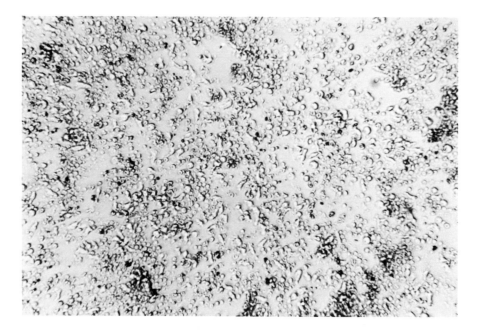

Figure 1. Example of a typical T cell clone 14 days after cloning. The T cells can be distinguished from the dead feeder cells by their larger bright appearance. (Magnification ×250).

through a 25× lens of an inverted phase contrast microscope with constant adjustment of focus. The cells forming a clone are usually scattered throughout the well (T_h), or concentrated at the edge of the well (Tc), and can be distinguished by their larger, sometimes irregular shape and bright appearance on phase (*Figure 1*).

Less than 12 positive wells/plate is acceptable, assuming Poisson distribution for the number of cells seeded.

6.2 Expansion of clones

In this step, a manageable number of clones (<30) is chosen from plates containing the lowest number of positive wells (<10/96).

(i)   Prepare APC (3000 rad; $2-3 \times 10^6$/ml) in complete medium containing 20% IL-2, and soluble antigen (100 μg/ml) for T_h clones.

(ii)   Plate out at 1.5 ml/well in 24-well Costar plates (Northumbria Biological).

(iii)   Transfer the growing clones to prepared wells.

(iv)   After 5−6 days add 0.5 ml of IL-2 (20%).

(v)   After a further 8−12 days, wells should be confluent. Re-stimulate with antigen/APC and transfer either to three wells in a Costar plate, or as 10 ml cultures in 50-ml upright flasks, using the same cell ratios.

(vi)   Thereafter, the expansion and feeding of T_h or Tc clones is determined by their growth rate.

(vii)   When established in flasks, return the T_h cell clones to the 'feed−starve−feed' cycle of the parental T_h line (Section 4.2), and add IL-2 only at the 'starve' phase.

Table 3. Suicide selection with bromodeoxyuridine.

1.	'Feed': APC and antigen (Ag a,b,c), 3 days.
2.	'Starve': APC alone, 8 days.
3.	Cross-stimulate: APC and antigen (Ag a,b,x), 2 days.
4.	Suicide: bromodeoxyuridine, 1 day.
5.	Expose to u.v. light.
6.	Repeat cycle: 1−5.
7.	Clone.

(viii) Test all new Tc and T_h cell clones for cytotoxic, or proliferative responses as soon as possible, and establish cell stocks in liquid nitrogen, preferably 3−4 days after antigen stimulation.

(ix) Maintain Tc cell clones in IL-2 throughout, but when clones are growing successfully, reduce the levels of IL-2 from 20% to 10%.

7. SUICIDE SELECTION FOR T_h OF A PRE-DETERMINED SPECIFICITY

T_h cell lines, raised against complex antigens such as viruses or parasites, consist of clones specific for a spectrum of antigenic proteins, and it may be necessary to focus on a single molecular species. Consider, as the initial immunogen, a virus (containing Ag a,b,c), which shares a minimum number of cross-reactive determinants with a related virus (Ag a,b,x). The suicide selection procedure (17), described here, provides a means for selecting Ag(c)-specific clones. It relies on the fact that T_h cells become arrested at the G_1/G_0 phase of the cell cycle in the absence of antigen for more than 6 days. Tc cell lines, on the other hand, require continuous exposure to IL-2, are perpetually 'in cycle', and cannot be used in this system.

T_h cells remain viable for 8−12 days in the absence of antigen, if provided with APC. At this time they have reverted from cycling lymphoblasts to small, resting lymphocytes. If cultures are now re-stimulated with a heterologous antigen (Ag a,b,x), T_h cells specific for Ag(a) and Ag(b) will enter the cycle and can be eliminated with an S phase-specific cytotoxic drug. The procedure is outlined in *Table 3*.

(i) and (ii) is the normal 'feed−starve' protocol for maintaining T_h lines (Section 4.2)

(iii) Re-stimulate the T_h cell line, as in (i), but substitute heterologous antigen at a concentration shown to be optimal for proliferation (Section 8.1).

(iv) Two days later add bromodeoxyuridine (15 μg/ml; Sigma).

(v) After 1 day harvest the cells, wash them twice with complete medium and resuspend them in 5 ml of PBS. Place them in a Petri dish and expose them to a u.v. light source (365 nm free) at a distance of 8 cm for 10 min. Do not use RPMI since toxic free radicals are generated. Wash and re-culture as (i).

(vi) Repeat (i)−(v).

(vii) Clone.

8. ASSAYS FOR T_h CELLS

T_h cell responses may be determined by measuring IL-2 release (48 h), or cellular proliferation (72 h) after re-stimulation with antigen and APC. To avoid high backgrounds, it is essential that T_h lines or clones are deprived of antigen for at least $6-8$ days before assay.

8.1 Proliferation assay

(i)   Prepare APC (3000 rad) at 4×10^6/ml in complete medium.

(ii)   Wash T_h cells twice in medium to remove residual antigen or IL-2. Resuspend in APC suspension at 4×10^5/ml.

(iii)   Plate out 100 μl/well in 96-well flat-bottomed microtitre plates.

(iv)   Prepare a range of antigen dilutions in complete medium $(1-300\ \mu$g/ml$)$ from frozen stocks (10 mg/ml in saline). Add 100 μl/well to (a minimum of) triplicate wells. Culture at 37°C.

(v)   After 72 h, add 25 μl of [methyl-^{3}H]thymidine (20 μCi/ml; sp. act. 5 Ci/mmol; Amersham International).

(vi)   After $6-8$ h, harvest the wells, either with a multichannel micropipette, or with an Automatic Cell Harvester, onto glass fibre filter paper (FG/A; Whatman).

(vii)   Wash the discs with distilled water and dry.

(viii) Add the filter discs to vials containing non-aqueous scintillation fluid and count.

(ix)   Express the results as arithmetic means of c.p.m./culture, or as stimulation indices, that is the ratio of c.p.m. in cultures given antigen + APC divided by the response to APC alone. A typical dose–response curve is shown in *Figure 2*.

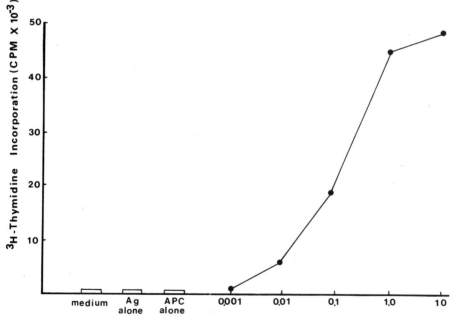

Figure 2. Dose–response curve of [^{3}H]thymidine uptake of an influenza virus (X31) specific T_h cell clone. Points on the curve represent c.p.m. incorporated by 2×10^4 T cells cultured with a range of concentrations of purified X31 virus plus APC. Control cultures with APC, antigen (Ag) or medium (med) alone gave background responses.

8.2 IL-2 assay

(i)   Culture cells as described in (i)−(iv) in Section 8.1.

(ii) After 48 h of culture, remove 100 μl of supernatant from individual wells with a multi-channel pipette, and transfer to a fresh microtitre plate.

(iii) Make serial dilutions of the supernatants in triplicate, and test their ability to support the growth of Con A blasts or the IL-2-dependent CTLL cell line as described in Chapter 10.

9. DETECTION OF CYTOTOXIC ACTIVITY

Cytotoxic activity of cells is estimated by measuring the release of sodium chromate (^{51}Cr) from labelled target cells. Lines of tumour cells make excellent targets for the demonstration of Tc cell activity, and the most commonly used murine lines are P815 (H-2^d), EL4 (H-2^b) and BW5147 (H-2^k). These are available from ECACC, PHLS, Porton Down, UK. MHC restriction analysis (Section 11) requires targets from recombinant mouse strains, and these may be TG-PEC (Section 2.5.1), or B or T cell lymphoblasts (Section 2.5.2). In general, bulk cultures are tested for Tc cell activity 4−6 days after the first *in vitro* stimulation, whereas lines and clones may be tested 3−8 days after antigenic stimulation. A typical example of target cell lysis mediated by an influenza virus-specific Tc cell clone is seen in *Figure 3*. This illustrates the lysis of histocompatible influenza-infected target cells, and also the low background levels of lysis on non-compatible, influenza-infected target cells, or uninfected control target cells.

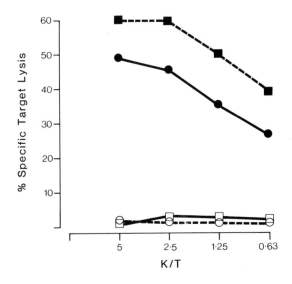

Figure 3. Analysis of lytic activity of an influenza virus-specific Tc cell clone, using ^{51}Cr-labelled target cells. The clone was derived from spleen cells of BALB/c mice primed intranasally with Type A influenza (A/X31). Stimulator cells were irradiated A/X31-infected BALB/c spleen cells. The ^{51}Cr release assay was 6 h, using the following targets: (■) P815 cells (H-2^d), infected with A/X31; (●) BALB/c (H-2^d) TG-PEC infected with A/X31; (○) EL4 cells (H-2^b) infected with A/X31; (□) uninfected P815 cells as controls. Spontaneous ^{51}Cr release varied between 12.2 and 15.4%.

9.1 Tc cell preparation

(i)   Centrifuge Tc cells (5 min, 200 g). Resuspend in 2 ml of complete medium and count.

(ii)   Dilute to 1×10^6 cells/ml (clone/line), or $2-4 \times 10^6$/ml (bulk culture), in complete medium.

(iii) Prepare 2-fold dilutions of Tc cells in complete medium. The target cell number remains constant, and the number of Tc cells/well is varied to give different killer/target ratios (K/Ts). The dilutions may be carried out in tubes and duplicate/triplicate 100 μl volumes of each dilution dispensed into 96 flat-bottomed well microtitre plates. Alternatively, make the dilutions in the plate using a multi-channel pipette.

(iv)   Incubate the plate(s) at 37°C.

9.2 ^{51}Cr labelling and preparation of target cells

(i)   Centrifuge 5×10^6 target cells (5 min, 200 g), and resuspend in $0.2-0.3$ ml of complete medium. (A small volume is essential for efficient ^{51}Cr labelling.) With TG-PEC use 1×10^7 cells, since some may be lost due to adherence to plastic at 37°C.

(ii)   Add 50 μCi ^{51}Cr (sp. act. $350-600$ μCi/μg chromium, Amersham International) per 5×10^6 cells. Incubate for 60 min at 37°C.

(iii) Add 10 ml of PBS, centrifuge (5 min, 200 g), and discard the supernatant into a radioactive waste sink. Repeat twice.

(iv)   Resuspend the pellet in 0.5 ml of complete medium, and count the number of viable cells.

(v)   Resuspend at 2×10^5/ml, and immediately plate out 100 μl/well onto the plate with the prepared Tc cells.

(vi)   Also plate out target cells into wells without Tc cells. To measure spontaneous ^{51}Cr release from target cells, add 100 μl of complete medium to four wells. To measure the maximum ^{51}Cr release from the target cells, add 100 μl of 2.5% (v/v) Triton X-100 to four wells.

(vii) Using plate carriers, centrifuge the plate(s) (1 min, 150 g). This gently pellets the Tc and target cells ready for interaction.

(viii) Incubate the plate(s) for $4-5$ h at 37°C.

9.3 Estimation of Tc cell activity

(i)   Centrifuge the plate(s) (5 min, 250 g).

(ii)   Immediately harvest 100 μl of supernatant/well, using a multi-channel pipette. Take care not to disturb the cell layer. Transfer the supernatants to LP2 tubes (Luckham).

(iii) Count the radioactivity in each sample in a gamma scintillation counter.

(iv)   Calculate the percentage killing as follows:

$$\left(\frac{\text{c.p.m. in presence of Tc} - \text{spontaneous } ^{51}\text{Cr release}}{\text{Total } ^{51}\text{Cr release} - \text{spontaneous } ^{51}\text{Cr release}} \right) \times 100$$

(v)   Ideally, spontaneous ^{51}Cr release by target cells should be less than 20%.

9.4 Additional notes

To measure virus-specific Tc cells, the virus infection of target cells may involve an overnight incubation step, which is then followed by the ^{51}Cr labelling as described. Alternatively, a virus such as influenza can infect the target cells during the ^{51}Cr labelling period, if serum-free RPMI is used (13).

10. T CELL SURFACE PHENOTYPING BY INDIRECT ROSETTING

In general, Class I-restricted Tc cells exhibit the L3T4$^-$, Lyt2$^+$ surface phenotype, while Class II-restricted T$_h$ cells are L3T4$^+$, Lyt2$^-$ (*Table 1*), although there are exceptions to this rule following *in vivo* activation. The indirect rosetting technique (18) is a convenient procedure for phenotyping cells, if a fluorescence activated cell sorter (FACS) is not available, and requires fewer cells.

T cell clones should be phenotyped more than 6 days after the last stimulation to allow sufficient time for expiry of feeder cells. Dead cells are removed by Metrizamide overlay (Section 2.4).

The reagents used are as follows:

(i)   monoclonal antibodies (MAb) to L3T4 or Lyt2 (Sera Labs);
(ii)   sheep or goat anti-mouse Ig (Ig fraction; Serotec, or Nordic);
(iii)   ox red blood cells (ORBC; Tissue Culture Services).

10.1 Coupling anti-mouse Ig to ORBC

(i)   Wash ORBC (stored in Alsever's solution for up to 4 weeks) three times with saline.
(ii)   Add 100 μl of packed ORBC to a 5-ml glass Bijou with 50 μl of anti-mouse Ig (5 mg/ml), previously dialysed against saline.
(iii)   Vortex while adding 500 μl of chromic chloride (0.1 mg/ml), dropwise. This is freshly diluted in saline from a 1 mg/ml stock solution, previously aged for more than 1 month and less than 12 months, with periodical adjustment to pH 5 by 1 M NaOH. (See also Chapter 2.)
(iv)   Layer 1 ml of saline onto the suspension and leave at 4°C overnight.
(v)   Wash the ORBC three times with PBS and resuspend to 5% (v/v) in 4 ml of complete medium.

Table 4. MHC restriction analysis of four T cell clones.

Mouse strain	H-2 subregion						Response of clone			
	K	A_α	A_β	E_β	E_α	D	1	2	3	4
CBA	k	k	k	k	k	k	+	+	−	−
BIO.AQR	q	k	k	k	k	d	+	+	−	+
BIO.A(4R)	k	k	k	k	b	b	+	−	−	−
BIO.A(5R)	b	b	b	b	k	d	−	−	−	+
BALB/c	d	d	d	d	d	d	−	−	+	+

10.2 **MAb binding to T cells**

(i)   Aliquot $1-2 \times 10^5$ T cells into plastic centrifuge tubes (LP3, Luckham) and centrifuge (5 min, 200 g).

(ii)   Resuspend the cell pellet in 100 μl of MAb (100 ng/ml) and incubate on ice for 30 min.

(iii)   Wash twice with 2 ml of RPMI.

10.3 **Rosette formation and counting**

(i)   Add 50 μl of anti-mouse Ig-coated 5% ORBC to MAb-treated T cells.

(ii)   Centrifuge (1 min, 200 g) and place on ice for 30 min.

(iii)   Gently resuspend the cells after adding 50 μl of AO/EB solution (Section 2.3.1).

(iv)   Using a fluorescence microscope, count the percentage of viable cells (green), forming rosettes (i.e. with four or more ORBC bound to each lymphocyte).

11. MHC RESTRICTION ANALYSIS

In general, T_h cells recognize foreign antigen only in association with MHC Class II antigens ($I-A$ or $I-E$ region gene products in the mouse), whereas Tc cells are restricted to Class I (K or D region) molecules. Restriction analyses are carried out on T_h cells using the proliferation assay (Section 8.1), and on Tc cells using the killing assay (Section 9), with APC or targets, respectively, from syngeneic, allogeneic or recombinant mouse strains (19). Only those APC or targets with the precise restriction element present will give a positive response. *Table 4* describes four clones 1, 2, 3 and 4 which are restricted to $I-A^k$, $I-E^k$, K^d and D^d regions, respectively.

12. REFERENCES

1. Fathman,G. and Fitch,F.W. (1982) *Isolation, Characterization and Utilization of T Lymphocyte Clones.* Academic Press, New York.
2. Arden,B., Klotz,J.L., Siu,G. and Hood,L.E. (1985) *Nature*, **316**, 783.
3. Fink,P.J., Matis,L.A., McElligott,D.L., Bookman,M. and Hedrick,S.M. (1986) *Nature*, **321**, 219.
4. Schwartz,R.H. (1984) *Annu. Rev. Immunol.*, **3**, 237.
5. Hansburg,D., Fairwell,T., Schwartz,R.H. and Appela,E. (1983) *J. Immunol.*, **131**, 319.
6. Berkower,I., Matis,L.A., Buckenmeyer,G.K., Gurd,F.R.N., Longo,D.L. and Berzofsky,J.A. (1984) *J. Immunol.*, **132**, 1370.
7. Manca,F., Clarke,J.A., Miller,A., Sercarz,E.E. and Shastri,E. (1984) *J. Immunol.*, **133**, 2075.
8. Townsend,A.R.M., Gotch,F.M. and Davey,J. (1985) *Cell*, **42**, 457.
9. Mills,K.H.G., Skehel,J.J. and Thomas,D.B. (1986) *J. Exp. Med.*, **163**, 1477.
10. Morgan,D.A., Ruscetti,F.W. and Gallo,R. (1976) *Science*, **193**, 1007.
11. Smith,K.A. (1989) *Immunol. Rev.*, **51**, 339.
12. Corradin,G., Etlinger,H.M., Chiller,J.M. (1979) *J. Immunol.*, **119**, 1048.
13. Townsend,A.R.M., Taylor,P.M., Melief,C.J.M. and Askonas,B.A. (1983) *Immunogenetics*, **17**, 543.
14. Farrar,J.J., Fuller-Farrar,J., Simon,P.L., Hilfiker,M.L., Stadler,B.M. and Farrar,W.L. (1980) *J. Immunol.*, **125**, 2555.
15. Von Boehmer,H. and Haas,W. (1985) In *Immunological Methods III*. Lefkovitz,I. and Pernis,B. (eds), Academic Press, New York, p. 245.
16. Shearer,G.M. (1974) *Eur. J. Immunol.*, **4**, 527.
17. Thomas,D.B., Skehel,J.J., Mills,K.H.G. and Graham,C.M. (1986) *Eur. J. Immunol.*, **16**, 789.
18. Mills,K.H.G. (1986) In *Methods in Enzymology*. Langone,J.J. and Van Vunakis,H. (eds), Academic Press, New York, Vol. 121, p. 726.
19. Klein,J., Fiueroa,F. and David,C.S. (1983) *Immunogenetics*, **17**, 553.

13. NOTE ADDED IN PROOF

Recent studies indicate that T_h cell clones can be divided into two populations, on the basis of the lymphokines they release following stimulation (1). T_{h1} cells produce IL-2, IL-3 and interferon-γ, whilst T_{h2} cells secrete IL-3 and IL-4 (B cell-stimulatory factor-1, see Chapter 10). The commonly used 'IL-2-dependent' cell lines HT2 and CTLL2 proliferate in response to both IL-2 and IL-4 (refs. 1−3), and hence can be used to measure activation of both subpopulations of T_h cells. In addition, cell lines which only respond to either IL-2 or IL-4 are now being developed in various laboratories (e.g. ref. 3).

1. Mosmann,T.R., Clerwinski,H., Bond,M.W., Giedlin,M.A. and Coffman,R.L. (1986) *J. Immunol.*, **136**, 2348.
2. Lichtman,A.H., Kurt-Jones,E.A. and Abbas,A.K. (1987) *Proc. Natl. Acad. Sci. USA*, **84**, 824.
3. Muller,W. and Vandenabeele,P. (1987) *Eur. J. Immunol.*, **17**, 579.

CHAPTER 7

Generation of human B lymphoblastoid cell lines using Epstein−Barr virus

ELIZABETH V.WALLS AND DOROTHY H.CRAWFORD

1. INTRODUCTION

1.1 The Epstein−Barr virus

The Epstein−Barr virus (EBV) is a human B-lymphotropic herpesvirus which causes infectious mononucleosis (1) and is also aetiologically associated with two human tumours: African Burkitt's lymphoma (2) and anaplastic nasopharyngeal carcinoma (3).

Primary infection of adolescents and adults with EBV can cause acute infectious mononucleosis whereas childhood infection is generally asymptomatic. The majority of the adult population worldwide (up to 90%) is seropositive for EBV (1). The virus, however, is not eradicated from the body after primary infection and biologically active EBV can be detected in saliva and throat washings taken from seropositive individuals. Replication of EBV occurs in epithelial cells lining the pharynx and a few virus-infected B lymphocytes are present in the circulation. In this carrier state a balance is maintained between the level of virus infection and the cellular and humoral immune responses which keep the infection controlled.

In vitro EBV can immortalize B lymphocytes giving rise to long-term cell lines which carry the viral genome and express restricted viral genes such as the nuclear antigens (EBNA) (4,5). B lymphocytes infected with EBV may also be polyclonally activated to proliferate and produce immunoglobulins (Ig) (6). Polyclonal B lymphocyte activation and B lymphocyte immortalization by EBV are both T lymphocyte-independent processes.

1.2 B lymphoblastoid cell lines

B lymphoblastoid cell lines (BLCL) established from normal blood or tissues, whether infected *in vitro* with EBV or spontaneously generated, are usually of polyclonal derivation and associated with EBV. Typically, the cells have a 'hand-mirror' shape and often grow in clumps (*Figure 1A*). The cells usually have a diploid number of chromosomes and the cytoplasm contains many free polyribosomes with poorly developed rough endoplasmic reticulum and Golgi apparatus. Phenotypically, BLCL express some normal B cell markers including HLA class I and class II antigens, CD19, CD20 and surface Ig, with or without cytoplasmic Ig and Ig secretion. Antigens characteristic of activated lymphocytes (not necessarily B cell-restricted) are present on BLCL such as CD23 (BLAST-2), PCA-1, an interleukin-2 (IL-2) receptor similar to that on T cells and receptors for transferrin (7). EBV-encoded antigens expressed by BLCL include the latent

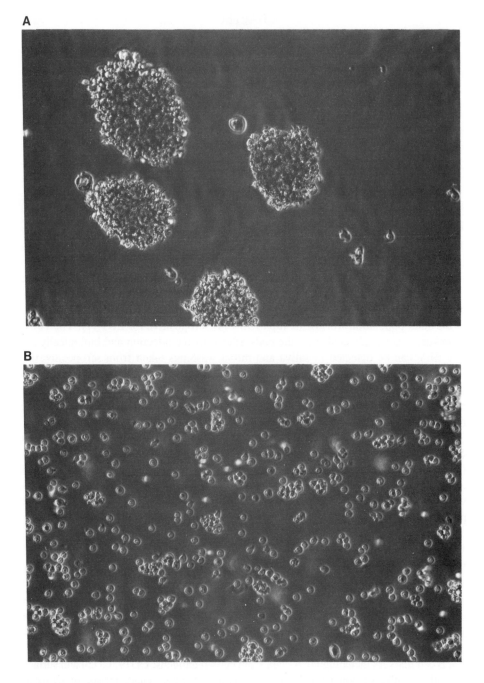

Figure 1. Photomicrographs of suspension cultures showing the morphology of lymphoblastoid B cell lines and Burkitt's lymphoma cell lines. (**A**) A lymphoblastoid B cell line derived by EBV immortalization of peripheral blood lymphocytes from a Burkitt's lymphoma patient. (**B**) An EBV-positive African Burkitt's lymphoma cell line (Raji).

membrane protein and EBNA complex; other virus-encoded proteins such as the early antigen and viral capsid antigen complexes are only expressed during lytic infections. Under standard culture conditions not more than 5% of EBV-immortalized B cells are undergoing lytic infection, thus virus production by such cultures is at a low level.

In contrast to BLCL, Burkitt's lymphoma (BL) cell lines are of neoplastic origin, capable of growing in soft agar and forming tumours in nude mice and also differ morphologically from BLCL (*Figure 1B*). BL cell lines are monoclonal, expressing surface Ig of one heavy chain isotype (usually IgM) and one light chain; they never have a normal diploid karyotype and characteristically carry one of three specific chromosomal translocations involving the c-*myc* gene: t8:14 or the variants t8:2 or t8:22 (8). Cell lines derived from the African type of BL carry the EBV genome, however, those isolated from sporadic cases of BL in other parts of the world are often EBV-negative. Like BLCL, some normal B lymphocyte surface antigens are expressed by BL cells such as HLA antigens: the common acute lymphoblastic leukaemia antigen, CD10, CD19, CD20 and surface Ig. Activation antigens are also present on BL cells including CD23, PCA-1 and receptors for IL-2 and transferrin (7).

2. PRINCIPLES

2.1 Production of virus

Infectious, wild-type EBV is present in the saliva or throat washings of infectious mononucleosis patients (9) and can be obtained intermittently from the same sources in normal seropositive individuals (10). In most laboratories, however, the cell line B95-8 is used to produce virus (11). This cell line was derived by *in vitro* infection of Cotton-topped marmoset peripheral blood mononuclear cells with wild-type virus isolated from an infectious mononucleosis patient. Under standard culture conditions around $1-10\%$ of cells are undergoing a lytic viral infection, but this percentage can be increased up to 80% following treatment with inducing agents such as phorbol esters (12) and sodium *n*-butyrate (13). Supernatants harvested from cultures at or approaching the stationary phase of their growth curves usually have an immortalizing titre of around 10^{-3} when used to infect human cord blood cells (Section 3.2). However, for some purposes it may be necessary to concentrate the virus by high-speed centrifugation, since increasing the virus dose does increase the number of cells infected (14 and Section 3.1.4).

2.2 Handling EBV in the laboratory

There is growing concern about safety precautions necessary for working with EBV and cell lines transformed by the virus. It must be remembered, however, that up to 90% of the adult population have already been infected with the virus and carry it as a lifelong infection in lymphoid cells, as well as intermittently secreting infectious virus particles into the oropharynx. Furthermore, EBV is of low infectivity and as yet no authenticated cases of laboratory-contracted infection have been reported. It is reasonable, therefore, to handle EBV-transformed cell lines (most of which produce small quantities of infectious virus) according to routine microbiological laboratory practice and to use a safety cabinet when handling concentrated virus preparations. EBV is a category 2 pathogen and basic precautions for working with the virus and immortalized cell lines will be described in Section 3.1.6.

2.3 EBV-B lymphocyte interactions

The receptor for EBV on B lymphocytes is a 140-kd glycoprotein (CD21) which also binds the complement component C3d, albeit at a different site from the virus (15). Recently it has been shown, using limiting dilution experiments, that although most peripheral blood B lymphocytes may be infected by EBV, only a subset (from 1 to 20%) are activated or immortalized *in vitro* (16,17). This may be a reflection of the inherent resistance of certain subpopulations of B lymphocytes to immortalization by EBV, or differences in growth requirements of these subsets after EBV infection (18,19).

2.4 Accessory and feeder cell requirements

It has been shown that activation of B lymphocytes by EBV to produce Ig is T cell-independent (6). However, immortalization of B lymphocytes by the virus does require feeder cells (20). Monocytes present in peripheral blood mononuclear cell preparations are efficient feeders for outgrowth of EBV-infected B lymphocytes. When purified B lymphocyte populations are infected with EBV feeder cells must be added to the cultures for optimal cell growth. The cellular interactions involved in this phenomenon are not fully characterized, but probably involve growth factor production. They are not genetically restricted since many allogeneic cells have been used successfully. Sources of feeder cells include fetal fibroblasts, allogeneic peripheral blood mononuclear cells and cord blood mononuclear cells, all of which are irradiated prior to culture. There is evidence that BLCL, once established, produce their own growth factors (21).

2.5 Regulation of the growth of EBV-infected B lymphocytes by T lymphocytes

Individuals seropositive for EBV (~90% of the adult population worldwide) possess circulating memory T lymphocytes which recognize autologous EBV-carrying B lymphocytes. These cells probably control growth of EBV-infected B lymphocytes *in vivo*, and give rise to specific cytotoxic cells when stimulated *in vitro* (22). Thus, in cultures of EBV-infected blood mononuclear cells from seropositive donors seeded at high density ($1-2 \times 10^6$/ml), proliferating foci of B lymphocytes regress after $3-4$ weeks and no cell lines are obtained. The problem of regression may be overcome in one of four ways:

(i)   cultures may be set up at low cell densities ($1-5 \times 10^5$/ml);
(ii)   mononuclear cells may be depleted of T lymphocytes by rosetting with sheep erythrocytes;
(iii)   T cell activation can be inhibited by cyclosporin A;
(iv)   phytohaemagglutinin may be added at the initiation of culture to inhibit specific T lymphocyte activation (23).

3. METHODOLOGY

3.1 Virus preparation

3.1.1 *Culture medium*

RPMI 1640 containing 100 IU/ml penicillin, 100 μg/ml streptomycin, 2 mM L-glutamine and 10% v/v heat inactivated, mycoplasma-screened fetal calf serum (FCS).

3.1.2 *Inducing agents*

(i) 12-O-Tetradecanoyl phorbol-13-acetate (TPA). Prepare a stock solution of 200 μg/ml TPA (Sigma) in dimethyl sulphoxide (DMSO), grade I, (Sigma) and store at $-20°C$; it is used at a final concentration of 20 ng/ml.

(ii) Sodium n-butyrate. Prepare a fresh solution of 3 M sodium *n*-butyrate (BDH) in water and sterilize by filtration. It is used at a final concentration of 3 mM.

3.1.3 *Culture of B95-8 cells*

Grow B95-8 cells in plastic tissue culture flasks at concentrations ranging from 1×10^5 up to 1×10^6 cells/ml in a 37°C incubator with a humid atmosphere of 5% CO_2 in air. Healthy cultures of B95-8 contain floating clumps of cells, while some cells adhere to the plastic surface so that flasks are usually kept flat to give the maximum surface area for adherence. When growing the cells for virus production, expand cultures up to 250 ml in a 175 cm^2 flask and once the cells have reached a density of 5×10^5/ml leave them for about $7-10$ days without replacing the medium. At this stage TPA or sodium *n*-butyrate may be added to the culture medium to increase virus production. The cells continue to proliferate and after 7 days the medium is harvested. When inducing agents are used, the EBV preparations contain TPA or sodium *n*-butyrate which may interfere with studies on B lymphocyte activation by the virus.

3.1.4 *Harvesting EBV from B95-8 cultures*

Centrifuge the culture supernatant at 400 *g* for 15 min at 20°C to remove most of the cells, then pass through a 0.45 μm pore filter, which retains cells and large particles of debris, but not the enveloped infectious virus particles. Supernatants from healthy cultures of B95-8 cells (at $\sim 1-2 \times 10^6$/ml) which have been prepared in this way should have an immortalizing titre of around 10^{-3} when used to infect human cord blood cells. Store EBV stocks in aliquots, usually 1 ml, at $-70°C$ since the viral infectivity declines if the preparations are kept above this temperature. Repeated freezing and thawing inactivates the virus. The B95-8 culture supernatant may be concentrated 50- to 100-fold by centrifugation at 27 000 *g* for 2 h at 4°C, the pellets are resuspended in culture medium and stored in 0.1 ml aliquots at $-70°C$. Concentrated EBV preparations are usually diluted 1:10 with fresh medium prior to infection.

3.1.5 *Titration of EBV preparations on cord blood mononuclear cells*

(i)   Prepare mononuclear cells from umbilical cord blood (Section 3.2) to assess the immortalizing titre of an EBV preparation; 10^7 cells are sufficient to test one batch.

(ii)   Prepare serial 10-fold dilutions of virus from neat culture supernatant to a $1:10^6$ dilution, using RPMI 1640/10% FCS medium (Section 3.1.1).

(iii) Dispense aliquots of 10^6 cord blood mononuclear cells into 12×75 mm plastic tissue culture tubes and pellet by centrifugation at 400 *g* for 10 min.

(iv)   Resuspend the pellets in 200 μl of each virus dilution, with controls of culture medium only and a batch of EBV with known immortalizing titre.

(v)   Incubate the cells at 37°C for 1 h, in a gassed incubator, agitating the tubes occasionally to keep the cells in suspension.

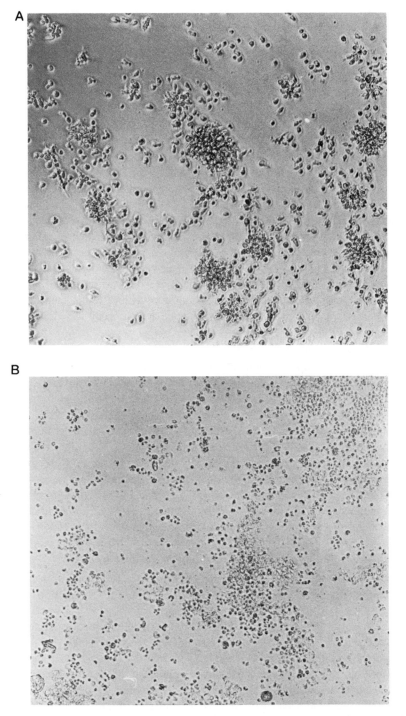

Figure 2. Photomicrographs of 3 week old cultures of cord blood mononuclear cells, **(A)** infected with EBV and **(B)** uninfected controls.

(vi)   Add 2 ml of wash medium (RPMI 1640/2% FCS, Section 3.2.1) to each tube, and centrifuge at 400 *g* for 10 min.

(vii)   Remove the supernatants, containing excess virus, and resuspend the cell pellets at 10^6/ml in RPMI 1640/10% FCS culture medium.

(viii)   Dispense five replicate 200 μl aliquots, containing 2×10^5 cells, for each virus dilution to a 96-well flat-bottom tissue culture plate and incubate for 4 weeks (37°C gassed incubator) before assessing immortalization.

(ix)   Feed the cultures at weekly intervals by removing half of the supernatant from each well and replacing it with fresh medium. It is important not to transfer cells or supernatant containing virus between wells.

Immortalization is usually assessed visually by examining the cultures using an inverted microscope. Proliferating foci of B lymphocytes can be seen 1−2 weeks after infection with EBV and large clumps of cells are usually macroscopically visible after 4 weeks, whilst only dying cells and debris remain in control cultures (*Figure 2*). The efficiency of immortalization is defined as the negative log to the base 10 of the virus dilution which induced immortalization in 50% of the cultures.

3.1.6 *Precautions for handling EBV and immortal cell lines*

(i)   When working with EBV preparations and immortal cell lines wear a laboratory coat, or disposable apron. Remove these and wash hands before leaving the laboratory.

(ii)   Gloves, preferably the close-fitting surgical types, may be worn but are not essential if manipulations are executed carefully.

(iii)   Never mouth-pipette.

(iv)   Render all waste material non-infective before disposal, either by autoclaving at 126°C for 30 min or by treatment with hypochlorite solutions such as 'Chloros' (sodium hypochlorite, 11% available chlorine content, Durham Chemicals Distributors Ltd).

(v)   Autoclave solid waste and small amounts of liquid waste, such as human sera and EBV preparations, in sealed containers.

(vi)   Aspirate liquid waste such as washing or culture media into a trap containing Chloros and allow to stand for 18 h (the final concentration of Chloros should not be less than 10% v/v). After decontamination the liquid waste may be flushed down a sink.

(vii)   Decontaminate glassware by soaking for at least 18 h in a 5% v/v solution of Chloros, the articles being completely immersed in the disinfectant.

(viii)   Clean up any spillages immediately and wipe the area with 10% v/v Chloros followed by 70% v/v alcohol.

3.2 Preparation of target cells for infection

3.2.1 *Washing medium*

RPMI 1640 containing 100 IU/ml penicillin, 100 μg/ml streptomycin, and 2% v/v heat inactivated, mycoplasma-screened FCS.

3.2.2 *Dextran sedimentation of cord blood erythrocytes*

(i)   Sterilize a solution of 6% w/v Dextran (250 000 mol. wt, Sigma) in 0.15 M sodium chloride by autoclaving at 110°C for 30 min.

(ii) Mix dextran solution and cord blood in a ratio of 1:4 (2.5 ml of dextran added to 10 ml of blood) and incubate in a 37°C water bath for 45 min.

(iii) Layer the erythrocyte-depleted supernatant onto a Ficoll density gradient to separate the mononuclear cells.

3.2.3 *Preparation of mononuclear cells and depletion of T lymphocytes*

Prepare mononuclear cells from heparinized blood, or from surgical specimens of tonsil and spleen by separation on a Ficoll gradient (Chapter 1). T lymphocytes can be removed from these preparations by rosetting with sheep erythrocytes followed by separation on a Ficoll gradient (Chapter 2). To obtain efficient immortalization of B cells from tonsils or spleens the specimens must be fresh.

3.3 Establishment of EBV immortalized cell lines

3.3.1 *Preparation of cyclosporine for use in cultures*

Cyclosporine, suitable for tissue culture may be obtained from Sandoz Ltd. Make a stock solution by dissolving the powder in injectable-grade alcohol to 1 mg/ml and dilute in culture medium to give a final concentration of $0.1-1$ μg/ml.

3.3.2 *EBV infection and culture*

(i)   Resuspend pellets of up to 10^7 cells (depending on the virus titre) in 1 ml of undiluted B95-8 culture supernatant and incubate at 37°C for 1 h in a CO_2 incubator, agitating the cells occasionally to keep them in suspension. Longer incubation periods (up to 24 h) can be used, although there may be a loss of viability of cells incubated at high density in the spent B95-8 culture medium.

(ii) Following incubation with EBV, wash the cells once with RPMI 1640 2% FCS, resuspend in culture medium at $1-2 \times 10^6$/ml and dispense 2 ml aliquots to 24-well flat-bottom tissue culture plates. If the cells were obtained from an EBV-seropositive donor and have not been depleted of T lymphocytes, then add cyclosporine to the culture medium to a final concentration of $0.1-1$ μg/ml.

(iii) Initially, feed the cells at weekly intervals by removing half of the supernatant and replacing it with fresh medium without disturbing the cell layer. Proliferating foci of B cells are usually microscopically visible $1-2$ weeks after infection with EBV and these will continue to proliferate on sub-culturing.

3.3.4 *Regression assay to demonstrate T cell-mediated immunity to EBV*

(i)   Culture EBV-infected mononuclear cells from seropositive donors in 200 μl flat-bottomed wells at doubling dilutions from 2×10^6 cells/ml to 2.5×10^5 cells/ml.

(ii) Plate ten replicate wells at each cell concentration, five of which contain cyclosporine.

(iii)   Culture for a total of 4 weeks and feed weekly.

After 1−2 weeks of culture, proliferating foci of B lymphocytes can be observed microscopically in all wells, but in the absence of cyclosporine these clumps usually regress after 3−4 weeks in wells seeded at high cell density. BLCL may be obtained from cultures seeded at lower densities ($2.5−5 \times 10^5$/ml). However, cells plated at both high and low densities in medium containing cyclosporine do yield BLCL which may be sub-cultured.

3.4 Expansion of cultures and cryopreservation of cell lines

3.4.1 *Freezing medium and ampoules*

RPMI 1640 containing antibiotics (see Section 3.1.1): 10% v/v DMSO and 20−50% v/v FCS. Ampoules — Nunc cryotubes.

3.4.2 *Expansion of BLCL*

EBV-carrying B cell lines vary with respect to their growth characteristics but are usually maintained at cell concentrations between 10^5 and 10^6/ml, having a doubling time of 24−72 h. Once immortalized, proliferating B cells may be transferred from 2 ml cultures in 24-well plates to 25 cm^2 tissue culture flasks, which are best kept upright initially. Thereafter cultures may be expanded into larger vessels, usually diluting the cells 1:2 every 3−7 days depending on their growth rate.

3.4.3 *Freezing and thawing lymphoblastoid cells*

(i)   Harvest cells from healthy cultures, pellet by centrifugation at 400 *g* and resuspend in cold freezing solution.

(ii)   Dispense the cells in 1 ml aliquots to freezing ampoules and freeze, either by incubation for 24 h at $-70°C$ in a block of expanded polystyrene (1 inch thick around each tube), or by more sophisticated methods of controlled cooling. Frozen cells are stored in the vapour phase above liquid nitrogen.

(iii)   To recover cells stored in liquid nitrogen, thaw ampoules quickly by incubating at 37°C.

(iv)   Transfer to a plastic universal tube, and dilute the cell suspension by adding 2 ml of warm washing medium dropwise with shaking and another 7 ml of warm medium slowly.

(v)   Pellet the cells, resuspend in medium and count.

(vi)   When culturing cells after freezing, it is advisable to seed them into a 24-well flat-bottom tissue culture plate at three or more concentrations ranging from 10^5 to 10^6/ml to ensure recovery of healthy, growing cells. Some cell lines require feeders such as irradiated (2000 rad) peripheral blood mononuclear cells at 0.5×10^6/ml.

3.5 Detection of EBNA by anti-complement immunofluorescence

3.5.1 *Reagents*

(i)   Prepare complement fixation test (CFT) veronal buffer pH 7.2 for washing cells and slides from Barbitone Diluent Tablets (Oxoid). The solution may be sterilized by autoclaving at 121°C for 20 min and stored at 4°C. Use with care — barbitone is poisonous.

(ii)   Prepare tri-sodium citrate, 0.95% w/v, and sterilize by filtration. This is used to resuspend cells for preparation of smears. Since it is slightly hypotonic, slight nuclear expansion occurs.

(iii)   Prepare a 1:1 (v/v) mixture of acetone and methanol.

(iv)   Heat-inactivate standard sera from known EBV seropositive and seronegative donors and store at −20°C.

(v)   Obtain fresh serum from a known EBV-seronegative donor as a source of complement. Store in aliquots at −70°C.

(vi)   Dilute goat anti-human C_3-FITC (fluorescein isothiocyanate) conjugate (Cappel) 1:30 in CFT for staining cells.

(vii)   Evans Blue, 0.1% w/v in distilled water, is used as a counterstain. Slides are mounted in a 1:1 mixture of CFT and glycerol.

(viii) Alcohol washed glass microscope slides, slide racks, Coplin jars, plastic boxes, soft paper tissues and magnetic stirrers are also required.

3.5.2 *Preparation of cell smears*

(i)   Wash the cells to be stained twice in CFT and resuspend at 5×10^6/ml in 0.95% w/v trisodium citrate. About 2.5×10^5 cells are required for each smear, thus 5×10^5 cells are sufficient for one positive and one negative slide. The BL cell lines Raji and Ramos can be used as EBNA positive and negative controls, respectively.

(ii)   Either place 50 μl aliquots of cell suspension on the microscope slides and allow them to dry in air, or prepare cytospin smears using 50 μl of cell suspension. Mark around the cell smears with a glass cutter and label the slides with pencil (not alcohol-soluble ink).

(iii)   For fixing the cells, the acetone−methanol fixative must be at or below −20°C otherwise the nuclear antigens may be lost. Either surround the Coplin jar of fixative with cardice, or pre-cool the vessel of fixative in a −70°C freezer. Fix the slides for at least 3 min at −20°C, during which time the jar of fixative is kept on cardice or in the −70°C freezer. Dry the slides at room temperature (20°C). They may be stored temporarily at 4°C (24 h), or for longer periods at −20°C prior to staining.

3.5.3 *Anti-complement immunofluorescence staining*

(i)   Prepare mixtures containing one part of positive or negative serum, one part of complement serum and eight parts of CFT and keep on ice.

(ii)   Dip the slides in CFT and wipe the slides around the smears with soft tissue; smears must not be allowed to dry out, so treat each slide individually in steps (iii) and (v).

(iii)   Place 20 μl aliquots of the diluted serum plus complement mixture on the cell smears, immediately place them in a moist box and incubate for 1 h at 37°C.

(iv)   Wash the slides twice for 10 min in CFT using a magnetic stirrer.

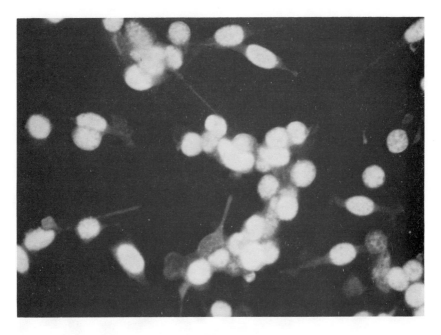

Figure 3. Anti-complement immunofluorescence staining for EBNA.

(v)   After drying around the smears with tissues, add 20 μl of the diluted goat anti-human C3 − FITC conjugate to each smear and incubate the slides in a moist box for 1 h at room temperature.

(vi)   Wash the slides twice for 10 min in CFT, with stirring.

(vii)   If the slides are to be counterstained, dip them briefly in distilled water and then incubate for 15 min in 0.1% w/v Evans Blue before again washing in CFT.

(viii) Mount the slides in CFT:glycerol mixture and store in the dark at 4°C before observing with a fluorescence microscope. Positively stained cells show speckled bright green nuclear fluorescence (*Figure 3*).

3.6 Immuno-peroxidase staining for EBNA

3.6.1 *Reagents*

(i)   Veronal buffer (CFT); tri-sodium citrate: acetone − methanol fixative: standard human sera: human complement and mounting solution prepared as described in Section 3.5.1.

(ii)   Peroxidase-conjugated rabbit anti-human C_3 (Dakopatts a/s) diluted 1:30 in CFT for staining.

(iii)   Phosphate-buffered saline (PBS) pH 7.2, as the substrate buffer and for washing the slides prior to incubation with the substrate.

(iv)   A fresh solution of 3,3′-diaminobenzidine tetrahydrochloride (DAB, Sigma), 0.5 mg/ml in PBS; add hydrogen peroxide to give a final concentration of 0.03% w/v (1 μl of 30% w/v hydrogen peroxide/ml).

(v)   Mayer's haematoxylin (Sigma) as a counterstain.

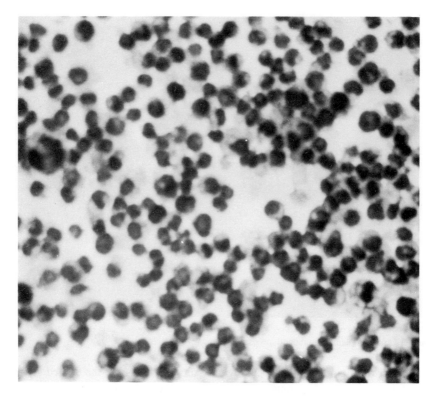

Figure 4. Anti-complement immunoperoxidase staining for EBNA.

3.6.2 *Procedure for anti-complement immunoperoxidase staining*

(i) Prepare and fix cell smears exactly as described in Section 3.5.2.

(ii) Incubate the cell smears with anti-EBNA positive and anti-EBNA negative serum plus complement mixtures and then wash as in Section 3.5.3(i−iv).

(iii) After drying around the smears with tissues, add 20 μl of the diluted rabbit anti-human C3−peroxidase conjugate to each smear and incubate the slides in a moist chamber for 30 min at 37°C.

(iv) Wash the slides once in CFT for 10 min and once in PBS for 10 min.

(v) Develop the peroxide label by immersing the slides in a freshly prepared DAB−hydrogen peroxidase solution for 5 min at room temperature.

(vi) Wash the slides in tap water several times before counterstaining for 3 min in Mayer's haematoxylin solution, which stains the nuclei blue.

(vii) After mounting, the slides are observed using a light microscope: positively stained nuclei are brown (*Figure 4*).

4. PROBLEMS

Although the techniques described in Section 3 are routinely used in several laboratories, difficulties are often encountered when initially attempting to generate BLCL. Potential problem areas will be described in this section.

4.1 Virus-related problems

Virus preparations with low immortalization titres can be detected by testing the batches on cord blood cells (Section 3.1.5). Low immortalization titres may result from harvesting the B95-8 culture supernatants too early; incorrect storage of the virus or even from mycoplasma contamination of the B95-8 cell line. Mycoplasma contamination of B95-8 cells and the EBV derived from them may have deleterious effects on the efficiency of B cell immortalization (24). Contamination of tonsil specimens by mycoplasma may also render them less susceptible to immortalization by EBV. It is advisable to have BLCL screened for mycoplasma and to fumigate tissue culture cabinets with formaldehyde on a regular basis.

4.2 Target cells

Fresh target cell preparations with a high percentage of viable cells are most efficiently immortalized by EBV. There is some evidence that 'resting' B cells are more susceptible to immortalization by EBV or have less stringent culture requirements than activated B cells (18,19). Generally, peripheral blood mononuclear cells are reproducibly immortalized by EBV, even after freezing, but problems may be encountered with surgical specimens of tonsil or spleen, especially after cryopreservation. When using lymphocytes from seropositive donors, the T cells must be removed or cyclosporine added to the cultures to avoid inhibition of B cell growth by the EBV-specific T cells. Preparations of cyclosporine should be checked for toxicity.

4.3 Detection of EBNA in cell lines

Occasionally EBNA staining is unsatisfactory. This may result from incorrect fixing of samples, which must be carried out at or below $-20°C$ using the acetone−methanol mixture given in Section 3.5.1. It is advisable to include Raji and Ramos cells as controls to check that the fixing was carried out correctly. Non-specific background staining may be a problem arising from the use of human sera on human cells. Some cells exhibit membrane staining, presumably due to the presence of membrane complement receptors, thus, staining with a control anti-EBV negative serum should always by included. Other problems may arise from inactivation of the complement during storage and from allowing the cell smears to dry out before adding various reagents.

4.4 Culture conditions

Generally media and supplements which support short-term activation or growth of human lymphoid cells are adequate for BLCL, but if possible they should be checked by limiting dilution cultures of established lines.

5. POTENTIAL USES OF BLCL

EBV-immortalized BLCL provide an unlimited supply of B lymphocytes which can be used in several ways (25). Biochemical studies of cell surface antigens require large numbers of relatively pure cells and BLCL, especially if they have been cloned, are an ideal source. The cell lines may also be used in the generation of rodent monoclonal antibodies specific for human B lymphocyte surface antigens and are particularly useful if antibodies to activation antigens are required. Since BLCL express HLA class I and class II antigens they can be used in tissue typing, both as stimulator cells in mixed lymphocyte cultures and as controls in serologic analyses.

EBV-immortalized B lymphocytes provide an infinite source of histocompatible feeder cells for T lymphocyte clones. They have also been used to demonstrate that B lymphocytes are capable of 'processing' soluble antigens and 'presenting' them to T lymphocytes in an antigen-specific, major histocompatibility complex-restricted manner (26).

Human monoclonal antibodies produced by EBV immortalization of antigen-specific B lymphocytes may be used in studies of human immune responses and, more importantly, could replace human antisera in the prevention and/or treatment of several diseases. Examples of the therapeutic uses of human antisera include the prevention of Rhesus haemolytic disease of the newborn; neutralization of bacterial toxins and snake venom; elimination of circulating drugs (overdoses); passive immunization of 'high risk' individuals against infections such as hepatitis, herpes simplex, varicella zoster, rubella and measles and the treatment of cytomegalovirus infections in immunodeficient individuals.

6. REFERENCES

1. Henle,G., Henle,W. and Diehl,V. (1968) *Proc. Natl. Acad. Sci. USA*, **59**, 94.
2. Epstein,M.A. and Achong,B.G. (1979) In *The Epstein–Barr Virus*. Epstein,M.A. and Achong,B.G. (eds), Springer, Berlin, p. 321.
3. Epstein,M.A. (1978) In *Nasopharyngeal Carcinoma: Aetiology and Control*. de-Thé,G., Ho,Y. and Davis,W. (eds), IARC, Lyon, p. 333.
4. Reedman,B.M. and Klein,G. (1973) *Int. J. Cancer*, **2**, 499.
5. Pattengale,P.K., Smith,R.W. and Gerber,P. (1973) *Lancet*, **II**, 93.
6. Rosen,A., Gergely,P., Jondal,M., Klein,G. and Britton,S. (1977) *Nature*, **267**, 52.
7. Crawford,D.H. and Ando,I. (1986) *Immunology*, **59**, 405.
8. Zech,L., Haglund,U., Nilsson,K. and Klein,G. (1976) *Int. J. Cancer*, **17**, 47.
9. Miller,G., Niederman,J.C. and Andrews,L.L. (1973) *N. Engl. J. Med.*, **288**, 229.
10. Golden,H.D., Chang,R.S., Prescott,W., Simpson,E. and Cooper,T.Y. (1973) *J. Infect. Dis.*, **127**, 471.
11. Miller,G., Shope,T., Lisco,H., Stitt,D. and Lipman,M. (1972) *Proc. Natl. Acad. Sci. USA*, **69**, 383.
12. zur Hausen,H., O'Neill,F.J., Freese,U.K. and Hecker,E. (1978) *Nature*, **272**, 373.
13. Luka,J., Kallin,B. and Klein,G. (1979) *Virology*, **94**, 228.
14. Zerbini,M. and Ernberg,I. (1983) *J. Gen. Virol.*, **64**, 539.
15. Nemerow,G.R., Siaw,M.F.G. and Cooper,N.R. (1986) *J. Virol.*, **58**, 709.
16. Tosato,G. and Blaese,R.M. (1985) *Adv. Immunol.*, **37**, 99.
17. Katsuki,T., Hiruma,Y., Yamamoto,N., Abo,T. and Kumagi,K. (1977) *Virology*, **83**, 287.
18. Aman,P., Ehlin-Henriksson,B. and Klein,G. (1984) *J. Exp. Med.*, **159**, 208.
19. Chan,M.A., Stein,L.D., Dosch,H-M. and Sigal,N.H. (1986) *J. Immunol.*, **136**, 106.
20. Pope,J.H., Scott,W. and Moss,D.J. (1974) *Int. J. Cancer*, **14**, 122.
21. Blazar,B.A., Sutton,L.M. and Strome,M. (1983) *Cancer Res.*, **43**, 4562.
22. Rickinson,A.B., Moss,D.J. and Pope,J.H. (1979) *Int. J. Cancer*, **23**, 610.
23. Crawford,D.H. (1981) In *Transplantation and Clinical Immunology XIII*. Touraine,J.T., Traeger,J., Betuel,H., Brochier,J., Dubernard,J.M., Revillard,J.P. and Triau,R. (eds), Excerpta Medica, Amsterdam, p. 48.
24. Doyle,A., Jones,T., Bidwell,J. and Bradley,B. (1985) *Hum. Immunol.*, **13**, 199.
25. Crawford,D.H. (1986) In *The Epstein–Barr Virus — Recent Advances*. Epstein,M.A. and Achong,B.G. (eds), W. Heinemann Medical Books, London, p. 250.
26. Lanzaveccia,A. (1985) *Nature*, **314**, 537.

CHAPTER 8

Limiting dilution analysis

HERMAN WALDMANN, STEVE COBBOLD and IVAN LEFKOVITS

1. INTRODUCTION

The immune response to any antigen involves the clonal expansion of pre-committed lymphocytes and the differentiation of clonal progeny to effector cells that, for example, produce antibody or kill appropriate target cells. For many purposes one can measure this response by simply quantitating the amount of final product, that is antibody or cytotoxicity. There are, however, many circumstances when one would like to know how many lymphocytes in a resting population participate in the response to a given antigen. For this purpose one needs a way to measure the frequency of such precursors. There is no simple way to identify which of the cells in a large population of lympho-cytes will go on to produce active clones. Precursors are rare and morphologically in-distinguishable from the silent majority of resting lymphocytes. Limiting dilution analysis (LDA) allows calculation of precursor frequencies as a retrospective process based on the measurement of the number of active clones generated from a given population of cells. As each active clone is derived from one precursor, then retrospectively one can estimate the frequency of precursors that gave rise to those clones. Estimation of the precursor frequency can be an end in itself. It can however be a necessary first step for analysing complex cellular interactions on a clonal level as will become apparent later.

In this chapter we will outline the theoretical basis for LDA, provide examples of experimental protocols that have been used in various areas of cellular immunology, and leave the reader with a user-friendly computer program based on previously described statistical methods for calculation of frequencies.

2. THEORETICAL CONSIDERATIONS

2.1 Single hit curves and calculation of frequency

There have been a number of previous reviews detailing the theory of LDA $(1-5)$. Here we will just briefly outline the essential principles. As an example we start with a population of T-lymphocytes taken from an animal immunized to keyhole limpet haemocyanin (KLH). Let us say that 1 per 20 000 of these cells was a helper T cell (T_h) with specificity to KLH. If we took, say, 10^6 cells and distributed them at random, with antigen, into 100 culture wells, together with a large excess of B cells and other vital accessory cells, then each culture well would, on average, receive 10^4 T cells. Because there is only one T_h per 2×10^4 T cells it is obvious that some culture wells would not have received a T_h cell. Those particular wells would score negative in an antibody readout at the end of the culture period. On the assumption that a single T_h

163

is sufficient to trigger a B cell clone to antibody production, we can perform the following calculation using the proportion or fraction of negative wells as the key. The proportion of negative cultures can be defined by the expression:

$$F_o = e^{-u}$$

where F_o is the fraction of negative cultures, e the base of the natural logarithm and u the average number of precursor cells (in this case T_h) per culture. This expression is the zero term of the Poisson distribution. The full distribution formula, its derivation and its relationship to the binomial distribution is considered in detail in ref. 1. In the example we have given the observed fraction of negatives substituted into the above formula should give an estimate of frequency.

In practice the situation is somewhat different. One does not know the frequency and want to measure it. It would be risky to conduct the one point exercise as above because you would not know what average number of T cells/well would give a workable proportion of negatives. For this and other reasons the conventional practice is to titrate the T cells so that one has a series of groups of cultures each with a different T cell input. As a result one generates a series of values of F_o for different T cell inputs. To be able to use these values we need to consider an alternative form of the equation above. The formula can be converted to its logarithmic form:

$$u = -\ln F_o$$

This conversion is necessary both because it yields an explicit expression of what we are trying to measure (u), and also because it can be represented graphically, providing a straight line in a semilog plot. In other words, the negative logarithms of the fraction of non-responding cultures is linearly proportional to the mean number of precursors per culture. The resulting straight line has two uses. First it allows the estimation of frequency by a variety of methods (see below). Second it acts as an internal control to validate that the system is measuring the activity of a single limiting cell type. A straight line means a single-hit curve which means that a single cell type is limiting. Deviations from linearity determined by use of appropriate statistical methods (see Section 4) would tend to invalidate that starting assumption, confound the estimate of frequency and preclude any further dependent analyses.

The reasons that a particular semilog plot may turn out as deviant (i.e. non-linear) are many. The culture conditions could, for example be suboptimal, or the readouts too insensitive to the products of a single clone. In the example of T cell help the readout depends on having excess B cells in all wells. If that requirement is not met then the semilog plot titration curves would level off (at high T_h input) to an asymptote reflecting the fraction of cultures that contained no antigen-specific B cells. Those familiar with these plots in radiobiology or virology will also recall 'multihit' and 'multitarget' curves. In an ideal world 'multitarget' reflects the need for two or more different particles to interact. In practice these curves are hard to exploit in cellular immunology due to the relatively small samples available. They serve, at best, to encourage experimental re-design to optimize culture conditions or to unravel cell interactions.

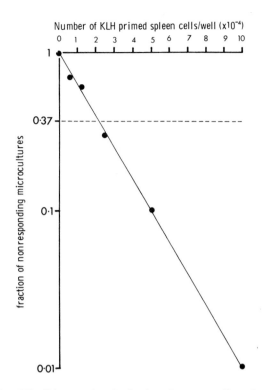

Figure 1. Semilog plot of T cell input against the fraction of non-responding cultures. T-enriched spleen cells from KLH-primed mice were added in increasing numbers to 'B cells' from the spleens of TNP-OVA primed mice. Groups of cultures (60/group) were challenged with TNP-KLH and the anti-TNP antibody response (in this case PFC) determined. In this single-hit curve the frequency of helper T cells for KLH can be interpolated from $F_o = 0.37$. The estimated frequency is about 1:20 000 T cells or 5×10^{-5}.

Back to our example. We have the semilog plot (*Figure 1*). We can apply statistical methods to test the goodness of fit of the data points with the single-hit Poisson model by calculating chi-squared statistics and confidence intervals for the slope (see Section 4). Let us assume we have the best fit line. We can from the plot make a reasonable estimate of the frequency by interpolating at the level of 37% non-responding cultures. This is best understood by substituting u = 1 into the zero term of the Poisson formula. We then derive:

$$F_o = e^{-u}$$
$$\text{Then } F_o = e^{-1} = 1/e = 0.37 \ (37\%)$$

There are more sophisticated ways of estimating frequency from calculations of the slope of the curve, and these are summarized elsewhere (5).

For our example the interpolation at $F_o = 0.37$ allows us to estimate the precursor frequency as about 1/20 000 cells or 5×10^{-5}.

2.2 **Partition analysis**

LDA is most frequently used to follow the behaviour of a single active cell type in a large heterogeneous population. It does seem possible to apply the same principles to examine interactions between different kinds of cell within a test population. To exemplify this we show a semilog plot of an experiment where the T-helper population contained two sorts of rare cell with opposing influences on B cell responses. This situation was contrived by mixing the same T_h cells as were used in *Figure 1* (H-2^k) with B cells that are only partially histocompatible (H-2^k × H-2^d). The T_h cell population is then composed of *bona fide* T_h cells as before, but also alloreactive cells (k anti-d). At low cell input these two sorts of cells would be expected to segregate randomly and independently of each other. At high T cell input many culture wells contain both cell types. This has a complex effect on the readout, since the B cells can be subject to both helper and inhibitory influences. In practice the demonstration of the 'reverse titration' or 'sawtooth' curve (*Figure 2*) in the quoted example was the first evidence that failure of T_h and B cells to cooperate over histocompatibility differences (even with sharing of Class II alleles) was a result of interference by alloreactive T cells (6). Analysis of such curves is not straightforward and various models have been offered (1,7,8). As indicated by Taswell (5) the validity of these models has yet to be established, but the soil is fertile for this type of application. For ease of communication we have referred to this more complex analysis as 'partition analysis' (1). It must be said

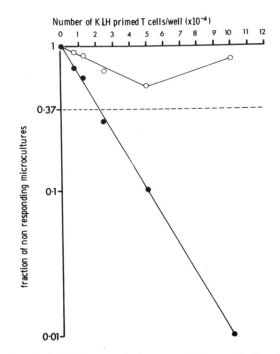

Figure 2. Deviation from single hit. The sawtooth phenomenon. The same T cells as in *Figure 1* (haplotype H-2^k) were analysed for help on a population of B cells that were F_1 (H-2^k × H-2^d). At high T cell input alloreactivity obscures help. At lower input T_h and alloreactive inhibitory cells segregate (O) or partition independently allowing expression of help in some wells.

that there has been a somewhat (in our opinion) precocious application of such analyses to phenomena that are ill understood. It is important for the experimenter to realize that we place great faith in at least two stages of the experimental process that may, in certain circumstances, be inappropriate. In particular the whole exercise is based on a readout that has to be re-coded as positive or negative. It is quite conceivable that at one input of test cells the readout may be reliable, while at a higher input of test cells the sensitivity may drop, resulting in an inappropriate score of negatives. Let us take a hypothetical example: we take T cells; plate them out in feeder cells at different inputs; stimulate with the polyclonal mitogen Concanavalin A (Con A) and then ask how many wells have helper clones by adding B cells after some suitable time. It is quite possible that, at a given T cell input, the Con A may have activated so many cells in that culture that the biological requirements for readout are compromised, for example the B cells make only small clones, and therefore less antibody. This may result in wells containing too little antibody to score positive, and consequently, sawtooth curves. This may be the sort of explanation for the bizarre results of Eichmann and collaborators (8, and many others). The message is not to underestimate the variables that can affect your experimental system: know the system; optimize the repeated reproducibility; and use strange curves only to give a qualitative feel of the biology, so that you can re-design experiments to test the new hypothesis.

3. METHODOLOGY

3.1 Introduction

LDA had been widely applied to many aspects of cellular immunology. Our major experience has been with the analysis of T-helper cell function in the secondary antibody response and for that reason we will confine ourselves in large part to methodology for measuring that function in the mouse model. The principles are really quite similar for other lymphocyte functions; and to avoid repetition and boredom we will simply provide the reader with a series of suitable references where recipes are well documented.

3.2 Limiting dilution analysis of T-helper cells

3.2.1 *T-helper cells*

Immunize CBA/Ca mice i.p. with $200-500$ μg of KLH in Freund's complete adjuvant (FCA). At any time after 4 weeks these animals can be boosted with 100 μg of soluble antigen in phosphate-buffered saline (PBS). One week after boost the spleen cells are an active source of T_h cells for both cognate and non-cognate help for B cells. The T cells are enriched by the nylon wool method (9) given below.

(i)   Pre-soak nylon wool in saline for 2 h at 37°C, rinse in distilled water and wash in double-distilled water at 37°C. Make three to four changes of water over 1 week, wring out the wool and dry at 37°C.

(ii) Make a column by packing 0.6 g of wool into the barrel of 12 ml plastic syringes.

(iii) Autoclave the syringes and before use rinse with a balanced salt solution [BSS containing 5% fetal calf serum (FCS)], and then drain off excess medium.

(iv) Load a total of $1-1.5 \times 10^8$ spleen cells in a volume of 2 ml onto the column, and after the cells have entered the wool overlay the sample by 1 ml of warm (37°C) BSS.

(v)   Incubate for 45 min at 37°C and then elute the cells with BSS.

(vi)   Collect the first 25 ml eluted; this routinely contains less than 5% B cells.

(vii)   This eluate contains red cells. For LDA experiments which depend on high T cell input, these can be inhibitory. Lyse the red cells by incubating in 2 ml of Gey's BSS where the sodium chloride has been replaced by ammonium chloride. After 10 min on ice, add excess BSS and remove residual ammonium chloride by washing and spinning through FCS. Our routine BSS is Eagle's medium without bicarbonate, rendered iso-osmolar with mouse cells by addition of sodium chloride, and buffered with 20 mM Hepes.

(viii) Incubate these T-enriched cells at 37°C with 40 μg/ml of mitomycin C (Sigma) in BSS for 20 min; wash the cells and then centrifuge through a layer of FCS to remove residual mitomycin C. This step is extremely important both because it prevents T and B cell division and thus enables one to focus on functions of single cells without any antibody production by residual B cells in the T inoculum, and because the background (no antigen added) antibody production of the readout B cells remains constant at any T cell input.

When using sensitive radioimmunoassay (RIA) or enzyme-linked immunosorbent assays (ELISA), increased background antibody production with increased T input can make the data deviate from single hit and confound interpretation.

3.2.2 *B-memory cells*

Immunize mice with $200-500$ μg of haptenated ovalbumin (TNP-OVA or NIP-OVA) in FCA followed by a boost with $100-200$ μg of soluble antigen after a further month. Spleen cells taken $7-17$ days after boost are a rich source of IgG memory cells. These cells cultured alone would generate 'background' responses in our sensitive assays. To reduce this the cells are routinely pre-treated with anti-Thy-1 antibody and complement. We presume that residual sequestered antigen (OVA conjugate) is released *in vitro* and if OVA-specific T cells are not removed they cooperate to give the 'background' response.

3.2.3 *Culture medium*

The optimal medium we have used is based on the original formula of Mishell and Dutton (10). For every 100 ml of Eagle's minimum essential medium (MEM) we add glutamine, pyruvate, non-essential amino acids, antibiotics, 20 mM Hepes, $5-10\%$ FCS and 5×10^{-5} M 2-mercaptoethanol.

3.2.4 *Cell cultures*

Cell mixes are established prior to dispensing cells into culture. For a standard titration of T_h cells the following procedure is adopted.

(i)   Add a constant aliquot of B cells to a series of sterile tubes.

(ii)   To this add a constant small volume of antigen (e.g. $0.01-0.1$ μg/ml TNP−KLH final concentration) and finally just prior to dispensing, a constant volume of T cells diluted to cover the expected dose range; that is a different T cell number per group in a constant volume. For this readout there will therefore be a different total number of lymphocytes in each treatment group: this does not affect derivation of single-hit curves. However, there are other circumstances where this would matter, and then addition of neutral 'filler' cells to make up the numbers is necessary. In our case they could be mitomycin-treated normal spleen cells, in other cases some other source of non-proliferating feeder cell.

(iii)   Dispense a volume of 15 μl to each of 60−120 wells per group in Terasaki type Falcon Microtest 3034 plates.

(iv)   To prevent dehydration, add about 4 ml of sterile water into the peripheral grooves of each plate, cover the plates and incubate in a humid sealed container at 37°C, in an atmosphere of 10% CO_2 in air or in 7% oxygen + 83% nitrogen.

(v)   Leave the cultures for 3 days.

(vi)   At this time flood the plates with 10 ml of fresh culture medium added from the edge so as not to disturb the cells.

(vii)   After gentle mixing of media, aspirate most of the excess medium leaving full wells and moist grooves. This procedure obviates the need for daily feeding and removes antibody produced over the early period from secreting cells transferred with the initial splenic inoculum. This is a further step to reduce background noise to help in the decision: positive or negative?

(viii)   Incubate these plates for a further 3−4 days.

(ix)   Aspirate the supernatants (10 μl) into 100−200 μl of assay diluent [1% bovine serum albumin (BSA), 5 mM EDTA, 0.1% sodium azide in PBS, pH 7.6] and store in a sealed box at 4°C until the assay is performed. Such samples can be stored for many months without loss of activity.

3.2.5 *Radioimmunoassay of culture supernatants*

A very convenient way to measure the response is by RIA of secreted antibody (11). ELISA assays would also be suitable.

(i)   Coat flexible polystyrene U-bottomed microtitre plates (Linbro-SMRC-96) with e.g. NIP_{15}−BSA or TNP_{13}−BSA.

(ii)   Leave 50 μl of conjugate in the wells overnight.

(iii)   Aspirate the unbound antigen for re-utilization in subsequent assays.

(iv)   Wash the plates well by flooding with PBS, and block with assay diluent (Section 3.2.4ix) for a further 2 h.

(v)   Wash the plates again and then add 20 μl of the dilute culture supernatants to the wells and incubate for 2 h.

(vi)   Wash the plates and then add radio-iodinated anti-mouse Ig antibody (IgG-specific) (20 μl/well, ~12 000 c.p.m.) and incubate for 3 h.

(vii)   Finally wash the plates six times with PBS, separate the wells with a hot wire and count in a gamma counter.

It is possible to perform 5−10 assays on the same sample by this method. *Figure 3* shows the reproducibility of duplicate assays performed months apart. In this particular experiment three groups of cultures were established; one had B cells but no T_h cells (*Figure 3a*); one had a high input of T_h (*Figure 3b*) and the last (*Figure 3c*) an intermediate input. This means that one can perform double sampling for responses

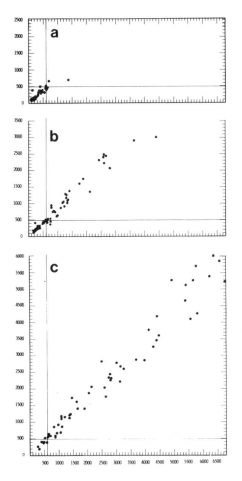

Figure 3. Radioimmunoassay. Reproducibility of the readout. Three groups of cultures were established. T cells were omitted from the control group (**a**), and added at 3×10^4/well (**b**), or 1×10^5/well (**c**). Supernatants were screened for anti-TNP antibody on two independent occasions weeks apart. The total c.p.m. were plotted and each point reflects the two independent readings. In the control group (**a**), lines were drawn to demonstrate the value below which 95% of the data points lay. This provides a satisfactory way of assigning cultures as positive or negative. At T cell inputs of 3 and 10×10^4 respectively an increasing number of wells scored positive with high reproducibility. This means that large experiments can be conducted with multiple sampling of supernatant antibody over prolonged periods of time.

to two different antigens with some degree of confidence (see Section 3.2.7). The advantages of using good anti-Ig antibodies cannot be understated. A convenient way to prepare anti-Ig antibodies with high specific activity is described in ref.11.

3.2.6 *Validity of the system*

If we are to apply LDA to T_h cells we need to be sure that the B cell inoculum has sufficient memory B cells in it so that every culture well will contain some. If that is the case we can be confident that a well scoring negative in a T_h titration contained no active T_h cells. To do this we perform T cell and B cell titrations in the same

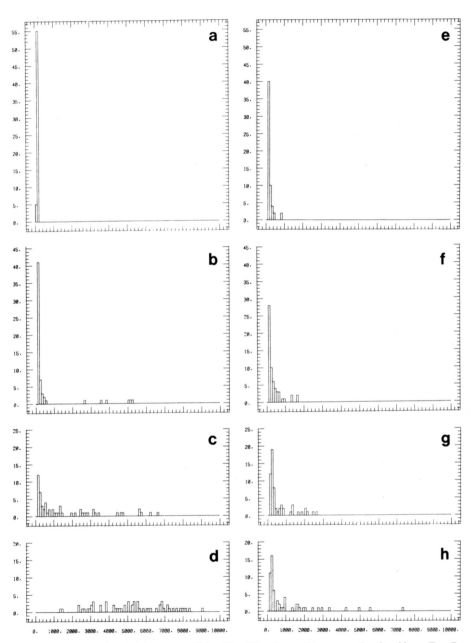

Figure 4. Demonstration that there are sufficient T and B cells to achieve saturation for either a T or B cell titration. In **a−d** are shown distribution histograms for the cultures with a constant 'excess' number of T cells (1×10^5) per well and increasing inputs of B cells. **a**: no B cells; **b**: 5×10^3/well **c**: 2×10^4/well and **d**: 1.5×10^5 B cells per well. Windows **e−h** show similar plots for titrations of T cells on constant 'excess' B cells. **e**: no T cells; **f**: 1.25×10^3; **g**: 2.5×10^5; and **h**: 5×10^5 T cells. Irradiated T cell-depleted spleen cells from unimmunized mice served as fillers for **a−d**; fillers were not necessary for **e−h**. The number of positives at low B and T cell inputs and the 100% positive wells at the highest cell input suggest that the system can be 'saturated' for either type of cell with the confidence that any negative is purely a reflection of segregation of the test cells, and not any of the accessory, filler or readout population.

171

experiment. Let us plot the raw data for this experiment (*Figure 4*). We start by group-ing counts in convenient blocks of $0-99$, $100-199$, $200-299$ and so on. Each of the 60 microculture wells is then accounted for within a particular block. We score on the ordinate the number of wells with counts in a particular block range (abscissa). If we start with *Figure 4a* we can see that the group with 1×10^5 T cells but no B cells contained no wells with counts above 200 c.p.m./well. As the B cell input increases we start seeing blocks appearing to the right, so that by 20 000 B cells/well only 18 wells out of the 60 fall into the blocks of less than 200 c.p.m. The addition of 1.5×10^5 B cells (*Figure 4d*) results in no wells having less than 1200 c.p.m. Clearly there must (from the Poisson formula) be more than five B-memory cells per well. *Figure 4e* shows the data for a high input of B cells (1.5×10^5) but no T cells. In this case there are eight wells with counts greater than 200 c.p.m. Here comes the first problem which is applicable to all limiting dilution systems: what do we score as positive? Is it any well over 900 c.p.m. (i.e. above the highest background block of two wells)? Should it be a value $2-3$ standard deviations (SD) above the mean? As the radioassay data of background do not show a normal distribution, the latter course does not seem suitable. We could analyse the data on the basis that 0, 1.7, 5 or 10% of the background cultures are 'positive'. For most purposes, given no outrageous outliers, these differ little. Therefore for convenience we often adopt a 5% cutoff to decide positive or negative. In other biological systems such as cell-mediated lympholysis (CML), $2-3 \times$ SD of background chromium release is widely used.

3.2.7 *Application of LDA to determine the life style of a single T cell: the monogamous T cell revisited*

With our ability to demonstrate single-hit curves and calculate frequencies we can ask questions of T_h statistically isolated by limiting dilution. One simple question was: how many B cells can a single T-helper cooperate with? Is it many, is it few, or is it even one? We actually found the number to be just one. For reasons that are hard to under-stand the finding $(6,12-15)$ made little impact on views about cooperation. The fact that cooperation was reckoned to occur by diffusible antigen-specific factors (now ob-solete!) probably led people to consider the finding artefactual or too contrived. In fact the likeliest conclusion, that monogamy implied a need for cell contact in cooperation was not really taken up; and it is only now some years later that the same conclusion has been reached by many other protocols. Most probably LDA attracted little interest at that time, and data derived using it were somehow not taken seriously.

Using the above system we established cultures containing two sets of B cells, some from TNP-OVA and some from NIP-OVA primed mice. We wished to determine how many culture wells scored positive for both anti-NIP and anti-TNP antibody when T_h cells were limiting. This meant performing T_h titrations, scoring wells for both TNP and NIP antibody, and assessing how these responses assorted. Obviously this sort of analysis depends upon a clear distinction between positive and negative wells. So that we did not select any arbitrary value as our cutoff, analyses were carried out assuming 0, 1.7, 5 or 10% of background values as positive. In the semilog plot shown in *Figure 5* it can be seen that the use of these different exclusion values made little difference to the frequency estimates of T_h cells. In *Figure 6(a−f)* are displayed the

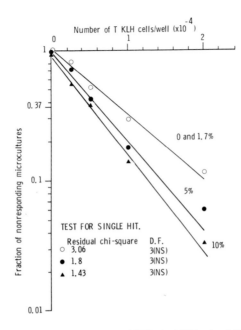

Figure 5. Semilog plot of T_h cells in the response of TNP- and NIP-primed B cells to NIP−KLH and TNP−KLH. A series of plots were constructed assuming that the highest 0, 1.7%, 5% and 10% of the values in the background (B cells alone) group were positive (from ref. 14). Significance tests for goodness of fit to single hit were performed and, on the basis of this, entry of data into double sampling analysis was undertaken (see *Table 1*).

results of those RIAs on supernatants derived from wells of all the groups, each well characterized by a value reflecting the anti-TNP (abscissa) and anti-NIP (ordinate) antibodies. The graphs show data from cultures with high T cell input (*Figure 6a*) down to those with no added T cells (*Figure 6f*). At high T cell input virtually all wells score positive for both anti-NIP and anti-TNP antibodies. At low T cell inputs most positive wells were positive for antibodies to one or the other, but not both, haptens.

Assuming that the number of T_h cells per well follows a Poisson distribution, and that there is a constant probability P_t that each opportunity for help is taken up by a TNP-specific B cell, and a complementary probability that $1-P_t$ that it is taken by a NIP-specific B cell, it is possible to derive expressions for 'expected' values for TNP^-NIP^-, TNP^+NIP^-, TNP^-NIP^+ and TNP^+NIP^+ frequencies in models where one T_h helps one B cell, or two B cells or . . . etc. One can test the goodness of fit of these models with the observed data by use of the G-test [a log-likelihood ratio test (16)]. The results of these analyses have been published (14,15) but to exemplify the process we present a matrix from a group containing 1×10^4 T cells/well using a 5% exclusion value (*Table 1*). It can be seen that in this extract from the experiment there was no significant difference between observed frequencies and those expected in a 1T:1B model, but a significant departure from what was expected on a 1T:2B model. *A fortiori* models with more B cells per T cell are not tenable.

This particular experiment has been performed often with the same result. It was discussed here in some detail because it is a useful example of the double (multiple)

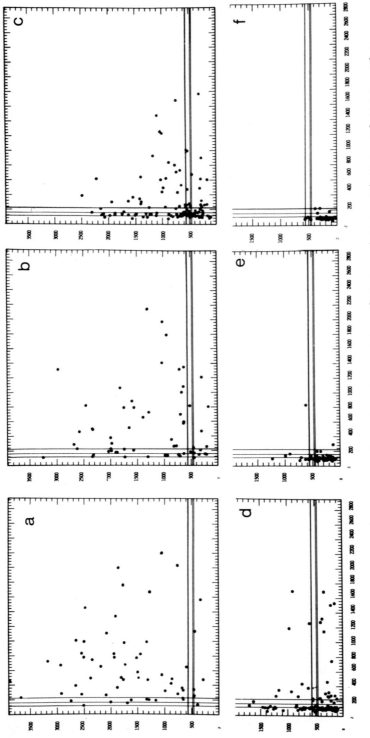

Figure 6. Distribution of NIP- and TNP-responsive wells with different T cell inputs. (**a**) 1×10^5, (**b**) 2×10^4, (**c**) 1×10^4, (**d**) 5×10^3, (**e**) 2.5×10^3, (**f**) zero T cells/well. Lines representing the 0, 1.7%, 5% and 10% exclusion limits are given. For anti-TNP responses these pass through 180, 159, 123 and 114 counts per 200 sec respectively. For anti-NIP these pass through 564, 559, 477, 453. Abscissa = anti-TNP (counts per 200 sec); ordinate = anti-NIP (counts per 200 sec). Readouts for the TNP and NIP were measured on different days. See sample analysis for various models of cooperation in *Table 1*.

Table 1. Observed and expected frequencies of anti-NIP and anti-TNP-producing wells.

		Observed			Expected (1T:1B)			Expected (1T:2B)	
		TNP			TNP			TNP	
	−	+	Total	−	+	Total	−	+	Total
NIP +	38	43	81	+ 40.5	40.5	81	+ 24.2	57.8	82
NIP −	22	17	39	− 19.5	19.5	39	− 32.5	5.6	38.1
Total	60	60	120	60	60	120	56.7	63.4	120.1

Residual chi-squared 0.95 df 1   Residual chi-squared 29.8 df 1

Each matrix represents the results from 120 wells of a group containing 1×10^4 T_h cells using a 5% exclusion value. Comparable matrices were constructed for all other groups. Goodness of fit was determined by G-tests except in some groups in the 1T:1B model when expected responses were small, in which case the G-test was supplemented by Fisher's exact test for 2×2 contingency tables (taken from refs. 14,15) (See *Figure 6*).

sampling strategy which is perhaps one of the major applications of LDA other than for measurement of frequencies. It provides a way to document the functions or specificities of single T cells or clones.

3.3 Overview of systems for application of LDA to other lymphocyte functions

It is not possible in a chapter this size to provide methodology for LDA of all other lymphocyte functions. Therefore we will simply list examples in the published literature and direct the reader to obtain methodological details from those selected references.

3.3.1 *Clonal aspects of B cell development*

The first major application of LDA in cellular immunology started with the paper of Lefkovits in 1972 (17). Since then a large number of papers concerned with B cell growth and development have accumulated, and these are quite fully reviewed elsewhere (1, 18,19). The application of a range of polyclonal activators that can trigger B cells at many different stages of development made it possible to evaluate the pre-committed frequency of B cells with any particular antigen specificity. Given that one can measure the precursor frequencies of B cells to many antigens quite easily, it has been possible to follow changes in frequency following exposure to tolerogens (20,21), antigens, and a range of growth and differentiation factors (1,22). It has also been possible to apply partition analysis to define interactions between B cells and other accessory cells (23).

3.3.2 *T-helper cells*

In the very first application of LDA to T_h cell function, attention was directed to so-called non-cognate help (24,25). Subsequent studies suggested that T_h cells of the non-cognate type could segregate independently from T_h cells capable of cognate or classical linked-recognition help (26−28). The demonstration that non-cognate help could be mediated by mitogen-triggered T cells (Sjoberg, unpublished; 22) made it possible to perform LDA of Con A-activated T cells with multiple sampling of culture supernatants for readout on many samples of B cells (29). These studies first suggested that there was a great deal of heterogeneity of T cell-derived factors and B cells responsive to them; findings quite predictive of the present situation.

A particularly elegant application of LDA has been its use in multiple sampling of T_h (cognate) for demonstration of T_h cells with distinct requirements for recognition of antigen with different major histocompatibility complex (MHC) products (30). Unlike the studies described in Section 3.2, the intention here was to allow the T_h memory cell to expand and produce a clone before multiple sampling of the progeny onto B cell readouts. Surprisingly no one has exploited this methodology to determine if helper cells can proliferate after they have donated help to a B cell.

3.3.3 *Suppressor cells*

Given the enormous literature on suppressor cells it is surprising that there is no documented LDA for them. If and when a suitable suppressor model puts itself to the test the theoretical frameworks have already been outlined in part. Experimental systems looking at negative allogeneic effects have provided model systems. It should be noted that in such studies it is worthwhile using semilog plots with the ordinate representing F_+, or the fraction of positive wells (1,7,31).

3.3.4 *Cytotoxic T cells and their precursors*

LDA of cytotoxic T cells is probably the most widely used of the applications of LDA in immunology. The major applications have been to determine frequencies of cells reactive to defined histocompatibility and conventional antigens as a way to study the immunological repertoire, its ontogeny and cellular basis, as well as a way to demonstrate clonal deletion in tolerance (21). The methodologies are well described for both mouse and man, and suitable references are: mouse, 2,21,32−37; man, 38−41.

3.3.5 *Monitoring T cells in therapy*

There are now an increasing number of therapeutic interventions involving T cell eradication that require one to be able to monitor depletion in a sensitive way. This is particularly the case in bone marrow transplantation where it is crucial to monitor depletion and to correlate residual T cells with subsequent clinical events such as graft-versus-host disease, graft failure and leukaemic relapse. LDA, combined with mitogens to generate observable growth of marrow T cells, has proven a sensitive and reliable indicator (42−44).

4. STATISTICAL METHODS

In analysing LDA data to calculate frequencies it is necessary to validate the curve as single hit as the first stage prior to an estimation of frequency. Validity testing to detect deviations from single hit has been well discussed by Taswell (5,45). These two articles are the best statistical treatments currently available on this subject. A number of computer programs based on Taswell formulae (2) are widely in use. We have appended a user-friendly program that adopts some of these principles (Appendix 1), which is a hybrid of an original written and kindly provided by Dr Klaus Heeg (Munich) with modifications by Dr B.Loveland and by us. We hope it will be useful for those who have access to BBC microcomputers (Acorn Computers, Cambridge, UK).

5. REFERENCES

1. Lefkovits,I. and Waldmann,H. (1979) *Limiting Dilution Analysis of the Immune System.* Cambridge University Press.
2. Taswell,C. (1981) *J. Immunol.,* **126**, 1614.
3. Lefkovits,I. and Waldmann,H. (1984) *Immunol. Today,* **5**, 265.
4. Waldmann,H. and Lefkovits,I. (1984) *Immunol. Today,* **5**, 295.
5. Taswell,C. (1987) *Cell Separation: Methods and Selected Applications.* Vol. 4, Academic Press, New York.
6. Waldmann,H. (1977) *Immunol. Rev.,* **35**, 121.
7. Corley,R.B., Kindred,B. and Lefkovits,I. (1978) *J. Immunol.,* **121**, 1082.
8. Eichmann,K. (1981) *J. Exp. Med.,* **152**, 477.
9. Julius,M., Simpson,E. and Herzenberg,L.A. (1973) *Eur. J. Immunol.,* **3**, 645.
10. Mishell,R.J. and Dutton,R.W. (1967) *J. Exp. Med.,* **126**, 432.
11. Newby,C.J., Hayakawa,K. and Herzenberg,L.A. (1986) In *Handbook of Experimental Immunology.* Weir,D. (ed.), Blackwells, Oxford, p.34.1.
12. Waldmann,H., Lefkovits,I. and Feinstein,A. (1976) *Immunology,* **31**, 353.
13. Phillips,J. and Waldmann,H. (1977) *Nature,* **268**, 641.
14. Waldmann,H., Kenny,G., Feinstein,A. and Brown,D. (1978) In *Cell Biology and Immunology of Leukocyte Function.* Quastel,M. (ed.), Academic Press, New York, p. 403.
15. Waldmann,H. and Phillips,J. (1980) *Springer Seminars Immunopathol.,* **3**, 129.
16. Sokal,R.R. and Rohlf,F.J. (1969) *Biometry: Principles and Practice of Statistics in Biological Research, 599.* Freeman, San Francisco.
17. Lefkovits,I. (1972) *Eur. J. Immunol.,* **2**, 360.
18. Quintans,J. and Lefkovits,I. (1974) *Eur. J. Immunol.,* **4**, 617.
19. Quintans,J. and Lefkovits,I. (1974) *J. Immunol.,* **113**, 1373.
20. Desaymard,C. and Waldmann,H. (1976) *Nature,* **264**, 780.
21. Good,M.F. and Nossal,G.J.V. (1983) *J. Immunol.,* **130**, 78.
22. Waldmann,H., Poulton,P. and Desaymard,C. (1976) *Immunology,* **30**, 723.
23. Kettman,J.R., Soederberg,A. and Lefkovits,I. (1986) *J. Immunol.,* **137**, 114.
24. Waldmann,H., Lefkovits,I. and Quintans,J. (1975) *Immunology,* **28**, 1135.
25. Lefkovits,I., Quintans,J., Munro,A. and Waldmann,H. (1975) *Immunology,* **28**, 1149.
26. Marrack,P. and Kappler,J.W. (1975) *J. Immunol.,* **114**, 1116.
27. Waldmann,H., Pope,H. and Lefkovits,I. (1976) *Immunology,* **31**, 343.
28. Waldmann,H. and Pope,H. (1977) *Immunology,* **33**, 721.
29. Lefkovits,I. and Waldmann,H. (1977) *Immunology,* **32**, 915.
30. Spoviero,J.F., Imperiale,M.J. and Zauderer,M. (1981) *J. Exp. Med.,* **152**, 920.
31. Waldmann,H., Pope,H. and Kenny,G. (1977) *Immunology,* **33**, 129.
32. Teh,H.-S., Phillips,R.A. and Miller,R.G. (1977) *J. Exp. Med.,* **146**, 1280.
33. Ryser,J.E. and MacDonald,H.R. (1979) *J. Immunol.,* **122**, 1691.
34. Langhorne,J. and Fischer Lindahl,K. (1979) In *Immunological Methods.* Lefkovits,I. and Pernis,B. (eds), Academic Press, New York, Vol. II, p. 221.
35. Stockinger,H., Bartlett,R., Pfizenmaier,K., Rollinghoff,M. and Wagner,H. (1981) *J. Exp. Med.,* **153**, 1629.
36. Reimann,J., Kabelitz,D., Heeg,K. and Wagner,H. (1985) *J. Exp. Med.,* **162**, 592.
37. Mizuochi,T., Munitz,T.I., McCarthy,S.A., Andrysiak,P.M., Kung,J., Gress,R.E. and Singer,A. (1986) *J. Immunol.,* **137**, 2740.
38. Moretta,A., Pantaleo,G., Moretta,L., Mingari,M.C. and Cerrottini,C. (1983) *J. Exp. Med.,* **158**, 571.
39. Moretta,A., Pantaleo,G., Moretta,L., Cerottini,J.C. and Mingair,M.C. (1983) *J. Exp. Med.,* **157**, 743.
40. Kabelitz,D., Herzog,W.R., Zanker,B. and Wagner,H. (1985) *Scand. J. Immunol.,* **22**, 329.
41. Sharrock,C.E., Man,S., Wanachiwanawin,W. and Batchelor,J.R. (1987) *Transplantation,* in press.
42. Martin,P.J. and Hansen,J.A. (1985) *Blood,* **65**, 1134.
43. Kernan,N.A., Collins,N.H., Juliano,L., Cartagina,T., DuPont,B. and O'Reilly,R.J. (1986) *Blood,* **68**, 770.
44. Rozans,M.K., Smith,B.R., Emerson,S., Crimmins,M., Laurent,G., Reichert,T., Burakoff,S.J. and Miller,R.A. (1986) *Transplantation,* **42**, 380.
45. Taswell,C. (1984) *J. Immunol. Methods,* **72**, 29.

6. APPENDIX 1

6.1 **Complete listing of BBC micro limiting dilution analysis programs**

Executable FILE !BOOT (allows program to start from Shift-BREAK):
Type in as follows:

```
*BUILD !BOOT
MODE7
CHAIN"$.MENU"
Escape
*OPT 4,3
```

The following are programs written in BBC BASIC and should be saved on
disk and then protected using *ACCESS filename L.

```
 10 REM PROGRAM $.MENU
 20 MODE7
 30*DIR D
 40*FX15,1
 50 I$=INKEY$(20):IF I$<>"" THEN GOTO 50
 60 PRINT'''" <LIMITING DILUTION ANALYSIS>"
 70 PRINT'"    STEVE COBBOLD APRIL 1986"
 80 PRINT'''" ENTER/ANALYSE DATA -PRESS 'D'"
 90 PRINT'" PLOT DATA FROM DISC-PRESS 'P'"
100 PRINT'" CHECK DATA ON DISC -PRESS 'C'";
110 I$=GET$
120 IF I$="P" THEN CHAIN"$.PLOT"
130 IF I$="D" THEN CHAIN"$.LIMIT"
140 IF I$="C" THEN CHAIN"$.CHECK"
150 GOTO 20
```

```
 10 REM PROGRAM $.LIMIT
 20 REM REQUIRES BBC MODEL>=B WITH FLOPPY DISK AND DFS
 30 REM CONFIGURED FOR EPSON COMPATIBLE PRINTERS
 40*FX5,1
 50*FX6,0
 60 VDU3
 70*DIR D
 80 ON ERROR GOTO 1840
 90*FX15,1
100 I$=INKEY$(20):IF I$<>"" GOTO 100
110 REM LIMITING DILUTION ANALYSIS
120 REM ORIGINATED FROM WAGNERS GROUP MAINZ, FRG
130 REM REWRITTEN TO BBC BASIC MARCH 1986 BY STEVE COBBOLD
140 MODE7
150 PRINT'"LIMITING DILUTION ANALYSIS"
160 PRINT'"DO YOU WANT A PRINTOUT (Y/N)":X$=GET$:P1S=0:IF X$="Y" OR X$="y"
THEN P1S=1:VDU2
170 REM INPUT DATA/OPEN FILES
180 PRINT'"LIMITING DILUTION ANALYSIS"
190 INPUT'"FILE NAME TO STORE DATA",NF$
200 IF LEN(NF$)>7 THEN PRINT"MAX SEVEN LETTERS":GOTO 190
210 NF=OPENOUT(NF$)
220 INPUT'"HOW MANY REPLICATES (NO OF WELLS)"'"PER DILUTION ";N
230 PRINT'"ARE THERE SERIAL (2-FOLD)"'"DILUTION STEPS (Y/N) ";:X$=GET$
240 IF X$="Y" OR X$="y" THEN GOTO 310
```

```
250 INPUT'"HOW MANY DILUTIONS ";P:IF P<3 THEN GOTO 250
260 X1$="HOW MANY RESPONDER CELLS (ABSOLUTE)"+CHR$(10)+CHR$(13)+"PER WELL
IN DILUTION "
270 Y1$="HOW MANY NEGATIVE WELLS    "
280 DIM RE(P):DIM NE(P):FOR I%=1 TO P
290 PRINT'X1$;I%;:INPUT RE(I%)
300 PRINT'Y1$;:INPUT NE(I%):NEXT:GOTO 370
310 INPUT'"HOW MANY DILUTION STEPS";P:IF P<3 THEN GOTO 310
320 INPUT'"HOW MANY RESPONDER CELLS (ABSOLUTE)"'"PER WELL IN FIRST
DILUTION";RE
330 X1$="HOW MANY NEGATIVE WELLS IN DILUTION "
340 RE=2*RE:DIM RE(P):DIM NE(P):FOR I%=1 TO P
350 PRINT X1$;I%;:INPUT NE(I%)
360 RE(I%)=RE/2:RE=RE(I%):NEXT:GOTO 370
370 PRINT'"DATA CHECK"'';N;"-FOLD DETERMINATION WITH"';P;" DILUTION
STEPS"
380 PRINT'"RESPONDERS";TAB(15);"NEG. WELLS"
390 FOR I%=1 TO P
400 PRINT;TAB(3);RE(I%);TAB(18);NE(I%):IF NE(I%)<1 THEN NE(I%)=1
410 NEXT
420 PRINT"INPUT CORRECT (Y/N) ?":X$=GET$
430 IF X$="N" OR X$="n" THEN GOTO 220
440 PRINT'"EVALUATION OF INDIVIDUAL POINTS"
450 DIM WN(P),CLI(P),F(P),NP(P),S(P):FOR I%=1 TO P
460 WN(I%)=NE(I%)/N:NP(I%)=WN(I%)*100
470 W=WN(I%):W=W*(1-W):S(I%)=SQR(W*N)
480 CLI(I%)=1.96*S(I%):CLI(I%)=1+INT(CLI(I%))
490 F(I%)=-LN(WN(I%)):F(I%)=F(I%)/RE(I%):NEXT
500 PRINT'"RESPONDERS";TAB(12);"NEGS 95%CL";TAB(30);"FREQ"
510 PRINT#NF,P,N
520 DIM E1(P),E2(P):FOR I%=1 TO P:E1(I%)=NE(I%)-CLI(I%)
530 IF E1(I%)<0 THEN E1(I%)=0
540 E2(I%)=NE(I%)+CLI(I%):IF E2(I%)>N THEN E2(I%)=N
550 PRINT RE(I%);TAB(12);E1(I%);" TO ";E2(I%);TAB(26);F(I%)
560 PRINT#NF,RE(I%),NE(I%)
570 NEXT
580 F=0:FOR I%=1 TO P:F=F+F(I%):NEXT
590 PRINT"AVERAGE FREQUENCY F=";F/P
600 PRINT"            OR F= 1/";P/F
610 Q1=10:DD=0.5:F1=F/P:PRINT'"PRESS ANY KEY":X$=GET$:VDU3
620 PRINT"EVALUATION BY CHI-SQUARE"
630 F=F1:Q=Q1
640 GOSUB 770
650 FR=F:CI=CH
660 GOSUB 820
670 IF CG>CI AND CK>CI THEN VDU3:PRINT"ITERATION RUNNING":GOTO 690
680 GOTO 1050
690 QA=Q:Q=Q-DD:C9=CG:C1=CK:F4=FK:F5=FG
700 GOSUB 820
710 PRINT "CHI(1)=";CK
720 PRINT "CHI(F)=";CI
730 PRINT "CHI(2)=";CG
740 IF CG<C9 AND CK<C1 THEN GOTO 690
750 IF CG>C9 THEN F2=F5 ELSE F2=F4
760 GOTO 890
770 CH=0
780 FOR K%=1 TO P
790 MM=F*RE(K%):A1=EXP(-MM)
800 A3=N*A1:A2=(NE(K%)-A3)^2:A4=1-A1:A5=A3*A4
810 A=A2/A5:CH=CH+A:NEXT:RETURN
820 F=FR*Q:FG=F
```

```
 830 GOSUB 770
 840 CG=CH
 850 F=FR/Q:FK=F
 860 GOSUB 770
 870 CK=CH
 880 RETURN
 890 PRINT'"READY":IF P1S=1 THEN VDU2
 900 PRINT'"CORRECTION FACTOR Q=";QA
 910 IF C9=CI AND C1=CI THEN 930
 920 GOTO 990
 930 D1=DD*100
 940 PRINT'"FREQUENCY ERROR IS SMALLER THAN";D1;"%"
 950 Q=1+1.2*DD
 960 PRINT'"ITERATION HAS TO RUN AGAIN":VDU3
 970 DD=DD/5:F=F2:GOTO 640
 980 F2=FR*Q
 990 PRINT"FREQUENCY F=";F2
1000 MM=INT(1/F2)
1010 PRINT"F=1/";MM;"+/-";DD*MM;"(ITERATION ERROR!)"
1020 PRINT'"DO YOU WANT THE FACTOR CALCULATED"'"5 TIMES MORE ACCURATELY
(Y/N)?":X$=GET$
1030 IF X$<>"Y" AND X$<>"y" THEN GOTO 1100
1040 Q=1+DD*5:F=F2:DD=DD/5:GOTO 640
1050 PRINT"INPUT FREQUENCY IS >= FACTOR 10 TIMES"
1060 PRINT"DIFFERENT FROM THE REAL VALUE;"
1070 PRINT"- FURTHER ITERATION NOT POSSIBLE"
1080 PRINT"FURTHER ITERATION FROM THIS DATA"'"NOT POSSIBLE"
1090 PRINT"PRESS ANY KEY TO ANALYSE MORE DATA":X$=GET$:CLEAR:GOTO 140
1100 VDU3:CLS:IF P1S=1 THEN VDU2
1110 PRINT"EVALUATION ACCORDING TO CHI-SQUARE"
1120 PRINT'"CALCULATED FREQUENCY: F=";F2;''" OR 1/";MM;"+/-";DD*MM;
"(ITERATION ERROR)"
1130 PRINT'"THE CHI-SQUARE VALUE IS ";CI
1140 DIM H(10):H(3)=3.8:H(4)=6:H(5)=7.8:H(6)=9.5:H(7)=11.1:H(8)=12.6:
H(9)=14.1:H(10)=15.5
1150 PRINT'"FOR ";P;" DILUTIONS & ";P-2;" DEGREES OF FREEDOM"
'"WITH P>0.05, CHI-SQUARE MUST BE <";H(P)
1160 DF=P-2:GOSUB 1690
1170 PRINT'"PROBABILITY ESTIMATION (n-2): P= ";PV
1180 H(2)=3.8:H(3)=6:H(4)=7.8:H(5)=9.5:H(6)=11.1:H(7)=12.6:H(8)=14.1:
H(9)=15.5
1190 PRINT'"FOR ";P;" DILUTIONS & ";P-1;" DEGREES OF FREEDOM"
'"WITH P>0.05, CHI-SQUARE MUST BE <";H(P)
1200 DF=P-1:GOSUB 1690
1210 PRINT'"PROBABILITY ESTIMATION (n-1): P=";PV
1220 IF CI<H(P) THEN GOTO 1250
1230 PRINT''"THE EXPERIMENT IS REJECTED!!!"
1240 GOTO 1270
1250 PRINT''"THE EXPERIMENT IS ACCEPTED***"
1260 GOTO 1270
1270 PRINT'"PRESS ANY KEY":X$=GET$:PRINT''"EVALUATION BY MAXIMUM
LIKELIHOOD":VDU3
1280 F=F2:Q1=2:Q=Q1:DD=.05:F1=F:GOSUB 1370
1290 GOSUB 1450:LL=L
1300 F1=F*Q:GOSUB 1450
1310 LG=L:IF LG<LL THEN VDU3:PRINT"ITERATION RUNNING":GOTO 1330
1320 Q=Q*2:GOTO 1300
1330 L2=LG:Q=Q-DD:F1=F*Q:GOSUB 1450
1340 LG=L:PRINT"L=";LL, "LG=";LG
1350 IF LG>L2 THEN GOTO 1330
1360 GOTO 1510
```

```
1370 DIM A5(P),A6(P),A7(P),A8(P):FOR I%=1 TO P
1380 A5(I%)=0:FOR J%=1 TO N
1390 A5(I%)=A5(I%)+LN(N):NEXT
1400 A6(I%)=0:FOR J%=1 TO NE(I%)
1410 A6(I%)=A6(I%)+LN(J%):NEXT
1420 A7(I%)=0:FOR J%=1 TO N-NE(I%)
1430 A7(I%)=A7(I%)+LN(J%):NEXT
1440 A8(I%)=A5(I%)-A6(I%)-A7(I%):NEXT:RETURN
1450 L=0:FOR I%=1 TO P
1460 A1=EXP(-F1*RE(I%)):A1=1-A1
1470 A2=N-NE(I%):A3=A2*LN(A1)
1480 A4=NE(I%)*F1*RE(I%)
1490 A9=A8(I%)-A4+A3:L=L+A9
1500 NEXT:RETURN
1510 F2=F1:IF P1S=1 THEN VDU2
1520 PRINT'"CALCULATED FREQUENCY F=";F2;'"          OR F=1/";1/F2
1530 PRINT'"ITERATION ERROR +/-";2*DD/F2
1540 PRINT'"DO YOU WANT THE FACTOR 5 TIMES MORE ACCURATELY (Y/N)?":X$=GET$
1550 IF X$="Y" OR X$="y" THEN F=F2:Q=1+4*DD:DD=DD/5:GOTO 1290
1560 VDU3:CLS:IF P1S=1 THEN VDU2
1570 PRINT'"EVALUATION BY MAXIMUM LIKELIHOOD"
1580 PRINT'"CALCULATED FREQUENCY: F=";F2;'" OR 1/";1/F2;" +/- 1/";
2*DD/F2;'"(ITERATION ERROR)"
1590 F=F2:L=0:FOR I%=1 TO P
1600 A1=EXP(-F*RE(I%)):A2=N-NE(I%)
1610 A3=A2*RE(I%)^2:A4=-A1*A3
1620 A5=(-1-A1)^2:A6=A4/A5:L=L+A6:NEXT
1630 V=-1/L:CL=SQR(V):CL=1.96*CL
1640 PRINT'"FREQUENCY F=";F;" +/-"';CL;" (95% CONFIDENCE LIMIT)"
1650 F1=F-CL:F2=F+CL
1660 PRINT''"OR FREQUENCY F=1/";INT(1/F);'"WITH 95% CL FROM 1/";INT(1/F1);
;" TO 1/";INT(1/F2)
1670 PRINT#NF,F,F1,F2:CLOSE#NF
1680 PRINT'"DO YOU WANT TO PLOT THE DATA (Y/N)?":X$=GET$:IF X$="Y" OR X$="y"
THEN CHAIN"$.PLOT":ELSE CLEAR:GOTO 140
1690 REM ALGORITHM FOR P VALUE FOR CHI SQUARE USING HAWKES NORMAL TAIL APPROX
1700 DEF FNPZG(X):IF X>1 THEN=EE ELSE=(1-X*(X-LN(EE+X)))/((1-X)^2)
1710 EE=10^-21
1720 IF DF=2 THEN PV=EXP(-0.5*CI):RETURN
1730 IF DF=1 THEN PZZ2=SQR(CI):GOSUB 1750:PV=P2TAIL:ELSE
PZZ2=(CI-DF+2/3-.08/DF)*SQR((1+FNPZG((DF-1)/CI))/(2*CI)):GOSUB 1750:PV=P1T
AIL
1740 RETURN
1750 PZZ=ABS(PZZ2)
1760 PZZ22=PZZ2^2
1770 IF PZZ>=2.2 THEN P2TAIL=.7978846*(1.184+PZZ)*EXP(-.5*PZZ22)/
(1.209+1.176*PZZ+PZZ22):GOTO 1800
1780 PZHT=PZZ*(1+PZZ22*(-.0075166+PZZ22*(3.1737E-4-PZZ22*2.9657E-6)))
1790 P2TAIL=(1-SQR(1-EXP(-.6366198*PZHT*PZHT)))
1800 P1TAIL=.5*P2TAIL
1810 IF PZZ2<0 THEN P1TAIL=1-P1TAIL
1820 RETURN
1830 END
1840 CLOSE#0:PRINT'"ERROR AT ";ERL:REPORT:PRINT'"PRESS ANY KEY TO RESTART":
X$=GET$:RUN

------------------------------------------------------------------------
10 REM PROGRAM $.CHECK
20 REM PRINTS DATA STORED IN A LIMITING DILUTION DATA FILE
30 REM ALL DATA FILES STORED IN DIRECTORY D
40 REM FREQUENCY RESULTS ARE THOSE OBTAINED BY MAXIMUM LIKELIHOOD
```

```
 50 ON ERROR GOTO 250
 60*DIR D
 70*FX5,1
 80*FX6,0
 90 CLS:PRINT'"    <PRINT LIMITING DILUTION FILE>"
100 PRINT''"DO YOU WANT A CATALOGUE (Y/N)?":I$=GET$:IF I$="Y" THEN *CAT
110 INPUT'"CHECK WHICH FILE",N$
120 NF=OPENIN(N$)
130 INPUT#NF,P,N
140 PRINT'"DO YOU WANT A PRINTOUT (Y/N)?":I$=GET$:CLS:IF I$="Y" OR I$="y"
THEN VDU2
150 PRINT''"FILE    : ";N$
160 PRINT';P;" DILUTIONS OF ";N;" WELLS"
170 PRINT'"RESPONDERS";TAB(12);"NO. NEG WELLS";TAB(28);"PROP NEGS"'
180 FOR M=1 TO P
190 INPUT#NF,RE,NE:PRINT;TAB(1);RE;TAB(15);NE;TAB(26);NE/N
200 NEXT
210 INPUT#NF,F,F1,F2
220 PRINT''"CALCULATED FREQUENCY BY"'"MAXIMUM LIKELIHOOD = 1/";INT(1/F);
'''"WITH 95% CONFIDENCE LIMITS"'"FROM 1/";INT(1/F2);" TO 1/
";INT(1/F1)
230 CLOSE#NF
240 VDU3:PRINT''"PRESS ANY KEY FOR MENU":I$=GET$:CHAIN"$.MENU"
250 IF ERR=222 THEN PRINT'"FILE NOT FOUND"
260 GOTO 230
```

```
 10 REM PROGRAM $.PLOT
 20 REM PLOTS LIMITING DILUTION DATA FROM FILES STORED ON DISK
 30 REM COMPATIBLE WITH LINEAR GRAPHICS PLOTMATE (PARALLEL INTERFACE) AND
 40 REM SCREENDUMP TO EPSON COMPATIBLE PRINTERS (EG FX-80/RX-80)
 50 MODE4
 60*DIR D
 70 ON ERROR GOTO 510
 80 MF=0
 90 VDU 28,0,1,39,0
100 PRINT"PLOT TO SCREEN OR PLOTMATE"'"PRESS 'P' OR 'S'";:I$=GET$:PRINT I$:
IF I$="P" OR I$="p" THEN POUT=1 ELSE POUT=0
110 INPUT'"MAX. NUMBER OF CELLS PER WELL",MC
120 MC1=MC:N=0:REPEAT N=N+1:MC1=MC1/10:UNTIL MC1<=10
130 MC=-((MC1<=2)*2+(MC1>2 AND MC1<=5)*5+(MC1>5 AND MC1<=10)*10)*10^N
140 VDU5
150 IF POUT=1 THEN *RUN"$.PLOTON":REM FILE $.PLOTON MUST CONTAIN PROGRAM
FOR ACTIVATING THE PLOTMATE INTERFACE (IF REQUIRED)
160 X=200:Y=700:IF POUT=1 THEN X=300
170 PLOT 4,X,Y:VDU5
180 FOR M=0 TO 1000 STEP 200
190 PLOT 5,X+M,Y:PLOT 5,X+M,Y+20:PLOT 5,X+M,Y
200 PLOT 4,X+M-12,Y+60:PRINT;MC*M/((10^N)*1000):PLOT 4,X+M,Y
210 NEXT M:PLOT 5,X,Y:PLOT 5,X-20,Y:PLOT 5,X,Y
220 FOR M=10 TO 1 STEP -1:M1=(1-LOG(M))*600
230 PLOT 5,X,Y-M1:PLOT 5,X-20,Y-M1:PLOT 5,X,Y-M1
240 PLOT 4,X-125,Y-M1+12:PRINT;M/10:PLOT 4,X,Y-M1
250 NEXT M
260 PLOT 4,X+80,Y+100:PRINT;"No. cells per well x 10";:PLOT 4,X+840,Y+110:
PRINT;"-";N
270 VDU 23,255,0,0,0,2,0,0,0,0
280 IF POUT=1 THEN PLOT 4,100,85:PRINT;"Freq of negative wells"
290 VDU 23,255,0,0,0,1,0,0,0,0
300 VDU4:INPUT"NAME OF FILE TO PLOT",N$
310 DATA "O","X","+","O","#"
```

```
 320 NF=OPENIN(N$):INPUT#NF,P,N
 330 READ XN$:VDU5:FOR M=1 TO P:INPUT#NF,RE,NE
 340 PLOT 4,X+(1000*RE/MC)-3,Y-(1-LOG(10*NE/N))*600+6:PRINT;XN$
 350 NEXT M
 360 INPUT#NF,F,F1,F2
 370 PLOT 4,X,Y
 380 PROCplot(F,0)
 390 VDU 23,255,0,0,0,0,0,0,MF*16,0
 400 PROCplot(F1,16):PROCplot(F2,16):CLOSE#NF
 410 PLOT 4,0,Y+250-MF*40:PRINT;"    FILE:      ";N$;"  ( ";XN$;" )"
 420 VDU4:IF MF<2:PRINT"PLOT ANOTHER FILE (Y/N)?";:I$=GET$:PRINT I$:
IF I$="Y" OR I$="y" THEN MF=MF+1:GOTO 300
 430 VDU5:IF MF=0 THEN PRINT"   FREQUENCY= 1/";INT(1/F);'"   WITH 95% CL
 FROM 1/";INT(1/F2);" TO 1/";INT(1/F1)
 440 VDU4:IF POUT=0 THEN PRINT"DO YOU WANT A SCREEN-DUMP?":I$=GET$:
IF I$="Y" OR I$="y" THEN *RUN M.SDUMP:REM FILE M.SDUMP MUST CONT
AIN MACHINE CODE FOR SCREEN DUMP TO PRINTER
 450 IF POUT=1 THEN CALL &C03
 460 CHAIN"$.MENU"
 470 END
 480 DEF PROCplot(FF,SO)
 490 PLOT 4,X,Y:M=0:REPEAT M=M+50:M1=Y-(1-LOG(3.7))*MC*FF*0.6*M:
PLOT 5+SO,X+M,M1
 500 UNTIL M>=1000 OR M1<=100:ENDPROC
 510 PRINT"ERROR AT ";ERL;" ";:REPORT
 520 IF ERR=222 THEN PRINT"FILE NOT FOUND"
 530 PRINT"PRESS ANY KEY";:I$=GET$:RUN
```

The following is a machine code dump in HEX suitable for generating a
screen-dump to EPSON FX/RX 80 or compatible printers. The file should be
called M.SDUMP. Users not familiar with entering machine code (via a BASIC
program for example) may prefer to obtain one of the many screen-dump
utilities available commercially for the BBC micro.

```
0000 4C E6 09 00 00 FF 03 00 L.......
0008 00 00 00 00 00 00 FF 03 ........
0010 4E 6F 74 20 67 72 61 70 Not grap
0018 68 69 63 73 0D 07 08 41 hics...A
0020 1B 03 C0 4C 1B 40 1B 04 ...L.@..
0028 00 00 00 00 00 00 FF 00 ........
0030 04 26 3F 00 10 84 49 66 .&?...If
0038 B9 6F FF 02 01 2D 09 04 .o...-..
0040 03 2F 09 08 06 33 09 00 ./...3..
0048 00 00 00 04 03 2D 09 08 .....-..
0050 06 33 09 A2 03 BD 0C 09 .3......
0058 9D 03 09 CA 10 F7 A9 1A ........
0060 20 EE FF A9 1D 20 EE FF  .... ..
0068 A2 03 A9 00 20 EE FF CA .... ...
0070 10 F8 A2 02 A9 01 20 EE ...... .
0078 FF BD 1E 09 20 EE FF CA .... ...
0080 10 F2 60 A9 87 20 F4 FF ..`.. ..
0088 98 8D 2A 09 C9 06 10 22 ..*...."
0090 C9 03 F0 1E 18 2A 2A AA .....**.
0098 BD 3B 09 8D 2B 09 BD 3C .;..+..<
00A0 09 8D 2C 09 BD 3D 09 8D ..,..=..
00A8 4B 0A BD 3E 09 8D 4C 0A K..>..L.
00B0 18 60 A0 00 B9 10 09 20 .`.....
00B8 E3 FF C8 C0 0E D0 F5 38 .......8
```

```
00C0 60 A2 01 A9 01 20 EE FF  '.... ..
00C8 BD 25 09 20 EE FF CA 10  .%. ....
00D0 F2 A2 18 A9 01 20 EE FF  ..... ..
00D8 A9 0A 20 EE FF CA D0 F3  .. .....
00E0 A9 03 20 EE FF 60 20 83  .. ..' .
00E8 09 90 01 60 A9 02 20 EE  ...`.. .
00F0 FF 20 53 09 A2 03 A9 01  . S.....
00F8 20 EE FF BD 21 09 20 EE  ...!. .
0100 FF CA 10 F2 A9 00 8D 28  .......(
0108 09 AD 2A 09 D0 08 AD 2C  ..*....,
0110 09 49 03 8D 2C 09 A9 04  .I..,...
0118 8D 27 09 A2 03 A0 09 A9  .'......
0120 09 20 F1 FF AD 2A 09 C9  . ...*..
0128 02 F0 0D C9 05 F0 09 AD  ........
0130 07 09 8D 08 09 4C 41 0A  .....LA.
0138 A2 07 A0 09 A9 0B 20 F1  ...... .
0140 FF AC 08 09 AD 28 09 29  .....(.)
0148 03 AA B9 33 09 E0 00 F0  ...3...
0150 05 6A 6A CA D0 FB 6A 2E  .jj...j.
0158 29 09 6A 2E 29 09 38 AD  ).j.).8.
0160 05 09 E9 04 8D 05 09 AD  ........
0168 06 09 E9 00 8D 06 09 CE  ........
0170 27 09 D0 A7 A9 01 20 EE  '..... .
0178 FF AD 29 09 20 EE FF 18  ..). ...
0180 AD 05 09 69 10 8D 05 09  ...i....
0188 AD 06 09 69 00 8D 06 09  ...i....
0190 EE 28 09 AD 28 09 CD 2C  .(..(..,
0198 09 F0 03 4C 16 0A 18 AD  ...L....
01A0 03 09 6D 2B 09 8D 03 09  ..m+....
01A8 AD 04 09 69 00 8D 04 09  ...i....
01B0 C9 05 F0 03 4C 04 0A A9  ....L...
01B8 00 8D 04 09 A9 01 20 EE  ...... .
01C0 FF A9 0A 20 EE FF 38 AD  ... ..8.
01C8 05 09 E9 10 8D 05 09 AD  ........
01D0 06 09 E9 00 8D 06 09 AD  ........
01D8 06 09 C9 FF F0 03 4C F4  ......L.
01E0 09 20 C1 09 60 ** ** **  . ..`...
```
----

7. APPENDIX 2

7.1 Example output from running the limiting dilution analysis program

(NB. Responses required from the keyboard are shown in BOLD.)

<LIMITING DILUTION ANALYSIS>

  STEVE COBBOLD APRIL 1986

ENTER/ANALYSE DATA -PRESS 'D'   COMMENT: This is the main
                                           menu screen.
PLOT DATA FROM DISC-PRESS 'P'

CHECK DATA ON DISC -PRESS 'C'

D

184

```
----------------------------------------------------------------------------

LIMITING DILUTION ANALYSIS

DO YOU WANT A PRINTOUT (Y/N) Y

LIMITING DILUTION ANALYSIS

FILE NAME TO STORE DATA? TEST

HOW MANY REPLICATES (NO OF WELLS)
PER DILUTION ? 96

ARE THERE SERIAL (2-FOLD)
DILUTION STEPS (Y/N) N
HOW MANY DILUTIONS ? 5

HOW MANY RESPONDER CELLS (ABSOLUTE)
PER WELL IN DILUTION 1? 100000

HOW MANY NEGATIVE WELLS    ? 12

HOW MANY RESPONDER CELLS (ABSOLUTE)
PER WELL IN DILUTION 2? 30000

HOW MANY NEGATIVE WELLS    ? 32

HOW MANY RESPONDER CELLS (ABSOLUTE)            COMMENT: This is the data
PER WELL IN DILUTION 3? 10000                           entry program.

HOW MANY NEGATIVE WELLS    ? 58

HOW MANY RESPONDER CELLS (ABSOLUTE)
PER WELL IN DILUTION 4? 3000

HOW MANY NEGATIVE WELLS    ? 78

HOW MANY RESPONDER CELLS (ABSOLUTE)
PER WELL IN DILUTION 5? 1000

HOW MANY NEGATIVE WELLS    ? 90

DATA CHECK

96-FOLD DETERMINATION WITH
5 DILUTION STEPS

RESPONDERS      NEG. WELLS
   100000          12
   30000           32
   10000           58
   3000            78
   1000            90
INPUT CORRECT (Y/N) ? Y

----------------------------------------------------------------------------

EVALUATION OF INDIVIDUAL POINTS

RESPONDERS   NEGS 95%CL       FREQ
   100000    5 TO 19      2.07944154E-5
```

185

```
30000   22 TO 42      3.66204096E-5
10000   48 TO 68      5.03905181E-5
 3000   70 TO 86      6.92131216E-5
 1000   85 TO 95      6.45385211E-5
```
AVERAGE FREQUENCY F=4.83113972E-5   Comment: This is simply
              OR F= 1/20699.0495   the arithmetic mean of the
                                        individual points.

PRESS ANY KEY Z

EVALUATION BY CHI-SQUARE   Comment: The iteration is
ITERATION RUNNING   repeatedly run until the desired
                                       accuracy has been achieved
READY

CORRECTION FACTOR Q=1.5
FREQUENCY F=3.22075981E-5
F=1/31048+/-15524(ITERATION ERROR!)

DO YOU WANT THE FACTOR CALCULATED
5 TIMES MORE ACCURATELY (Y/N)? Y
ITERATION RUNNING

READY

CORRECTION FACTOR Q=1
FREQUENCY F=3.22075983E-5
F=1/31048+/-3104.8(ITERATION ERROR!)

DO YOU WANT THE FACTOR CALCULATED
5 TIMES MORE ACCURATELY (Y/N)? Y
ITERATION RUNNING

READY

CORRECTION FACTOR Q=1.04
FREQUENCY F=3.09688445E-5
F=1/32290+/-645.8(ITERATION ERROR!)

DO YOU WANT THE FACTOR CALCULATED
5 TIMES MORE ACCURATELY (Y/N)? N

EVALUATION ACCORDING TO CHI-SQUARE   Comment: Output of results
                                       from evaluation by minimum
CALCULATED FREQUENCY: F=3.09688445E-5   chi-square

 OR 1/32290+/-645.8(ITERATION ERROR)

THE CHI-SQUARE VALUE IS 39.4339097

FOR 5 DILUTIONS & 3 DEGREES OF FREEDOM
WITH P>0.05, CHI-SQUARE MUST BE <7.8

PROBABILITY ESTIMATION (n-2): P= 3.06344784E-9

FOR 5 DILUTIONS & 4 DEGREES OF FREEDOM   Comment: Checking for
WITH P>0.05, CHI-SQUARE MUST BE <9.5   goodness of fit

PROBABILITY ESTIMATION (n-1): P=7.94134996E-9
```
```

THE EXPERIMENT IS REJECTED!!!

PRESS ANY KEY Z

COMMENT: This particular
example did not fit the single
hit model

NOTE THAT, ALTHOUGH THE EXPERIMENT HAS BEEN REJECTED ON THE BASIS OF
NOT FITTING THE SINGLE-HIT MODEL, THE PROGRAM DOES NOT ABORT, BUT
CONTINUES TO ESTIMATE FREQUENCIES BY MAXIMUM LIKELIHOOD. THESE MUST
THEN, OF COURSE, BE TREATED WITH EXTREME CAUTION.

EVALUATION BY MAXIMUM LIKELIHOOD
ITERATION RUNNING

CALCULATED FREQUENCY F=3.25172868E-5
OR F=1/30752.8732

ITERATION ERROR +/-3075.28732

DO YOU WANT THE FACTOR 5 TIMES MORE ACCURATELY (Y/N)? Y
ITERATION RUNNING

CALCULATED FREQUENCY F=3.31676327E-5
OR F=1/30149.8756

ITERATION ERROR +/-602.997512

DO YOU WANT THE FACTOR 5 TIMES MORE ACCURATELY (Y/N)? Y
ITERATION RUNNING

CALCULATED FREQUENCY F=3.33666386E-5
OR F=1/29970.0552

ITERATION ERROR +/-119.880221

DO YOU WANT THE FACTOR 5 TIMES MORE ACCURATELY (Y/N)? N

EVALUATION BY MAXIMUM LIKELIHOOD

CALCULATED FREQUENCY: F=3.33666386E-5
OR 1/29970.0552 +/- 1/119.880221
(ITERATION ERROR)

FREQUENCY F=3.33666386E-5 +/-
9.78333686E-6 (95% CONFIDENCE LIMIT)

COMMENT: This is the data
which is stored on
disk and used in the plot.

OR FREQUENCY F=1/29970
WITH 95% CL FROM 1/42402 TO 1/23174

DO YOU WANT TO PLOT THE DATA (Y/N)? Y

THE EXAMPLE DATA IS SHOWN PLOTTED AND SCREEN-DUMPED IN THE FOLLOWING
FIGURE.

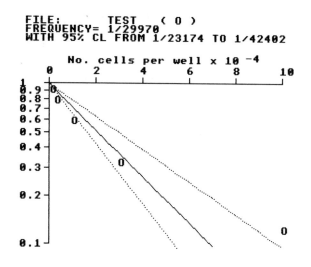

CHAPTER 9

Lymphocyte proliferation assays

STELLA C.KNIGHT

1. INTRODUCTION

There has been progressive miniaturization of cultures used for assessing lymphocyte proliferation. Cultures of 1 ml volumes in tubes were replaced by 200 μl samples in microplates following the advent of appropriate automated harvesting procedures (1,2). Lymphocytes can now be cultured in 20 μl hanging drops and stimulated with mitogens, antigens or allogeneic leukocytes. The proliferation can be measured from the uptake of [^{3}H]thymidine by using a harvesting device where the radiolabelled cultures are simply blotted onto filter discs which are then washed and processed for scintillation counting (3). This further miniaturization of the culture system has the dual advantages of using 5 − 10 times fewer cells and a simplified and rapid harvesting technique. The technique is patented through the British Technology Group in London.

The theoretical considerations concerning lymphocytes in culture cannot be considered in depth here. However, the dynamic nature of lymphocyte proliferation dictates the way in which the assays should be designed if interpretable results are to be obtained. For example, 'bell-shaped' response curves result when the number of antigen-presenting cells, the number of responding lymphocytes, the concentration of antigen or the culture period are increased (4). These factors also interact (*Figure 4*) and may interact with other experimental variables under consideration (5,6). The majority of work using the larger 100 − 200 μl culture systems has relied on the use of limited 'standardized' culture conditions. These may identify 'enhanced' or 'reduced' responses but such alterations can reflect changed dynamics of the responses. There may, for example, be a changed requirement for antigen-presenting cells, responder cells, antigen dose or culture period. The 20 μl hanging drop technique was devised as a practical solution to the need for multifactor experiments to identify the nature of any changes in lymphocyte proliferation.

Lymphocytes from humans and animals can be cultured successfully in 20 μl hanging drops in Terasaki plates. Compared with the larger cultures, the 20 μl technique demands more careful attention to the maintenance of a suitable pH during handling procedures and to the humidity within the incubator during culture. However, the harvesting procedures for these small cultures are very simple. To harvest a plate of 60 cultures the 20 μl drops are blotted onto filter discs and washed in a process that takes less than 2 min per plate. The technique makes it possible to perform multifactor experiments to look at the dynamics of lymphocyte growth in different experimental systems and has been used successfully for measuring the proliferation of lymphocytes in response to non-specific mitogens, antigens and in mixed leukocyte reactions.

A consequence of the capacity for performing multifactor experiments provided by this technique is the necessity for new methods of analysing the data. Analysis of variance is a useful tool for this (6). The 20 μl culture technique, and its use for studying stimulation of lymphocytes by various agents, and the methods for analysing the dynamic data obtained will, therefore, be described.

2. THE BASIC HANGING DROP CULTURE TECHNIQUE

2.1 **Culture substrate**

2.1.1 *Medium*

The use of the Dutch modification of RPMI 1640 (Flow Laboratories) which incorporates both bicarbonate and Hepes buffers is recommended. Eagle's medium and Dulbecco's modification of Eagle's are adequate for culture of human and rabbit lymphocytes. However, RPMI 1640, a medium specifically developed for lymphocyte culture, is excellent for lymphocytes from most species and will also support growth of mouse and rat cells. The most labile component of these media is the glutamine and it is advisable to add this shortly before use. In mouse cultures 1×10^{-5} M 2-mercapto-ethanol is required to permit satisfactory growth and for rat cultures half this amount of 2-mercaptoethanol will suffice. Penicillin (100 units per ml) and streptomycin (100 μg/ml) inhibit infections and have little effect on lymphocyte stimulation. Bicarbonate is needed in these cultures and medium buffered only with bicarbonate can be used. Some of the work described (e.g *Figures 1 − 5*) used bicarbonate-buffered medium. However, the cultures are of 20 μl volumes and additions of some cell suspensions may be of 5 or 10 μl, so that it is impossible to prevent a rise in pH during the setting up of cultures. This effect is difficult to see from the colour change in the indicator in such small volumes. The addition of Hepes buffer to help the maintenance of a suitable pH for a longer period during handling procedures may, therefore, be advisable and the Dutch modification of RPMI 1640 is appropriate in these circumstances. Lymphocyte stimulation in 20 μl hanging drops can also be achieved in a serum-free medium which is based on that of Iscove and Melchers and contains transferrin, delipidated albumin and soybean lipids as serum substitutes (7).

2.1.2 *Serum supplements*

Serum supplements are required to obtain lymphocyte growth in 20 μl cultures in RPMI 1640 medium as described for the larger volume cultures (4,8). For cultures of human lymphocytes, 10% autologous human serum or pooled AB serum can be used. The latter should not include serum from individuals who have received blood transfusions, or from multiparous women since these may contain blocking or stimulatory antibodies. Rabbit serum (10%) is suitable for rabbit lymphocytes, but mouse serum except at levels of less than 2% is unsuitable for the culture of mouse lymphocytes. Fetal calf serum (FCS) at between 5 and 10% is almost universally used for allowing lymphocyte stimulation. Batches should be screened to find those causing low 'background' stimulation, but permitting lymphocyte growth in response to stimulants.

High 'background' lymphocyte proliferation in the presence of FCS may result from

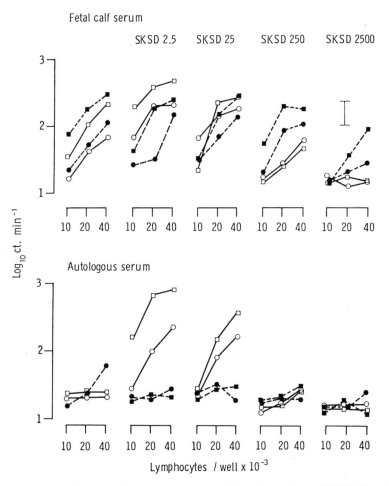

Figure 1. Stimulation of human PBL with the antigen streptokinase/streptodomase (SKSD). Lymphocytes from defibrinated human peripheral blood from two individuals were separated using sedimentation with 1% gelation (4): 20 000−40 000 cells were cultured in duplicate in bicarbonate-buffered medium (50% Dulbecco's, 50% RPMI 1640) containing 10% FCS or 10% autologous serum. Some cultures were stimulated with different doses of SKSD (in U/ml) as indicated. Cultures were pulsed for 2 h with [³H]thymidine (1 μl to give final concentration 1 μg/ml of 1 Ci/mmol) on day 3 or day 5. The bar lines indicate differences significant at $P = 0.001$. (O———O) Individual 1, day 3; (□———□) individual 1, day 5; (●---●) individual 2, day 3; (■---■) individual 2, day 5.

the presence of xenoantigens acquired by antigen-presenting cells which are then presented to lymphocytes in culture and the kinetics of this proliferation are similar to those for stimulation with mitogens and antigens. An example is shown in *Figure 1*. Human peripheral blood lymphocytes were cultured at 10 000−40 000 cells per well in the presence of 10% FCS or 10% autologous human serum. Cultures of 40 000 cells in FCS gave [³H]thymidine incorporation of up to 300 c.p.m. on day 5 whereas the values never went above 30 c.p.m. in autologous serum.

2.2 **Hanging drop cultures**

2.2.1 *Setting up 20 μl cultures*

(i)   Use Hamilton repeating syringes dispensing volumes of 1, 5 and 10 μl. Culture plates are the 60-well tissue-typing plates (Terasaki plates) with wells designed to hold 10 μl (e.g. Nunc, Gibco Ltd).

(ii)   Add cell suspensions in supplemented medium containing appropriate concentrations of cells (which will be discussed for the different types of stimulant) into the wells of the Terasaki plates and add the stimulant (e.g. mitogens, Section 3.2; antigens, Section 3.3, or allogeneic cells, Section 3.4).

(iii)   Although the wells are designed to hold 10 μl, the final volumes of the cultures should be between 15 and 23 μl. If less than 15 μl is used the cells will not be sufficiently proud of the rims of the wells when the plates are inverted. If more than 23 μl is used the cultures may coalesce if the plates are shaken during handling. Some workers reported that volumes of greater than 15 μl could not be used because of the problem of coalescence (9,10), although this has not been our experience where cultures of up to 23 μl are commonplace.

(iv)   Take great care that the pH does not rise to damaging levels; it may be necessary to re-gas between additions to the cultures. A safety cabinet with a fierce flow of air may increase the pH problem and can also lead to some drying. Thus, if a 1 μl aliquot of a stimulant is used it will be necessary to add this after addition of a larger volume of medium, or of the cell suspension to avoid drying.

(v)   After adding all the components invert the plates. A beneficial effect of culturing lymphocytes in inverted Terasaki plates with the cells resting on the meniscus was observed when compared with conventional cultures in the bottom of the wells (11,12).

2.2.2 *Culturing*

(i)   Use a 37°C incubator gassed with 5% CO_2 in air which is well-humidified. Wash plastic boxes with loosely fitting lids thoroughly in hot water, rinse with alcohol and add sterile saline. Place in the incubator and add cultures when the temperature of the saline has equilibrated. A grid or upturned Petri dish slightly deeper than the saline supports the inverted Terasaki plates. The cultures are thus suspended in a well-humidified atmosphere just above the saline (*Figure 2*). In incubators with well-regulated humidity the saline may be unnecessary.

(ii)   There have been few sterility problems using this procedure, but more stringent precautions to ensure sterility may be required in areas rich in fungal contaminants. Clean the boxes between each experiment and do not add further sets of plates to boxes before the end of an experiment, since this can result in severe problems of contamination.

(iii)   Check the amount of drying in cultures by adding medium containing [³H]-thymidine to blank wells and measure the activity in a 5 μl aliquot before and after culture. An increase in the counts indicates drying. Successful proliferative responses have still been obtained where a loss of volume of up to 20% over 7 days in culture or where a gain up to 12% was recorded.

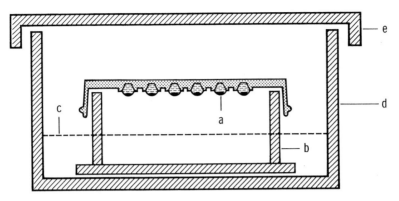

Figure 2. Culture system for 20 μl hanging drops. (**a**) Cultures of 20 μl hanging drops in inverted Terasaki plates with cells on the meniscus. (**b**) Support for Terasaki plate. (**c**) Saline to help maintain humidity. (**d**) Box with loosely fitting lid (**e**) allowing gassing of cultures.

2.3 Use of [³H]thymidine

Use a 2 h pulse time with 1 μg/ml thymidine (sp. act. 2 Ci/mmol, Amersham International) (8). This provides freely available thymidine without causing too much radiological damage and gives an accurate reflection of the level of lymphocyte stimulation. If alterations are made in this procedure two major factors are relevant — the amount of thymidine used and its specific radioactivity (6,13).

2.3.1 *Amount of thymidine added*

The addition of thymidine provides an alternative nucleotide which can be incorporated into the DNA synthesized. It is unlikely that there is any other significant source of thymidine in most cultures so that the amount added will effectively be the amount available. Sufficient thymidine must, therefore, be added to be freely available otherwise the technique will reflect not only the amount of DNA synthesis but also the availability of the precursor. Two major factors will reduce the amount of thymidine available in the cultures. The first is the amount taken into the stimulated cells and the second is the breakdown of the thymidine (13). Breakdown to thymine is increasingly significant after 4−6 h in culture. Thus, the maximum c.p.m. obtained by pulsing a lymphocyte culture for 24 h with [³H]thymidine is substantially lower than that obtained by pulsing the cultures every 6 h. Thymidine at 0.5−1 μg/ml is sufficient to be freely available even in highly stimulated cultures if the pulse time is 2 h. This is 10 times less than the amount of thymidine needed to cause a significant block in DNA synthesis.

2.3.2 *The specific activity of the [³H]thymidine*

A specific activity of [³H]thymidine of 2 Ci/mmol gives significant incorporation into DNA with a minimal amount of radiological damage. The short emission path of the isotope means that damage to cells will be effectively confined to those cells which incorporate the [³H]thymidine. The usual rule that the amount of damage is a reflection of the total radioactivity present irrespective of specific activity does not, therefore, apply in cultures with freely available [³H]thymidine. Instead, the amount of damage

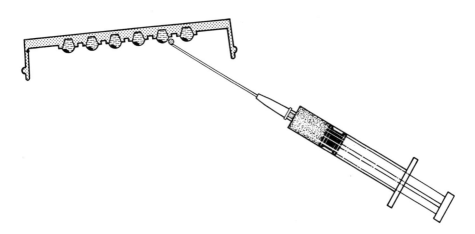

Figure 3. Addition of [³H]thymidine to cultures. Thymidine (1 μl to give a final concentration of 1 μg/ml at 2 Ci/mmol) is added from a repeating syringe. The culture plate can be held at a slight angle so that the thymidine can be added more easily without disturbing the cell pellet. The thymidine is first expelled onto the end of the 25 gauge needle and can be seen to merge with the hanging drop.

is directly proportional to the specific activity of the [³H]thymidine, since this influences the proportion of the thymidine in the cell that is radioactive. High specific activity [³H]thymidine (e.g. >10 Ci/mmol) if freely available in culture can be used to kill dividing cells. To use [³H]thymidine to measure DNA synthesis the specific activity must be as low as possible to minimize radiological damage.

Fortunately, the degree of damage is directly proportional to the specific activity of the [³H]thymidine used, and this effect does not interact with any of the culture variables (e.g. cell concentration in culture, the dose of stimulant or the period in culture) (6). When the thymidine is freely available, the uptake of [³H]thymidine is reduced by radiological damage, but nevertheless reflects the biological effects of the stimulant and not the limitations of the assay procedure.

2.3.3 *Addition of [³H]thymidine to the cultures*

(i)   To add the [³H]thymidine to the cultures use a Hamilton repeating syringe delivering 1 μl and fitted with a 25-gauge needle.

(ii)   Hold the plate at a very slight angle to give a larger area of the meniscus so that the thymidine can be added without disturbing the cell pellet.

(iii) Expel a 1 μl drop of [³H]thymidine onto the tip of the needle and bring the tip of the needle up towards the side of each culture until the drop disappears into the culture (*Figure 3*).

2.4 Harvesting procedure

2.4.1 *Cutting the filter discs*

The harvesting plate has 60 recessed wells for holding filter discs and beneath each well there is a hole for applying suction (*Figure 4*). Place a piece of fibreglass filter paper (Titertek, Flow Laboratories) above the harvesting plate and cut 60 filters. In

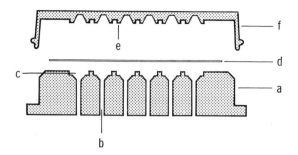

Figure 4. Cutting filter discs in the harvester plate. The harvester plate (**a**) is a polycarbonate block with holes (**b**) which open into wells (**c**) to hold filter discs. A fibre-glass filter (**d**) is placed above the wells and the rims (**e**) of the wells of a Terasaki plate (**f**) are used to cut 60 filter discs.

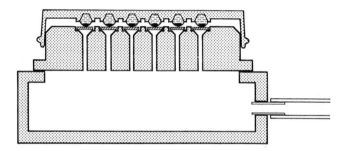

Figure 5. Harvesting cultures. The harvester plate with the filters (diagonal hatching) is sealed onto a vacuum box, which is attached to a simple tap pump, and suction applied. The Terasaki plate is lowered onto the harvester plate so that the cells on the miniscus of each 20 μl hanging drop are trapped onto the filter discs. The Terasaki plate is then removed and the filters washed with 20 ml saline, 5% TCA and methanol delivered from wash-bottles. The filters can then be transferred with a needle to beta scintillation counting vials.

the original version of the harvester made at the Clinical Research Centre, the rims of the wells of Terasaki plates (either Nunc or Falcon) are used as cutting edges to cut the 60 filter discs (*Figure 4*). The base plates thus require precise engineering for each make of Terasaki plate to allow cutting of filter discs − although cultures from any make of the standard format plates can be harvested on any harvesting plate. In the version of the harvester produced by Flow Laboratories a metal cutting plate cuts the filter discs.

2.4.2 *Harvesting the cultures*

(i)   Place the harvesting plate holding the filter discs over the vacuum suction box and seal with grease or with a bayonet lock.

(ii)   Prepare wash bottles of saline, 5% trichloroacetic acid (TCA) and methanol.

(iii) Moisten the filter discs with saline and apply gentle suction via a vacuum pump. A simple tap pump provides sufficient vacuum. If the filters are all moist this will prevent uneven suction through the filters as the cultures are harvested.

(iv)   Lower the culture plate onto the harvester so that the 60 cultures are blotted onto the filter discs (*Figure 5*). Once the cultures are on the discs the suction can be increased and material is not dislodged from the filters, even if the harvester plate is flooded with wash fluids.

(v)   Wash the filters with saline, TCA and finally with methanol (10−20 ml of each fluid per plate). Many harvesting procedures for larger cultures (200 μl) use only distilled water for washing. In tests with this 20 μl system, the use of saline followed by TCA increased the counts significantly, particularly when higher concentrations of cells were used (e.g. >20 000). If samples contain some red cells the methanol wash decolourizes the filters so preventing significant colour quenching on scintillation counting. Methanol also dries the discs.

(vi)   Use a needle to transfer the filter discs to plastic beta vials, add 0.5 ml of scintillant; either count directly or place in glass vials and count using a liquid scintillation counter.

2.5 Experimental design and analysis of data

To examine several variables simultaneously in cultures, levels of each factor are used in combination with every level of the other factors in a symmetrical fashion. Such experiments are then amenable to analysis of variance (6,14−16). This allows individual effects and their interactions to be measured so that the influence of the various technical and experimental factors on lymphoproliferation can be assessed. In many experiments most variables will be fixed factors (such as the numbers of cells, the dose of stimulants, times in culture, types and doses of additives) and only replication will be random (16). Raw data should be $\log_{10}$ transformed before analysis (14). With large multifactorial lymphocyte stimulation experiments, the data then give a near-normal distribution and analysis of variance can be performed (6,15,16). This can be done with the aid of a Fortran subroutine from the general subroutine library of the Clinical Research Centre, written by M.J.Healy (CRSTAT 14). This produces a table of the marginal means for each factor and combination of factors, as well as calculating the sums of squares of deviations from the mean for these factors. The sums of squares can be divided by the appropriate degrees of freedom to give the mean squares of the deviation for each component (e.g. *Table 2*). These variance components can be tested for significance using a mean square ratio (F test). If replication is present, this ratio can use the error variance obtained by combining all the terms containing replication, and dividing by the total number of degrees of freedom for these terms. This will test for effects significantly greater than the variability due to replication. In experiments with many variables, the highest order interaction can be used as the error variance for testing significance. Another program, BMDP 8V (BMDP Statistical Software Inc., University of California) produces a complete analysis of variance. Once the error variance in any experiment has been found, any two marginal means can be tested for significant differences using the Student t test:

$$t = \frac{\bar{x}_1 - \bar{x}_2}{\sqrt{\dfrac{2 \times \delta^2}{n}}}$$

where t is Student's t with the degrees of freedom of the residual error variance at the required probability level, $\bar{x}_1$ and $\bar{x}_2$ are the two marginal means to be compared;

Table 1. Effects of dendritic cells on the proliferative response to Con A.

Con A	Cells (10^{-3})	No dendritic cells added				+ 1000 dendritic cells			
		Plate 1		*Plate 2*		*Plate 1*		*Plate 2*	
No mitogen	0	32	24	36	54	26	28	48	20
	20	50	58	58	50	56	48	56	42
	40	82	86	90	90	82	78	72	74
	80	142	96	152	162	130	118	176	154
	160	158	180	230	474	192	160	256	246
0.1 μg/ml	0	30	46	44	48	36	26	32	68
	20	96	78	92	74	142	138	150	120
	40	114	128	158	158	202	216	192	216
	80	180	150	184	194	424	312	482	454
	160	294	208	346	482	630	980	818	662
1 μg/ml	0	26	28	32	38	28	34	26	202
	20	116	124	136	138	372	338	388	108
	40	130	138	470	304	796	878	794	762
	80	323	319	414	294	290	274	420	344
	160	646	697	594	910	134	156	222	244

CBA mouse lymph node cells (numbers $\times 10^{-3}$ are shown on left) were cultured in RPMI 1640 (Dutch modification) and low doses of Con A and dendritic cells added as indicated (17). The experimental points were in duplicate and the whole experiment was repeated on two plates. The c.p.m./culture are shown. The boxed numbers indicate where two cultures had co-mixed during handling.

δ^2 is the residual variance and n is the number of observations contributing to each marginal mean.

If factors do not cause significant effects, data can be pooled and graphs showing significant effects can be drawn using the appropriate marginal means. If $\log_{10}$ data are plotted, a single bar line can show differences significant at a chosen level obtained from the Student t test (*Figure 1*).

3. RESULTS

3.1 Reproducibility of the technique

The data in *Table 1* are from an experiment where replication was not particularly good: it was chosen to show the problems that can occur using this technique. The experiment was to test the accessory effect of adding dendritic cells to cultures of mouse lymphocytes stimulated with low doses of Concanavalin A (Con A). In 20 μl cultures of rabbit peripheral blood lymphocytes with sub-optimal doses of Con A, the addition of dendritic cells causes more sensitive responses that occur with lower responder cell numbers in culture (17). Mouse lymph node cells at five different concentrations were stimulated with two different doses of mitogen. The cultures were in duplicate and the whole experiment, which was contained on one plate, was also repeated on a second plate. This allowed the study both of replication within each plate and of reproducibility between plates.

In this experiment two wells co-mixed during the handling as indicated. There are also some examples of poor replication within plates (e.g. 230 and 474, 594 and 910), and between plates (e.g. 130 and 138 on plate 1 and 470 and 304 on plate 2). In many experiments there are no significant differences between plates, but in this experiment the counts on plate 2 were higher than those on plate 1. This difference was significantly greater than the variability between the duplicates ($P = 0.01$ using analysis of variance). Such effects can also occur between plates when using 200 μl cultures when this sensitive method of analysis is used. In the experiment shown, despite the overall increase in counts on plate 2, there were no significant differences between the plates in the effects of changing cell concentration, mitogen dose or adding dendritic cells. This was ascertained by analysis of variance, since there were no significant interactions between the effect of culturing in different plates and of changing cell concentrations ($P = 0.20$), between the effect of plates and the mitogen dose ($P = 0.27$), or between the plate effect and that of adding dendritic cells ($P = 0.37$). In addition, most effects studied are likely to be highly significant ($P < 0.001$) using this analysis so that the variability between plates is not necessarily a problem. However, it may be advisable to make important comparisons within plates if possible. If this is not possible and small effects are being studied, the use of replicates on different plates could be indicated. It seems probable that, when harvesting several plates, slight variations in the timings of addition of thymidine and harvesting may contribute to the variations observed, since the pulse time is only 2 h. More precise attention to details of this type may minimize these problems.

A further problem demonstrated in *Table 1* concerns the counting of blank filters. The wells with no responder cells or dendritic cells gave counts ranging from 24 to 54 c.p.m. This is very high and was seen only using one of the scintillation counters available. Using other counters, blanks remain less than 10 c.p.m. In this miniaturized system, it is important to avoid high 'blank' values if possible.

In a recent trial we used this 20 μl hanging drop technique to study stimulation of mouse lymph node lymphocytes with Con A, using five different types of well-humidified, microprocessor-controlled, gassed incubators. Successful results were obtained in each of these incubators. Since experimental points in this study were in quintuplet the variability across the plates could be examined. There was no evidence of variability and no 'edge-effects' of the type frequently reported in 200 μl cultures.

3.2 Responses to mitogen

Responses of lymphocytes from various species to different mitogens stimulating B or T lymphocytes can be obtained. The responses of mouse lymph node lymphocytes to low doses of Con A have already been described in the previous section (*Table 1*). An example of the responses of human peripheral blood lymphocytes (PBL) to Con A, phytohaemagglutinin (PHA) and pokeweed mitogen (PWM) is shown in *Figure 6* where arithmetic data are plotted. The first two of these mitogens initially stimulate T lymphocytes, although in cultures of mixed cells B cells become involved particularly later on. PWM has more effect on B lymphocytes (4,8). There is a requirement for higher numbers of PBL in culture to see optimal responses to PWM: in the experiment shown in *Figure 6* no peak response was seen even with 80 000 cells/culture. This requirement for more cells probably reflects the smaller proportion of B cells than T cells in peripheral blood. A similar relationship with the numbers of potentially responsive cells present in culture was observed in cultures of mouse lymphocytes from

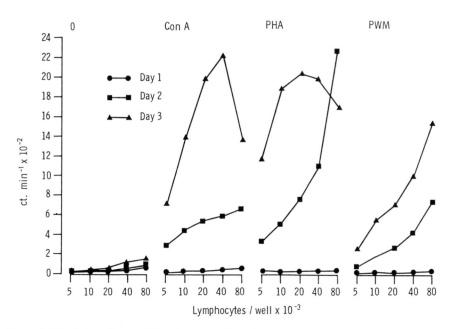

Figure 6. Stimulation of human PBL with mitogens. Lymphocytes were separated and cultured as described in *Figure 1* in medium supplemented with 10% autologous serum. Cells at different concentrations were cultured from 1−3 days with Con A (5 μg/ml), PHA, (Wellcome, unpurified, at a final dilution of 1 in 120) or PWM (Difco, 1 μg/ml). Differences of 0.32 of a $\log_{10}$ unit were significant at $P = 0.001$.

different sources using 200 μl cultures (18). The dynamics of responses are indicated further in *Figure 7*. In this experiment data were $\log_{10}$ transformed. Here, the peak response on day 2 to a single dose of PHA was seen with 40 000 or 80 000 cells initially put into culture. After 3 days the best responses occurred with a starting population of 10 000 or 20 000 lymphocytes. By day 4 the peak response was obtained with 5000 initial cells. A similar relationship between the numbers of cells and the dose of stimulant is also shown in *Figure 7*. The maximum responses were seen with fewer cells in culture when higher doses of mitogen were used. These effects are similar to those already reported for the cultures in larger volumes (4,8). Analysis of variance of this type of experiment using different concentrations of cells, different doses of mitogen and different times in culture, demonstrated that these three factors each affect the stimulation ($P < 0.001$) and also interact significantly ($P < 0.001$). These experiments used only duplicate cultures for each experimental point. The bar lines show the differences required for effects significant at $P = 0.001$ using the Student t test. The dynamics of lymphocyte proliferations are shown more graphically in the data from lymphocytes stimulated with antigen (*Figures 8 and 9*), since the principal interactions between the culture factors apply to all types of proliferative responses described in this Chapter.

3.3 Responses to antigen

Responses of lymphocytes from antigen-primed individuals to re-stimulation with antigen *in vitro* can be obtained in 20 μl hanging drops. The effect of different sera on the

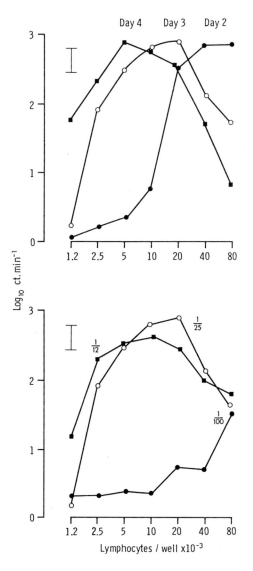

Figure 7. Stimulation of human PBL with PHA. Human PBL were cultured as in *Figure 6* and were stimulated with PHA (Wellcome, unpurified), diluted 1 to 12, 1 to 25 or 1 to 100, (as indicated) in medium before addition of 1 μl to 20 μl cultures. Results from days 2, 3 and 4 in culture using the intermediate dose of mitogen (**top**) and the day 3 results with the three doses of mitogen (**bottom**) are shown. Bar lines indicate the differences required for points to differ significantly at the level $P = 0.001$.

responses of human PBL to stimulation with streptokinase/streptodomase (SKSD; Varidase, Lederle) has already been described (*Figure 1*). *Figure 1* also emphasizes the need for sensitization of the lymphocyte donor with antigen to allow detection of responses: donor 2 gave no response to the antigen and this presumably reflected the lack of recent sensitization. *Figure 8* shows a more thorough study of the stimulation of human lymphocytes with SKSD. The figures describe the responses to different doses

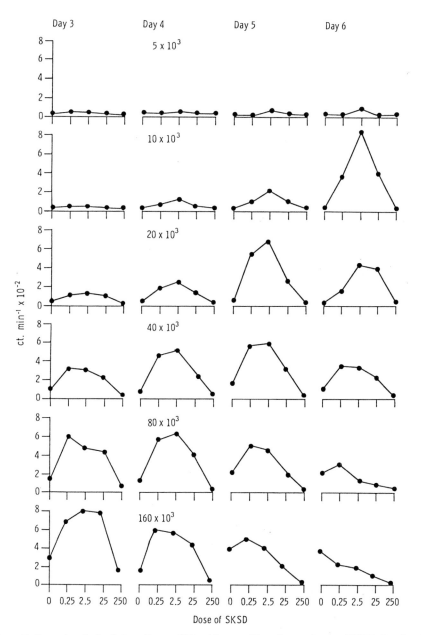

Figure 8. Dynamics of stimulation of human PBL with streptokinase/streptodomase (SKSD). Details of the separation and culture technique are as in *Figure 1* and 10% autologous serum was used. Cultures contained 5000 – 160 000 cells and different doses of SKSD (in U/ml). Duplicate cultures were pulsed with [³H]thymidine for 2 h on days 3, 4, 5 and 6 of culture.

of antigen using 5000 – 160 000 peripheral blood cells cultured for 3 – 6 days. The uptake of [³H]thymidine increased, reached a plateau and decreased when each of these parameters was varied. The 'background' turnover increased with the higher cell

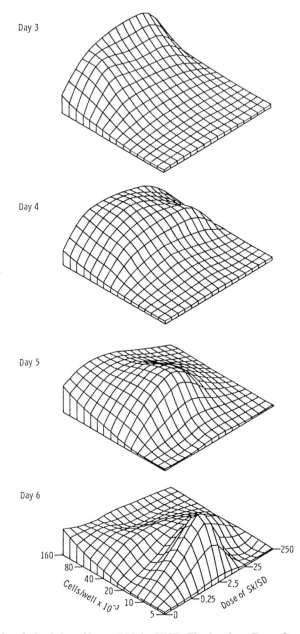

Day 3

Day 4

Day 5

Day 6

160
80
40
20
10
5

Cells/well x 10⁻³

250
25
2.5
0.25
0

Dose of SkISD

Figure 9. Dynamics of stimulation of human PBL by SKSD. The data from *Figure 8* are shown by three-dimensional computer graphics. The height of the 'mountains' indicates the level of the response in c.p.m. Smooth surfaces were generated and plotted using an algorithm for surface fitting by bivarate interpolations (21) and the Ginosurf surface plotting package (Computer-Aided Design Centre, Cambridge).

concentrations and the longer times in culture. The dynamic nature of the response is emphasized by the three-dimensional depiction of these same data in *Figure 9*.

Primary stimulation to some antigens, particularly contact sensitizers can be obtained

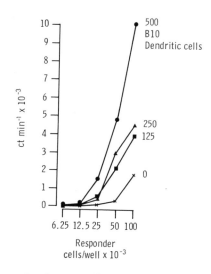

Figure 10. Responses of mouse lymphocytes to allogeneic dendritic cells (MLR). Lymph node lymphocytes from CBA mice were cultured at different concentrations in RPMI 1640 medium (Dutch modification) with 10% FCS and 10^{-5} M 2-mercaptoethanol. Syngeneic or allogeneic (B10) dendritic cells were isolated (19) and 125–500 added to cultures. These numbers of syngeneic dendritic cells taken from specific pathogen-free animals cause no significant stimulation. The stimulation with allogeneic dendritic cells is shown.

in culture and this has been studied in mouse lymph node cells using picryl chloride or fluorescein isothiocyanate (19).

3.4 Mixed leukocyte reactions (MLR)

The major cells stimulating allogeneic lymphocytes in the normal MLR are the dendritic cells. Responses are initiated following the clustering of lymphocytes around dendritic cells and as few as one dendritic cell per 3000 allogeneic cells can cause significant uptake of [^{3}H]thymidine. *Figure 10* demonstrates the stimulation of lymph node cells from a CBA mouse with 125–500 allogeneic (B10) dendritic cells. The same numbers of syngeneic dendritic cells cause no significant syngeneic MLR, when the cell donors are specific pathogen-free mice (17). In this system significant stimulation of thymidine uptake can be obtained with as few as 25 allogeneic dendritic cells added to 50 000 or 100 000 lymph node cells.

Responses in the 20 μl hanging drop technique can be detected earlier than in the 200 μl culture system, and this is particularly true in MLR. *Figure 11* shows a primary and secondary response of human PBL to stimulation with cells of a B cell line. This experiment demonstrates both the detection of early responses and the use of primed lymphocytes to see typing effects. The cell line used for priming was from an individual homozygous for the histocompatibility antigen, HLA DW2 (HOM1) and these cells were treated with mitomycin C (Sigma) at 50 μg/ml for 25 min and washed twice before use. Lymphocytes were primed in bulk in 25 cm² tissue culture flasks in 10 ml of Dulbecco's medium with 15% autologous serum and contained 8×10^6 mitomycin-treated stimulators and 40×10^6 PBL. An equal number of lymphocytes was cultured in a flask without stimulators. After 6 days the cultures were fed with a further 10 ml of medium and after a further 4 days the cells were collected, put into fresh medium

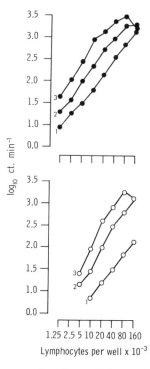

Lymphocytes per well x 10⁻³

Figure 11. Secondary mixed leukocyte reactions. Human PBL separated using Ficoll gradients were primed in bulk cultures (see text) using mitomycin-treated cells from a B-cell line homozygous for HLA-DW2. Primed cells (**top**) and non-primed cells (**bottom**), were cultured at different cell concentrations for 1, 2 or 3 days with 80 000 mitomycin-treated cells from the B-cell line homozygous for DW2. Further details are discussed in the text.

and re-stimulated with mitomycin-treated stimulator cells in 20 μl cultures. *Figure 11* shows the responses on days 1, 2 and 3 of culture to re-stimulation of the primed and non-primed cells with mitomycin-treated cells homozygous for DW2 (HOM1). The increased sensitivity to stimulation after priming is evident from the requirement for fewer primed cells in culture to obtain responses. With low numbers of responder cells the response also occurred earlier. In this experiment re-stimulation with another cell line homozygous for DW2 (PGF) gave similar responses. A DW4 cell line (PRIESS) was also used as a third party cell to re-stimulate the cultures and on the third day of culture the stimulation was not significantly different using the primed and the non-primed cells (data not shown).

The technique has been used for MLR with normal PBL as stimulator cells (10,20). An experiment examining the capacity of the PBL of two siblings to respond to mitomycin-treated cells from different members of the family and to unrelated cells is shown in *Table 2* and *Figure 12*. The siblings had been tissue-typed for HLA-A, B, C and DR antigens and found to be identical. The purpose of this experiment was to test if the two siblings responded in the same way to cells from the different family members. It was anticipated that they would since they were HLA-identical.

204

Table 2. Analysis of variance of mixed leukocyte cultures.

Factors:

A   Replication − duplicates

B   Responder lymphocyte concentrations (CONC): 5, 10, 20, 40, 80, 160 $\times$ 10^3 per well

C   Source of stimulator cells (STIM): unrelated, maternal, paternal, Sib 1, Sib 2

D   Source of responder lymphocytes (SIBS): Sib 1, Sib 2

E   Day of harvest (DAY) 3, 4 and 6 of culture

Source of variation	Sums of squares	Degrees of freedom	Mean square	F	P
CONC	11.0100	5	2.2020	210.82	<0.001
STIM	5.1853	4	1.2963	124.11	<0.001
SIBS	2.3980	1	2.3980	229.59	<0.001
DAY	22.8130	2	11.4065	1092.07	<0.001
CONC/STIM	1.2937	20	0.0647	6.19	<0.001
CONC/SIBS	0.3807	5	0.0761	7.29	<0.001
CONC/DAY	21.2319	10	2.1232	203.28	<0.001
STIM/SIBS	0.0442	4	0.0111	1.06	>0.25 NS
STIM/DAY	0.1838	8	0.0230	2.20	<0.05
SIBS.DAY	0.1502	2	0.0751	7.19	<0.005
CONC/STIM/SIBS	0.3376	20	0.0169	1.62	>0.05 NS
CONC/STIM/DAY	1.4601	40	0.0365	3.49	<0.001
CONC/SIBS/DAY	0.8576	10	0.0858	8.21	<0.001
STIM/SIBS/DAY	0.0738	8	0.0042	<1.00	>0.25 NS
CONC/STIM/SIBS/DAY	0.5353	40	0.0134	1.28	>0.1 NS
POOLED ERROR	1.8801	180	0.0104		

This experiment used bicarbonate and Hepes-buffered RPMI-1640 medium and 10% FCS. This latter produced some 'background' stimulation but the genetic effects are still identifiable. The experimental conditions are indicated in *Table 2*, where the analysis of variance is shown in detail. The siblings (SIBS) responded to stimulatory cells from the different family members (STIM) in a similar fashion, since there is no significant interaction between STIM/SIBS. This was true when different responder cell concentrations (CONC) were used, since the interaction CONC/STIM/SIBS was not significant. The same answer was obtained on different days of culture (DAY), as STIM/SIBS/DAY also showed no significant effects. The MLR 'typing', therefore, confirmed the similarity between the two responder populations. Since the two siblings gave similar responses to the different stimulator cells these effects are shown for one sibling on day 3 of culture in *Figure 12*. The response of these cells to stimulation with cells from the other sibling was not significantly different from the stimulation with syngeneic cells. The greatest response was to the cells from the unrelated individual and the proliferation initiated by maternal and paternal cells was intermediate (the latter are not shown).

The experiment provides considerable further information. As expected from the

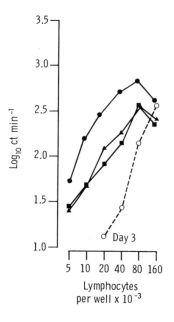

Figure 12. Human mixed leukocyte reactions. Graph showing some data from the experiment described in the analysis of variance (*Table 2*). Lymphocytes were separated using Ficoll gradients and cultures were in RPMI 1640 medium (Dutch modification) with 10% FCS. Different numbers of lymphocytes were cultured on their own (○—○), or with 80 000 mitomycin-treated lymphocytes, ■—■ autologous stimulator cells, ▲—▲ stimulator cells from an HLA-identical sibling, ●—● stimulator cells from an unrelated donor.

previous discussions (Sections 3.1 and 3.2), the concentration of responder lymphocytes and the time in culture affected the proliferation and also were interdependent: the effects CONC, DAY and CONC/DAY were all significant ($P < 0.001$). The source of the stimulator cells influenced the response, and affected requirements for the numbers of responder cells and time in culture (STIM, CONC/STIM, CONC/DAY, CONC/STIM/DAY were all significant, $P < 0.001$). The fact that the siblings respond overall in a significantly different way is at first surprising (SIBS, $P < 0.001$). Further examination shows that this reflects a different cell concentration requirement and time course for cells from two sibs (CONC/SIBS, $P < 0.001$; SIBS/DAY, $P < 0.005$; CONC/SIBS/DAY, $P < 0.001$).

This 20 μl culture technique can, therefore, be used to obtain MLR with human PBL which reflects the genetic differences between responder and stimulator cells. The responses are more easily obtained at earlier culture periods than those in 200 μl cultures. The analysis of variance can be used to distinguish different sources of variability in the cultures. For example, from *Table 2*, the effects of individual variations between the siblings in the dynamics of the lymphocyte responses (i.e. in the overall cell numbers required for stimulation and the kinetics of the responses) can be identified separately from the genetic influences within the MLRC.

4. ACKNOWLEDGEMENTS

I am grateful to my colleagues for their kindness in allowing me to present data from collaborative work. The work presented in *Table 2* and in *Figures 11* and *12* are taken from Stephen Burman's M.Phil thesis (1981, Council for National Academic Awards) where further details of these studies can be found. Tissue typing for the study described in *Table 2* and *Figure 12* were done by Peter Hall. I am also indebted for other data to Steven Macatonia, Jacqueline O'Brien and Penelope Bedford. The assistance of the Medical Illustration Department at the Clinical Research Centre and of Kathleen Jameson who prepared the manuscript are greatly appreciated. The harvester is patented through the British Technology Group, Newington Causeway, London.

5. REFERENCES

1. Thurman,G.B., Strong,D.M., Ahmed,A., Green,S.S., Sell,K.W., Hartzman,R.J. and Bach,F.H. (1973) *Clin. Exp. Immunol.*, **15**, 289.
2. Bondeuik,H., Helgesen,A., Thoresen,A.B. and Thorsby,E. (1974) *Tissue Antigens*, **4**, 469.
3. O'Brien,J., Knight,S., Quick,N.A., Moore,E.H. and Platt,A.S. (1979) *J. Immunol. Methods*, **27**, 219.
4. Ling,N.R. and Kay,J.E. (eds) (1976) *Lymphocyte Stimulation*. North Holland, Amsterdam.
5. Knight,S.C. (1982) *J. Immunol. Methods*, **50**, R51.
6. Farrant,J., Clark,J.C., Lee,H. and Knight,S.C. (1980) *J. Immunol. Methods*, **33**, 301.
7. Farrant,J., Newton,C.A., North,M.E., Weyman,C. and Brenner,M.K. (1984) *J. Immunol. Methods*, **68**, 25.
8. Hume,D.A. and Weidemann,M.J. (eds) (1980) *Mitogenic Lymphocyte Transformation*. Elsevier/North Holland, Amsterdam.
9. Traill,K.M., Chandler,P. and Krammer,P.H. (1981) *J. Immunol. Methods*, **40**, 17.
10. Taylor,G.M., Jones,H., Hughes,G., Harris,R. and Dyer,P.A. (1984) *Tissue Antigens*, **24**, 129.
11. Fainboim,L. and Festenstein,H. (1979) *Transplant Proc.*, **11**, 700.
12. Pena-Martinez,J. and Festenstein,N.H. (1975) *Transplantation*, **20**, 26.
13. Cleaver,J.E. (ed.) (1967) *Thymidine Metabolism and Cell Kinetics*. North Holland, Amsterdam.
14. Dei,R. and Urbano,P. (1977) *J. Immunol. Methods*, **15**, 169.
15. Knight,S.C., Harding,B., Burman,S. and Mertin,J. (1981) *Clin. Exp. Immunol.*, **46**, 61.
16. Felder,M., Dore,C.J., Knight,S.C. and Ansell,B.M. (1985) *Clin. Immunol. Immunopathol.*, **37**, 253.
17. Knight,S.C., Balfour,B.M., O'Brien,J., Buttifant,L., Sumerska,T. and Clarke,J. (1982) *Eur. J. Immunol.*, **12**, 1057.
18. Thorpe,P.E. and Knight,S.C. (1974) *J. Immunol. Methods*, **5**, 387.
19. Macatonia,S., Edwards,A. and Knight,S.C. (1986) *Immunology*, **59**, 509.
20. Knight,S.C. and Burman,S. (1981) *Transplant. Proc.*, **13**, 1637.
21. Akima,H. (1974) *Commun. ACM*, **17**, 26.

CHAPTER 10

Assays for interleukins and other related factors

ANNE S.HAMBLIN and ANNE O'GARRA

1. INTRODUCTION

During the last 20 years an astonishing number of soluble factors have been described which influence leucocytes involved in immune and inflammatory responses. Since the introduction of the term lymphokine [non-antibody proteins or glycoproteins generated by lymphocyte activation that act as intercellular mediators of the immunological response (1,2)] there have been continuous efforts to classify the various factors which have been grouped under this umbrella term. Thus cytokine, monokine (3) and interleukin (4) were added to the vocabulary to underline the principle that not all the activities are derived from lymphocytes. Many are derived from other lymphoid cells, as well as from cells of non-lymphoid origin. In addition, early evidence suggested that the same factor could be derived from a variety of cell sources and that the same factor could affect multiple target cells (5). Recombinant DNA technology has provided the means to determine the primary amino acid sequences of lymphokines and a source of homogeneous material for laboratory assays.

Amongst the lymphokines of which the primary amino acid sequences are known are the interleukins, IL-1, IL-2, IL-3, IL-4 and IL-5. IL-1 and IL-2 are essential for T cell stimulation and IL-4 and IL-5 for B cell stimulation. IL-3 promotes the differentiation and self-renewal of bone marrow-derived multi-lineage progenitor cells. Experiments with recombinant interleukins have shown that, in addition to their principal effects, the interleukins are indeed pleiotropic, influencing a number and sometimes many different target cells. Here we deal with the principal assays for interleukins and related factors which affect T and B lymphocytes and refer briefly to their other reported activities. In addition we have included an assay for IL-3 to complete the current interleukin series.

1.1 Interleukins acting on T lymphocytes

The mechanism by which antigens stimulate the clonal expansion of T lymphocytes involves antigen processing and presentation by monocytes/macrophages, together with the release of IL-1 by monocytes and IL-2 by T lymphocytes. IL-1 is an essential requirement for antigen-presenting cell activation of T lymphocytes (6), and facilitates both IL-2 production by T lymphocytes (7), and IL-2 receptor expression (8). Once activation signals have been received by T lymphocytes, antigen and IL-1 are no longer necessary. The interaction of IL-2 with its receptor then progresses the resting lymphocyte through the cell cycle (9), and the IL-2 responsive cell will continue to proliferate in the presence of IL-2 (see reviews 10 and 11). In addition to the above roles of IL-1 and IL-2 in antigen-driven T lymphocyte activation, both these lymphokines exert other biological activities. IL-2 is required for proliferation of natural killer (NK) cells (12), and lymphokine-activated killer (LAK) cells (13), and for induction of cytotoxic T cell activity (14). To date IL-2 is made only by T cells and most of the biological effects of IL-2 seem to be on T or T-related (NK, LAK) cells; thus, assays for IL-2 rely on its growth-promoting activity for T cells. In contrast, IL-1 has a remarkably wide range of targets. IL-1 acts on B cells to cause their clonal expansion and maturation, hepatocytes to cause acute phase protein release, chondrocytes to release a variety of enzymes, osteoclasts to cause bone resorption, endothelial cells to cause their proliferation and brain to cause fever and somnolence. IL-1 seems to be identical with leucocyte endogenous mediator (LEM), catabolin and endogenous pyrogen (EP) (see reviews 15−17). Complete characterization of IL-1 may therefore rely on the demonstration of one or more of the activities listed here, together with the 'definitive but not specific' (18) mouse thymocyte assay.

1.2 Interleukins acting on B lymphocytes

It is now clear that the helper function of T cells in antibody responses can be explained by their production of growth and differentiation factors that act on B cells. These soluble factors were functionally divided into two groups: B cell growth factors (BCGF), thought to be involved in B cell proliferation, and B cell differentiation factors (BCDF), responsible for maturation of activated B cells into immunogloblin-secreting cells (19−22).

This classification now needs to be re-examined in the light of recent evidence. Thus, the cloning of cDNA encoding murine IgG_1 induction factor (IL-4) (23) has shown that recombinant IL-4 has both BCGF and BCDF activities. It not only affects B cells, but also T cells and mast cells (23,24). Another well characterized B cell factor (BCGF-II) was initially described as a growth factor for a murine B cell lymphoma (BCL_1) (25). It also causes both DNA synthesis and antibody secretion (IgM and some IgG) in pre-activated normal mouse B cells (26). The availability of recombinant murine BCGF-II has revealed that this factor also has T-cell-replacing factor (TRF) activity, and the factor has therefore been designated IL-5 (27). This factor has also been shown to cause the differentiation of bone marrow cells into mature eosinophils (EDF activity, ref. 28).

A third molecule is a 20-kd human BCDF (now called B cell-stimulating factor-2, BSF-2), which induces antibody secretion in both Epstein−Barr virus (EBV)-transformed human B cells and pre-activated normal cells, but thus far has not been shown to cause normal B cells to proliferate. The cDNA for this molecule has also now been cloned (29), although its murine homologue has not yet been identified. Recently it has been shown that BSF-2 is identical to interferon-β_2 (30), and with a hybridoma/plasmacytoma growth factor (HPGF) (31). The molecule qualifies as a B cell growth and differentiation factor, but has little if any anti-viral activity, despite original evidence suggesting this. Interestingly, this lymphokine is the only one of these three factors which so far seems only to act on B cells. Various other less well-defined factors acting on B cells have been described, but these will not be discussed here.

2. INTERLEUKIN 1

Interleukin 1, formerly known as lymphocyte activating factor (LAF), was first described by Gery *et al.* (32) as a factor which was found in the culture supernatant of adherent human blood leucocytes which promoted mouse thymocyte proliferation. It has now been shown that IL-1 is released by stimulated monocytes, monocyte/macrophage cell lines, large granular lymphocytes (LGL), dendritic cells, endothelial cells, neutrophils, fibroblasts, astrocytes and epithelial cells as well as unstimulated B cell lines and an adult T cell leukaemia line (16). IL-1 affects a variety of target systems (see Section 1).

Data from cDNA cloning of both human (33,34) and murine (35) sources have indicated two distinct forms of IL-1, known as IL-1α and IL-1β. Both have a molecular weight of 17 kd, but differ in their pI (IL-1α, pI 5.0; IL-1β, pI 7.0). The differential biological activity of these two forms of IL-1 have yet to be fully determined.

The 'definitive but not specific' assay for IL-1 is the mouse thymocyte bioassay (18). In this assay the ability of IL-1 to replace the accessory effect of intact macrophages in T cell proliferation is assessed. Further assays for IL-1 rely on the ability of this interleukin to stimulate IL-2 production by cell lines (36), or to stimulate IL-1-sensitive cell lines to proliferate (8). More recently a commercial radioimmunoassay (RIA) for measuring IL-1 has become available (Cistron Biotechnology).

2.1 Sources

IL-1 is most readily prepared by activation of monocytes and macrophages from blood or other tissues with lipopolysaccharide (LPS), particles such as a silica, or phorbol myristic acetate (PMA). Described below is a method for preparing IL-1 from human blood monocytes (37). Alternatively IL-1 may be obtained from the sources indicated above. Commercial IL-1 may be obtained from a number of companies (e.g. Cistron Biotechnology; Genzyme Corp.) in both native or recombinant forms.

2.2 Preparation of IL-1 from human peripheral blood monocytes

(i)   Prepare a sample of peripheral blood mononuclear cells by Metrizoate−Ficoll separation as described in Chapter 1. Resuspend cells at 1×10^6/ml in RPMI 1640 medium containing 5×10^{-5} M 2-mercaptoethanol.

(ii)   Place 1 ml of cell suspension in each well of a 24-well plate (Nunclon Delta; Gibco). To one culture add LPS (*Escherichia coli* 055 B5; Difco) in RPMI to a final concentration of 10 μg/ml, and to another add an equal volume of RPMI.

(iii)   Incubate at 37°C in 5% CO_2 in air.

(iv)   After 24 h recover the culture supernatant by centrifugation at 400 *g* for 8 min at room temperature; sterilize by membrane filtration (0.2 μm) and store at −20°C.

A bulk preparation prepared as above may be used as a laboratory standard. The technique may be modified for monocytes and macrophages from other tissues and other species.

2.3 Mouse thymocyte assay for IL-1

In this assay dilutions of a sample thought to contain IL-1 are cultured with mouse thymocytes, usually in the presence of suboptimal concentrations of mitogens like phytohaemagglutinin (PHA), or concanavalin A (Con A) (co-mitogenic assay). IL-1 samples may also be added directly to the thymocytes (direct assay), although responses are less readily seen by this method (37). Mouse lymphocytes will respond to IL-1 from human or other species. A number of controls and technical points must be considered. Thymocytes obtained from many mouse strains respond to LPS, so mice are usually selected which are LPS-unresponsive (C3H/HeJ strain). The thymocytes will also respond to IL-2 and mitogens: samples being tested for IL-1 must therefore be checked for the presence of IL-2 or mitogens. Supernatants prepared as in Section 2.2 should not contain IL-2. However, samples from other sources may do so.

(i)   Prepare a suspension of thymocytes as described in Chapter 1.

(ii)   Adjust the cell suspension to 12×10^6 viable lymphocytes/ml in RPMI medium containing 10% fetal calf serum (FCS) and 2-mercaptoethanol at 5×10^{-5} M (complete medium).

(iii) Prepare serial 2-fold dilutions of the test samples and control samples. Appropriate controls include samples from mononuclear cells incubated without LPS, and a laboratory standard of IL-1. Aliquot 50 μl of each dilution in two separate sets of three wells in a 96-well round-bottomed microtitre plate (e.g. Costar, Northumbria Biologicals).

(iv)   To one set of dilutions add 50 μl of purified PHA (Wellcome Diagnostics) at 3 μg/ml in complete medium and 50 μl of medium to the other set.

(v)   Add 50 μl of thymocyte suspension to each culture and incubate at 37°C in 5% CO_2 in air for 48 h.

(vi)   At the end of the culture period, add 50 μl [^{3}H]thymidine (methyl [^{3}H]-thymidine, sp. act. 185 GBq/mmol, Amersham International) solution at 1 μCi/ml and incubate for a further 20 h.

(vii) Determine the radioactivity incorporated by harvesting the cultures onto filter paper using an automated harvester (e.g. Skatron), drying the filters and counting in a liquid scintillation counter.

(viii) Express the results as stimulation indices as follows:

$$\frac{\text{d.p.m. thymidine incorporated in the presence of IL-1}}{\text{d.p.m. thymidine incorporated in cultures of medium alone}}$$

Do this for cultures containing PHA plus IL-1, and IL-1 alone. In this way the direct and co-mitogenic activity of the samples can be evaluated. A significant response may be determined from a stimulation index of greater than 3.0 in an assay showing a response to an IL-1 standard (37).

3. INTERLEUKIN 2

Interleukin 2 (IL-2), formerly T cell growth factor (TCGF), was first described in 1976 (38) as a factor promoting growth of T lymphocytes from normal human bone marrow. This inducible glycoprotein of mol. wt 15 000 is synthesized and secreted by T lymphocytes following their activation with antigens and mitogens. It is required for the growth of T cells following their exposure to antigen and is required for the maintenance of T cells in long-term culture (reviewed in 10, see Chapter 6). The sequence of amino acids has been derived by examination of cDNA from transformed and non-transformed human T cells: the mature protein is an 133 amino acid protein with a single disulphide bond which is essential for bioactivity (39).

IL-2 is assayed by its ability to promote the growth of T cell lines of human (HT-2), or mouse (CTLL-2) origin (available from American Type Culture Collection), or to maintain the growth of polyclonally activated T lymphocytes. Growth of the cells is measured by thymidine incorporation (40), or a modified MTT method (41). More recently a commercial enzyme-linked immunosorbent assay (ELISA) has become available for assaying human IL-2 (Genzyme Corporation). Below is described the maintenance of the CTLL-2 cell line and its use to assay IL-2, and the assay of IL-2 on human blast cells.

3.1 Sources

IL-2, together with many other lymphokines, is generated when T lymphocytes are stimulated with antigens and mitogens (42). Mononuclear cells prepared from peripheral blood or from lymphoid organs (Chapter 1) are stimulated with optimal concentrations of antigens and mitogens (e.g. Chapter 6). After $24-48$ h in culture, the supernatants are collected and stored at $-20°C$, and may be assayed for IL-2. In addition IL-2 is produced by a number of T cell lines as well as T cell tumours (e.g. EL4, Chapter 6) and hybridomas (10,11). Commercial IL-2 may be obtained from a number of companies (e.g. Genzyme Corporation, Amgen Biologicals) in native or recombinant forms.

3.2 Assay of IL-2 on CTLL cells

3.2.1 *Maintenance of mouse CTLL cells*

(i)   Maintain continuously proliferating CTLL cells in complete medium (Section 2.3), containing IL-2 (recombinant IL-2 at ~ 10 U/ml, or laboratory prepared IL-2, see above).

(ii) Culture the cells in 2 ml volumes in individual wells of 24-well plates, covered with loose-fitting plastic lids.

(iii) Passage the cells when they have achieved a density of $1-3 \times 10^5$/ml (usually every $3-4$ days).

(iv) Establish new cultures by seeding 5×10^3 viable cells/ml in fresh medium.

(v)   Wash cells twice in complete medium prior to the assay to remove any remaining IL-2.

3.2.2 *Assay*

(i)   Prepare at least five serial 2- or 4-fold dilutions of assay samples in complete medium. Lymphocyte culture supernatants prepared as above are normally used at a final concentration of 1:4 downwards. In addition prepare serial 2- or 4-fold dilutions of a laboratory standard preparation of IL-2.

(ii) Distribute 100 μl aliquots in $3-4$ replicate wells for each dilution into individual wells of round-bottomed 96-well culture plates.

(iii) Add 100 μl washed CTLL cells to each well at 2×10^4 viable cells/ml in complete medium and cover with gas-permeable plate sealing tape or a loose

lid. Incubate at 37°C in a humidified atmosphere of 5% CO_2 in air for 24 h.
(iv)   Add 50 μl of [^{3}H]thymidine (Section 2.3) containing 2 μCi/ml in complete medium to each well and re-incubate for 20 h.
(v)   Harvest the cultures as in Section 2.3. Samples containing IL-2 give dose-related stimulation of thymidine incorporation.

3.3 Assay of IL-2 on human blast cells (modified from 43)

3.3.1 *Preparation of human blast cells*

(i)   Separate blood on Metrizoate–Ficoll to obtain mononuclear cells (Chapter 1).
(ii)   Resuspend cells at 1×10^6/ml in 10% autologous plasma in RPMI 1640.
(iii) Place the cell suspension in 80 cm^2/260 ml tissue culture flasks (e.g. Nunclon) with 20 μg/ml PHA-R (Wellcome) or 20 μg/ml Con A (Pharmacia). Lay flasks on their side with loose-fitting caps in a humidified atmosphere of 5% CO_2 in air at 37°C for 3 days.
(iv)   Wash the cells with RPMI twice and count.

3.3.2 *Percoll gradients for separating blast cells (modified from 44)*

(i)   Add Percoll (Pharmacia) to 10 times concentrated RPMI 1640 (at a ratio of nine parts Percoll to one part RPMI. This is referred to as 100% Percoll and has a density of 1.1294 g/ml.
(ii)   Dilute this solution further with $1 \times$ RPMI to 70% (1.090 g/ml), 60% (1.077 g/ml), 50% (1.067 g/ml), 40% (1.056 g/ml) and 30% (1.043 g/ml). Make these up so there is 2 ml of each dilution for every gradient.
(iii) Resuspend cells in 2 ml of 30% Percoll with no more than 50×10^6 cells/gradient.
(iv)   Prepare a layered gradient of Percoll solutions in tissue culture tubes (16 × 125 mm, Falcon) starting with 100% and finishing with the cells in 30% Percoll.
(v)   Spin at 450 g for 17 min at room temperature.
(vi)   After spinning the cells will be seen at the various density interfaces. The fraction most enriched for blast cells is at the interface of 40–50% Percoll. Remove this layer with a Pasteur pipette into a sterile Universal container and dilute with 20 ml of RPMI 1640.
(vii) Spin at 200 g for 10 min. Wash twice more.
(viii) Place the cells in 80 cm^2/260 ml tissue culture flasks at 1×10^6/ml in RPMI containing 10% heat-inactivated horse serum (Gibco). Culture at 37°C in a humidified atmosphere at 5% CO_2 in air for 4 days.
(ix)   Wash the cells twice and resuspend in RPMI containing 20% horse serum at 2.5×10^5 viable blast cells/ml.

3.3.3 *Blast cell assay*

(i)   Prepare serial 2-fold dilutions of both unknown and standard IL-2 samples in complete medium.
(ii)   Place 100 μl of cell suspension in each well in a 96-well flat-bottomed tissue culture plate and to this add 100 μl of IL-2 dilution. Set up 3–4 replicate cultures

for each dilution and appropriate controls without IL-2.

(iii)   Incubate in a humidified atmosphere of 5% CO_2 in air for 37°C for 3 days. Then add 20 μl of [^{3}H]thymidine at 25 μCi/ml (74 GBq/mmol, Amersham International) to each well.

(iv)   Determine the radioactivity incorporated.

Samples containing IL-2 give dose-related stimulation of thymidine incorporation. Since human blast cells respond to mitogen, samples thought to contain mitogens as well as IL-2 should be assayed on mitogen-unresponsive cell lines such as CTLL-2.

4. INTERLEUKIN 3

This is one of a number of colony stimulating factors (CSF) that are known to regulate haematopoiesis (45–47). The factor is produced by mitogen- or antigen-activated T lymphocytes and by a number of continuous cell lines (48,49). IL-3 is involved in regulating the growth and differentiation of pluripotent stem cells, leading to the production of all the major cell types. Recombinant murine IL-3 has mast cell growth factor (MCGF) activity, and supports the growth and differentiation of progenitor cells committed to monocytic, granulocytic, erythroid and megakaryocytic cell lineages and the growth of pluripotent precursor cells (50). A human cDNA clone coding for IL-3 has now been isolated which also has multipotent colony stimulating activity for normal human bone marrow cells (51). It has been suggested that the partially purified factors designated as burst-promoting activity, P cell-stimulating factor, multi-lineage CSF, haematopoietic cell growth factor and MCGF may be identical to IL-3 (52–54), although direct evidence is lacking. At present, it remains uncertain how many molecular species share similar biological properties. Purification of factors from various sources and amino acid sequence analysis of the purified proteins, plus molecular cloning based on expression of functional products may establish whether all these activities may be attributed to IL-3. This approach was successfully demonstrated recently with the cloning of murine granulocyte/macrophage CSF (55).

IL-3 may be assayed using factor-dependent cell lines (49,56,57) that differentiate along erythroid, neutrophil–granulocyte and basophil/mast cell pathways after appropriate stimulation *in vitro*. We describe one such standard assay and in addition an *in vitro* colony assay to demonstrate its CSF activity.

4.1 Sources

IL-3 may be obtained from antigen or mitogen-stimulated T cells. A useful source is the WEHI-3 cell line which constitutively produces the factor (48). The factor can be readily obtained and purified from WEHI-3 conditioned medium (58).

4.2 Cell line proliferation assay

The 32-D cell line is a haematopoietic progenitor cell line which was established from non-adherent cell populations taken from continuous mouse bone marrow cultures (59).

(i)   Maintain the 32-D cells in RPMI 1640 supplemented with 10% FCS and 10% (v/v) conditioned medium from the WEHI-3 line (48).

(ii)   Plate out 50 μl aliquots of serial dilutions (in RPMI + 5% FCS) of the

Table 1. Composition of Dulbecco's modified double strength Eagle's medium.

Components	Volume (ml)
Eagle's minimal essential salts × 10	100
NaHCO$_3$ (2.8%)	80
Eagle's MEM vitamins × 100	10
Eagle's MEM amino acids A × 100	10
Eagle's MEM amino acids B × 100	10
Glutamine solution (200 mM)	10
Sodium pyruvate (2.2%)	5
Fetal calf serum	100
L-serine (21 mg/ml)	1
Penicillin (200 000 U/ml)	0.58
Streptomycin (200 mg/ml)	0.38
Phenol red (%)	2
Double glass distilled water	135

      supernatants under test into round-bottomed microtitre plates.

(iii)   Wash 32-D cells twice and suspend at 2×10^5/ml, in RPMI + 5% FCS. Aliquot 50 μl of the cell suspension into the microwells.

(iv)   Incubate for 24 h at 37°C, in a humidified atmosphere of 5% CO_2.

(v)   Add 0.5 μCi of [^{3}H]thymidine per well, for the last 4 h of the culture and then harvest and count incorporated [^{3}H]thymidine as described in Section 2.3.

4.3 Colony-stimulating factor assay (60)

(i)   Prepare a mouse bone marrow cell suspension as described in Chapter 1.

(ii)   Prepare the agar culture medium by mixing equal volumes of 2 × Dulbecco's modified medium (*Table 1*) and freshly boiled 0.6% Bacto-Agar (Difco) in water; equilibrate to 37°C.

(iii)   Place 100 μl of test supernatants in 35-mm tissue culture dishes.

(iv)   Resuspend bone marrow cells (7.5×10^4) in 1 ml of the agar culture medium. Mix well and dispense into the 35-mm dishes containing the test supernatants; allow the agar to solidify.

(v)   Incubate the cultures at 37°C in a humidified atmosphere of 10% CO_2 in air for 7 days, when colonies of cells should be visible.

(vi)   Count colonies (clones containing >50 cells) under a binocular dissecting microscope.

5. INTERLEUKIN 4

Interleukin 4, formerly known as BSF-1 or BCGF I, has multiple activities. Initially the factor was described by its ability to synergize with sub-mitogenic concentrations of anti-immunoglobulin antibodies (anti-Ig) to induce DNA synthesis in small resting B cells (63–66). By itself it induces resting B cells to enter a transitional activation state characterized by expression of high levels of Class II MHC (I-A and I-E in the mouse) antigens (67,68). IL-4 can also act as a rather selective B cell differentiation factor in that it promotes the secretion of IgG$_1$ and IgE antibodies by B cells pre-activated by LPS (3). The recombinant molecule has also been shown to induce the proliferation of both mast cell lines and T cells.

We describe the assay conditions for testing these biological activities. The assays for both IL-4 and IL-5 apply to the mouse, although the human cDNA sequences for both factors have now been isolated (61,62). For all these B cell assays in the following sections use RPMI 1640, made with pyrogen-free water (or specially distilled water) supplemented with 5×10^{-5} M 2-mercaptoethanol, 2 mM glutamine, 1 mM pyruvate, non-essential amino acids, penicillin, streptomycin, and 5% FCS, unless otherwise indicated. Pre-select FCS for low backgrounds in all the proliferation assays described, and for supportiveness in the assays for B cell differentiation into antibody-secreting cells.

5.1 Sources

A wide variety of T cells produce IL-4. A convenient source, which is easy to maintain is the EL4 thymoma. This line produces significant amounts of both IL-4 and IL-5, when stimulated with 5 ng/ml PMA for 24 h, at 37°C (see Chapter 6). However, EL4 cells like many other T cell lines, produce a range of lymphokines, which are extremely difficult to separate from each other, or from residual PMA (which has effects on B cells, *per se*). Thus, T cell hybrids are an alternative source, since they may be selected for the production of a limited range of activities, due to their unstable phenotype. The methods for constructing these hybrids are described elsewhere (69).

5.2 Co-stimulator assay

(i)   Prepare spleen cell suspensions, for example from (CBA $\times$ C57Bl)F$_1$ mice, and deplete T cells with anti-Thy 1 antibodies and complement (Chapter 2).

(ii) Prepare gradients of Percoll as follows. Dilute 100% Percoll (Section 3.3.2) to 85, 75 and 50% by mixing with 0.15 M saline or Dulbecco's PBS A. Carefully layer 2.5 ml of 85%, 2.5 ml of 75%, followed by 2.5 ml of 50% Percoll in a round-bottomed centrifuge tube. Avoid mixing of the layers.

(iii) Layer 1 ml of T-depleted spleen cell suspensions on the top of the gradient (maximum of 5×10^7 cells per gradient), and centrifuge at 1300 g for 15 min at 4°C with brake off. These conditions apply to a Beckman J6-B centrifuge. Optimal conditions for other centrifuges must be determined empirically. Collect the small dense B cells from the 85/75% interface, wash once in RPMI/5% FCS and repeat the procedure.

(iv) Wash the B cells three times in RPMI/5% FCS to remove all traces of Percoll. Spin the cells the first time at 800 g and then at 400 g for the next two washes.

(v)   For definitive experiments adherent cells may be depleted by filtering the B cells through two consecutive columns of Sephadex G-10 (Chapter 1). These B cell preparations should contain more than 90% surface Ig-positive cells and no Thy-1 positive cells.

(vi) Add 100 μl of serial dilutions (in the same medium), of the factor under test into flat-bottomed 96-well microtitre plates.

(vii) Some wells also receive a submitogenic dose of anti-Ig. (Controls do not.) This may be rabbit or goat anti-mouse Ig (both commercially available) or a monoclonal anti-mouse IgM, for example, Bet-2 (70). If rabbit anti-mouse Ig is used, it is advisable to use the $F(ab')_2$ fragments (71).

(viii) Adjust the concentration of B cells to 5×10^5 cells/ml and plate out 100 μl.

(ix) Incubate for 3 days, at 37°C, in a humidified atmosphere of 5% CO_2 in air; add 0.5 μCi/well of [^{3}H]thymidine.

(x) After 4 h harvest and count the cultures as described in Section 2.3.

IL-4 containing supernatants or anti-Ig should not induce DNA synthesis individually, but when applied together give at least a 10-fold increase in DNA synthesis, at the appropriate concentrations, as compared to the controls.

5.3 Increase in Ia expression

(i) Prepare small dense B cells as described in Section 5.2, for example from CBA/Ca mice.

(ii) Culture B cells at 10^6/ml in 16 mm wells with or without factor, or with 10 μg/ml anti-Ig as a positive control, for 24 h.

(iii) Wash the cells twice with PBS/0.1% BSA/0.1% sodium azide and then stain at 4°C with an appropriate fluorescein-conjugated monoclonal anti-I-A or anti-I-E antibody (hybridomas available from the American Type Culture Collection).

(iv) Determine the fluorescence profiles by flow cytofluorography (Chapter 2) using log-transformed data. Data can be expressed as changes in median fluorescence intensities of stimulated versus control cultures, expressed in channel numbers.

5.4 Induction of IgG$_1$ production (23)

(i) Culture aliquots of 10^5 T-depleted spleen cells in 0.2 ml of supplemented RPMI 1640 plus 15% FCS and 50 μg/ml LPS, in triplicate, at 37°C in a humidified atmosphere of 5% CO_2.

(ii) On day 1, add supernatants to be tested.

(iii) On day 6 or 7 pool the cultures and determine the number of Ig-secreting cells using the protein A reverse plaque assay (Chapter 5).

(iv) Use rabbit anti-mouse IgG$_1$, IgG$_3$ or IgG$_{2b}$ as developing antisera (available commercially) to determine the (elevated) levels of IgG$_1$ induced by IL-4, and the suppression of IgG$_3$ and IgG$_{2b}$ responses in LPS-stimulated cultures.

(v) The specificity of the antisera should be tested. This can be done using plasmacytoma cells as secretors (available from the ATCC) (22). Alternatively, harvest the culture supernatants at the appropriate time by centrifugation at 1500 g, and freeze until assay, by an isotype-specific ELISA, as in Section 5.5.

5.5 Induction of IgE production

(i) Culture T-depleted spleen cells (from BALB/c or C57Bl.10 mice) at 5×10^5 cells/ml in round-bottomed 96-well plates in 100 μl of supplemented RPMI containing 10% FCS and 4 μg/ml LPS.

(ii) Dilute T cell supernatants to be tested in 100 μl of RPMI + 10% FCS and add to the cultures 1 day later.

(iii)   Harvest culture supernatants 7 days after the initiation of the cultures and freeze until they are to be assayed using an isotype-specific ELISA assay (72).

5.6 Mast cell growth factor activity

(i)   The cloned mast cell line MC/9 (73,74) is obtainable from the ATCC. Growth factor activity may be determined using [^{3}H]thymidine incorporation (50), or by a colorimetric assay (75), both described below.

(ii)   Culture MC/9 (or other mast cell line) in flat-bottomed microtitre plates at 10^4 cells/well in a volume of 100 μl supplemented RPMI + 4% FCS, containing dilutions of test supernatants. Serial dilutions may be made directly in the plate in complete medium. In this case, add the cells in 50 μl of complete medium at 2×10^5 cells/ml.

(iii)   After 20 h incubation at 37°C, in a humidified atmosphere of 5% CO_2 either:

      (a)   add 0.5 μCi of [^{3}H]thymidine per well for 4 h and harvest and count as in Section 2.3, or

      (b)   add 50 μl of 3-(4,5-dimethylthiazol-2-yl)-2,5-diphenyltetrazolium bromide (Sigma) in 10 μl of PBS to each well. After 4 h, add 0.1 ml of 0.04 M HCl in isopropanol to solubilize the coloured formazan reaction product. Read the absorbance at 570 nm (reference 630 nm) on a Dynatech Microelisa Autoreader (MR580).

5.7 T cell growth factor activity

(i)   Determine T cell growth factor (TCGF) activity using the HT-2 line (74), or the CTLL-2 line as for the IL-2 assay described in Section 3.

(ii)   Culture the T cell line at 5×10^3 cells/well under the same conditions as for the mast cell line, and use identical procedures for determining TCGF activity, as described for the MCGF assay.

6. INTERLEUKIN 5

Recombinant IL-5 has been primarily defined by induction of proliferation and IgM secretion by the BCL$_1$ leukaemic B cell line, and by induction of secondary anti-dinitrophenol (DNP) IgG antibody synthesis by DNP-primed T-depleted spleen cells (TRF assay) (27). The observation that TRF had BCGF II activity had been previously made when the former was purified to homogeneity (76). Also, as previously mentioned, IL-5 acts as an eosinophil differentiation factor (EDF). We also describe the assay systems for determining its effects on normal B cells. Sources of IL-5 are the same as for IL-4.

6.1 Effects of IL-5 on the BCL$_1$ lymphoma

6.1.1 *Maintenance of the BCL$_1$ lymphoma*

Maintain this line (soon to be obtainable from the ECACC, Porton Down, Salisbury, UK) by injecting 5×10^6 BCL$_1$ cells obtained from the spleens of BALB/c mice, previously injected i.p. with the tumour (4−6 weeks after inoculation). Use the tumour cells for experiments at any time between 1 week after the appearance of the tumours and the death of the animals (6−8 weeks after inoculation). Examine the mice regularly, since they are prone to become very sick and die quite suddenly.

6.1.2 *Assays for IL-5 on BCL₁ cells*

(i)   For the BCL_1 assays, remove spleens from tumour-bearing mice (recoveries vary from 8×10^8 to 1.3×10^9 cells per mouse), and prepare a cell suspension (Chapter 1).

(ii)   Deplete T cells: resuspend one spleen in 10 ml of RPMI + 5% FCS, 5 ml of 1:3 guinea pig complement, and 0.5 ml of a pre-titrated anti-Thy-1 monoclonal antibody. Incubate for 45 min at 37°C.

(iii)   Wash the cells three times in supplemented medium and count.

(iv)   Proliferation assay: resuspend the cells at 2.5×10^5 cells/ml in the same medium, and plate out 100 μl volumes into 96-well microtitre plates.

(v)   Add a further 100 μl of RPMI + 5% FCS, containing the factor(s) to be tested.

(vi)   Incubate for 2 days at 37°C and then assay for DNA synthesis as in Section 2.3.

(vii)   Antibody production: culture $2-4 \times 10^5$ BCL_1 cells in a volume of 0.5 ml in 24-well Costar plates with and without the factor(s) to be tested.

(viii) Incubate the plates at 37°C, in a humidified atmosphere of 5% CO_2 in air.

(ix)   After 2−5 days, collect the cells and determine the IgM-secreting cells by the reverse plaque assay (77) (Chapter 5).

6.1.3 *Standardization of the BCL₁ assay*

A frozen stock of BCL_1 cells may be used for the assays.

(i)   Prepare the BCL_1 cell suspension and T cell deplete, using the methods described above.

(ii)   Wash the cells three times, and then resuspend in cold freezing mixture (RPMI containing 20% FCS and 10% dimethyl sulphoxide), at a final concentration of 10^7 cells/ml, in freezing ampoules.

(iii)   Freeze in a programmable liquid nitrogen vapour freezing cabinet at 1°C/min. If this apparatus is not available use a special container (available with most liquid nitrogen tanks), which can be held at the top of a liquid nitrogen tank, so that cells are frozen down at an appropriate rate.

(iv)   Store indefinitely in a liquid nitrogen tank.

(v)   For use in an assay, thaw an ampoule quickly by standing it in a waterbath at 37°C.

(vi)   Immediately dilute the cell suspension to 9 ml with supplemented RPMI + 5% FCS and centrifuge at 400 g for 7 min.

(vii)   Resuspend in 5 ml of medium and count. Use in assays as above.

6.2 **Effects of IL-5 on normal B cells**

IL-5 acts on pre-activated B cells (probably at a late stage in the G_1 phase of the cell cycle), but has no detectable effects on resting B cells, unlike IL-4 (cf. Section 5 and ref. 26). Thus, IL-5 will cause proliferation of large naturally occurring B cells, which have presumably been pre-activated *in vivo*, and induce their maturation into IgM- and IgG-producing cells (26). As previously discussed the factor also has TRF activity, enabling B cells to make specific antibody responses *in vitro*. A detailed description of the experimental systems used to determine the responses of normal B cells to the factor is given below.

6.2.1 *Assays of IL-5 on large B cells*

For assaying proliferative responses carry out the following.

(i)   Prepare spleen suspensions, for example from (CBA × C57Bl)F$_1$ mice, and T cell deplete, using anti-Thy 1 antibodies and guinea-pig complement (Section 6.1.2).

(ii)   Prepare solutions of Percoll (Section 5.2), at 85, 80, 75, 70, 65 and 50%, and construct a six-step gradient. Load the cell suspension on to the gradient and centrifuge as in Section 5.2.

(iii)   Collect the cells from the 65/50% interface. One such gradient is sufficient to obtain large B cells. For initial experiments the cells obtained from other interfaces may be tested, in order to compare the proliferative effect of the factor(s) on the different cell densities.

(iv)   Do not attempt to deplete adherent cells using Sephadex G-10, since activated B cells, such as these large B cells, are also lost by this method.

(v)   Wash the B cells three times in RPMI + 5% FCS. Spin the cells the first time at 800 *g*, and then at 400 *g* for the next two washes. Resuspend in complete medium and count.

(vi)   Dilute the cells to 5×10^5 cells/ml and plate out 100 μl into flat-bottomed 96-well microtitre plates.

(vii)   Add a further 100 μl of the same medium, containing the factor under test. It is often more convenient to add this to the plate before the cells, especially if the supernatant to be tested is to be titrated.

(viii) Incubate for 3 days and assay for DNA synthesis as described in Section 5.2.

For assaying antibody secretion, the following procedure can be used.

(i)   Culture large B cells at 10^5/well, under the same conditions for 5 days.

(ii)   Harvest the cells and assay for IgM-producing cells using the reverse plaque method described in Chapter 5.

(iii)   To measure IgG-secreting cells incubate the large B cells similarly, but in supplemented RPMI + 15% FCS for 7 days.

(iv)   Remove 100 μl of medium on day 4, and replace with fresh medium containing the relevant additives and/or factor(s).

(v)   On day 7 harvest the culture and test for IgG-producing cells by reverse plaque assay.

In both cases, LPS (10 μg/ml) may be used as a positive control. If the supernatants under test contain IL-5 they will produce substantial levels of IgM, and lower but reproducible levels of IgG-secreting cells. The actual number of plaque-forming cells may vary from one experiment to the next, although the differential values should stay the same.

6.2.2 *T cell-replacing factor (TRF) assay*

TRF is defined by its capacity to replace T cells in T-dependent antibody responses. The TRF activity of IL-5 has been substantiated in a number of systems. We shall describe assays for determining its effects in:

(i)   anti-hapten (DNP) IgG responses of DNP-primed B cells, using the hapten coupled to a heterologous carrier (78).

(ii)   anti-sheep red blood cell (SRBC) IgM responses of B cells from unprimed mice.

   For induction of anti-DNP IgG responses carry out the following steps.

(i)   Inject BALB/c mice i.p. with 100 μg of DNP−keyhole limpet haemocyanin (KLH) in 4 mg of aluminium hydroxide gel, plus 1×10^9 *Bordetella pertussis* and boost with 20 μg of DNP−KLH in saline 8−12 weeks later.

(ii)   Prepare spleen cells from the mice 4−7 days after the booster injection, and deplete T cells as described above.

(iii)   Add 0.5 ml of the T-depleted cells (5×10^6/ml) in complete RPMI (10% FCS) to 0.5 ml of the test supernatants. To these cell suspensions add 10 μl of DNP−KLH to a final concentration of 40 ng/ml.

(iv)   Plate out 300 μl of the cell suspension, in triplicate into the wells of a microtitre plate and culture for 5 days, at 37°C in a humidified atmosphere of 5% CO_2.

(v)   Assay anti-DNP IgG plaque-forming cells (Chapter 5).

   Alternatively, the effects of TRF-containing supernatants can be assayed in primary anti-SRBC antibody responses using a mini Mishell−Dutton culture system (Chapter 5): here T-depleted spleen cells from unimmunized (or SRBC-primed) mice are cultured at 10^6 cells/200 μl culture. IgM antibody-forming cells are measured by a conventional plaque assay on day 4.

6.3 Eosinophil differentiation factor activity

IL-5 stimulates the differentiation of eosinophils from committed eosinophil progenitor cells. The most sensitive assay for EDF is the production of eosinophils in bulk bone marrow cultures (79). It is important to remember that normal mice have very few eosinophil progenitors: to increase the sensitivity of the assay, bone marrow from mice with induced eosinophilia should be used. A convenient way of doing this is to infect mice with the tetrahydridia (second stage larvae) of the cestode *Mesocestoides corti* (80). The larval form is passaged by i.p. injection and, under strict laboratory conditions, should be unable to complete its life cycle, and thus not able to infect other mice. This parasite also has very low, if any infectivity for man.

6.3.1 *Maintenance of M. corti*

(i)   Inject approximately 100 μl of packed *M. corti* tetrahydridia i.p. into BALB/c mice, using a 0.8 mm diameter needle. The tetrahydridia increase in number throughout several months, and although the mice become distended with parasites and ascites in the peritoneum, they do not seem to suffer any other effects from the infection, and can be maintained for months as a source of the parasite.

(ii)   Kill the mice and collect the larvae by removing the skin over the abdomen and opening the peritoneal cavity so that the contents can be collected in a Petri dish containing sterile PBS.

(iii) Transfer to a sterile tube and wash by allowing the parasite larvae to settle and removing the supernatant. (The larvae survive for months in PBS at 4°C, providing the fluid remains sterile.) Viability can be checked by placing a drop on a microscope slide, allowing it to warm slightly, and looking for movement under low power magnification.

6.3.2 *The EDF assay*

(i) Kill the mouse 10−18 days after infection (maximum number of eosinophil progenitors present in the bone marrow).

(ii) Remove both femurs and prepare a bone marrow cell suspension as described in Chapter 1.

(iii) Pellet the cells and resuspend at 10^6/ml in supplemented RPMI + 15% FCS, containing 10^{-6} M hydrocortisone.

(iv) Plate out 100 μl of cell suspension in round-bottomed microtitre wells, containing 10 μl of test supernatants and incubate in a humidified atmosphere of 5% CO_2 at 37°C for 5−7 days.

(v) Assay for eosinophils either by cell count or by eosinophil peroxidase (81) as described below.

6.3.3 *Eosinophil cell count*

(i) Harvest each replicate and count.

(ii) Smear the cell suspension on a slide, cytocentrifuge, and stain in dilute Giemsa (the nucleus should only be lightly stained and eosinophil granules should be prominent).

(iii) Count the number of eosinophils per well in test replicates as compared with controls.

6.3.4 *Eosinophil peroxidase assay*

(i) Remove most of the medium from the bone marrow cultures.

Table 2. Reagents for eosinophil peroxidase assay.

Stock solutions
0.05 M Tris-HCl buffer, pH 8.0
10% (v/v) Triton X-100
20 mg/ml *O*-phenylenediamine (OPD, Sigma)
30% (w/v) hydrogen peroxide

Peroxidase solution
(Make up fresh for assay)
50 ml of Tris-HCl buffer
0.5 ml of Triton X-100 stock solution
0.5 ml of OPD stock solution
6 μl of hydrogen peroxide solution

(ii)   Add 100 μl of peroxidase solution (*Table 2*) and leave at room temperature for 30 min.

(iii)   Stop the reaction by adding 50 μl of 4 M sulphuric acid.

(iv)   Read the absorbance in an automatic microplate spectrophotometer (blank the instrument against control cultures containing medium only).

A linear relationship exists between eosinophil peroxidase measured by this assay and eosinophil number (81). It is advisable to pool the bone marrow from a number of mice for the peroxidase assay, since this may vary between individual mice.

6.4 Concluding remarks

Neither the BCL_1 assay for BCGF II activity, nor the EDF assay are specific for IL-5. Thus, BCL_1 cells appear to synthesize DNA in response to IL-4, but this factor can be distinguished from IL-5 by the various assays described in Section 5, in which IL-5 does not score. Similarly, IL-3 causes eosinophil differentiation, but can be distinguished by the use of with IL-3-dependent cell lines, as described in Section 4.

7. B CELL-STIMULATING FACTOR-2

BSF-2 (BCDF) induces IgG and IgM secretion in EBV-transformed human B cell lines without any effect on cell growth, and in addition induces IgM and IgG secretion in *Staphylococcus aureus* Cowan I-activated normal B cells (82). We describe here the standard assays used for measuring these parameters.

7.1 Sources

BSF-2 may be obtained from purified protein derivative (PPD)-stimulated pleural lymphocytes (83), or from PHA-stimulated tonsillar mononuclear cells (84). Although human T cell hybridomas which secrete the factor have been described, they are usually unstable and do not produce BSF-2 in amounts sufficient for chemical characterization or isolation (85). An excellent source is a human T cell leukemia virus-transformed T cell line, TCL-Nal, which secretes relatively large amounts of BSF-2 (85). In addition, the bladder carcinoma cell lines, T24, Rt4 and 5637, also constitutively secrete a molecule with BSF-2 activity (86,29).

7.2 Induction of Ig production in normal B cells

(i)   Separate human peripheral blood lymphocytes by Metrizoate − Ficoll gradient centrifugation, or prepare a cell suspension from tonsils obtained by tonsillectomy (Chapter 1).

(ii)   Wash three times with minimal essential medium (MEM) containing 5% FCS and resuspend in supplemented RPMI containing 10% FCS.

(iii)   Use SRBC treated with 2-aminoethylisothiouronium bromide hydrobromide (AET) to separate the T cells from the B cells, as described in Chapter 1 (and ref. 87).

(iv)   Resuspend the B cell fraction in RPMI 1640. This should contain 30−60% Ig-positive cells.

(v)   Partially deplete monocytes by either passing through a Sephadex G10 column

(Chapter 1), or by adherence to a plastic Petri dish. The resultant B cell preparation should contain less than 1% T cells (by E rosetting) and less than 1% monocytes by latex bead phagocytosis.

(vi)   Culture B cells (1×10^6/ml) with *S. aureus* Cowan strain (0.0025%, v/v) for 3 days in flasks.

(vii)   Separate the low-density blast cells on a gradient of 30%: 40%: 50%: 60% Percoll in PBS, centrifuged at 1280 *g* for 12 min at 4°C.

(viii)   Recover the blasts from the 40/50% interface and culture at 5×10^5 cells/ml in 200 μl of supplemented RPMI 1640, containing 10% FCS and the factor under test for 3 days.

(ix)   Determine the concentration of Ig in culture supernatants by an ELISA (88), or antibody-secreting cells by a reverse plaque assay as described in Chapter 5.

7.3 Induction of Ig production in EBV-transformed cell lines

The SKW6-CL4 (89) or the CESS (90) EBV-transformed cell lines may both be used to assay BSF-2. Generation of EBV-transformed B cell lines is described in Chapter 7.

(i)   Culture 4×10^3 SKW6-CL4 cells or 6×10^3 CESS cells in 200 μl cultures in the presence of 3-fold dilutions of the test factor.

(ii)   After 3 days determine the concentrations of IgM in the supernatants for SKW6-CL4 cells, and IgG for CESS cells by an ELISA (88).

8. STANDARDIZATION OF LYMPHOKINE ASSAYS

The above methods rely on the biological effects of interleukins on cells. Such assays will be particularly subject to day-to-day variations in assay performance. It is therefore essential that assays of interleukin activity are standardized as much as is possible to minimize within-assay and between-assay variation. All assays should include a standard interleukin preparation, firstly to assess the responsiveness of the cells within an assay and secondly so that the activity of unknown preparations can be expressed in terms of a standard. Activities should then be expressed in a unitage which is acceptable internationally. With such a procedure results within one laboratory can be easily compared to each other and with those of other laboratories.

Various approaches have been taken to applying standards within assays for the calculation of activity of IL-2 (40,91) and other lymphokines (92,37). The Lymphokine Standardisation Committee of the International Union of Immunological Societies (IUIS) has begun to assess products which may be developed as international reference preparations of IL-1 and IL-2 and other lymphokines will follow (see 93). In setting up the assays described the reader is then urged to consider the inclusion of a positive control standard interleukin in each assay, and the use of such standards to measure lymphokine activity.

9. REFERENCES

1. Dumonde,D.C., Wolstencroft,R.A., Panayi,G.S., Matthew,M., Morley,J. and Howson,W.T. (1969) *Nature*, **224**, 38.
2. Dumonde,D.C. and Hamblin,A. (1983) In *Immunology in Medicine*. 2nd edition. Holorow,E.J. and Reeves,W.G. (eds), Academic Press, London and New York, p. 121.

3. Cohen,S. *et al.* (1977) *Cell Immunol.*, **33**, 233.
4. Aarden,L.A. *et al.* (1979) *J. Immunol.*, **123**, 2928.
5. Cohen,S., Pick,E. and Oppenheim,J.J., eds (1979) *The Biology of The Lymphokines*. Academic Press, London and New York.
6. Scala,G. and Oppenheim,J.J. (1985) In *Lymphokines*. Pick,E. and Landy,M. (eds), Academic Press, London and New York, Vol. 12, p. 39.
7. Smith,K.A., Lachman,L.B., Oppenheim,J.J. and Favata,M.F. (1980) *J. Exp. Med.*, **151**, 1551.
8. Kaye,J., Gillis,S., Mizel,S.B., Shevach,E.M., Malek,T.R., Dinarello,C.A., Lachman,L.B. and Janeway,C.A. (1984) *J. Immunol.*, **133**, 1339.
9. Sekaly,R.P., Macdonald,H.R., Zaech,P. and Nabholz,M. (1982) *J. Immunol.*, **129**, 1407.
10. Smith,K.A. and Ruscetti,F.W. (1981) *Adv. Immunol.*, **31**, 137.
11. Gillis,S., Mochizuki,D.Y., Conlon,P.J., Hefeneider,S.H., Ramthun,C.A., Gillis,A.E., Frank,M.B., Henney,C.S. and Watson,J.D. (1982) *Immunol. Rev.*, **63**, 167.
12. Henney,C.S., Kuribayashi,K., Kern,D.E. and Gillis,S. (1981) *Nature*, **291**, 335.
13. Grimm,E.A., Ramsey,K.M., Mazumder,A., Wilson,D.J., Djeu,J.Y. and Rosenberg,S.A. (1983) *J. Exp. Med.*, **157**, 884.
14. Gillis,S., Union,N.A., Baker,P.E. and Smith,K.A. (1979) *J. Exp. Med.*, **149**, 1460.
15. Gery,I. and Lepe-Zuniga,J.L. (1984) In *Lymphokines*. Pick,E. and Landy,M. (eds), Academic Press, London and New York, Vol. 12, p. 109.
16. Oppenheim,J.J., Kovacs,E.J., Matsushima,K. and Duram,S.K. (1986) *Immunol. Today*, **7**, 45.
17. Kluger,M.J., Oppenheim,J.J. and Powanda,N.C., eds (1986) *The Physiologic, Metabolic and Immunologic Actions of Interleukin 1*. Alan R.Liss, New York.
18. Oppenheim,J.J. and Gery,I. (1982) *Immunol. Today*, **3**, 113.
19. Howard,M., Nankanishi,K. and Paul,W.E. (1984) *Immunol. Rev.*, **78**, 185.
20. Kishimoto,T.A. (1985) *Immunol. Rev.*, **3**, 133.
21. Isakson,P.C., Pure,E., Vitetta,E.S. and Krammer,P.H. (1982) *J. Exp. Med.*, **155**, 734.
22. Bergstedt-Lindqvist,S., Sideras,P., MacDonald,H.R. and Severinson,E. (1984) *Immunol. Rev.*, **78**, 25.
23. Noma,Y., Sideras,P., Naito,T., Bergstedt-Lindqvist,S., Azuma,C., Severinson,E., Tanabe,T., Kinashi,T., Matsuda,F., Yaoita,Y. and Honjo,T. (1986) *Nature*, **319**, 640.
24. Lee,F., Yokota,T., Otsuka,T., Meyerson,P., Villaret,D., Coffman,R., Mosmann,T., Rennick,D., Roehm,N., Smith,C., Zlotnik,A. and Arai,K.-I. (1986) *Proc. Natl. Acad. Sci. USA*, **83**, 2061.
25. Swain,S.L. and Dutton,R.W. (1982) *J. Exp. Med.*, **156**, 1821.
26. O'Garra,A., Warren,D.J., Holman,M., Popham,A.M., Sanderson,C.J. and Klaus,G.G.B. (1986) *Proc. Natl. Acad. Sci. USA*, **83**, 5228.
27. Kinashi,T., Harada,N., Severinson,E., Tanabe,T., Sideras,P., Konishi,M., Azuma,C., Tominaga,T., Bergstedt-Lindqvist,S., Takahashi,M., Matsuda,F., Yaoita,Y., Takatsu,K. and Honjo,T. (1986) *Nature*, **324**, 70.
28. Sanderson,C.J., O'Garra,A., Warren,D.J. and Klaus,G.G.B. (1986) *Proc. Natl. Acad. Sci. USA*, **83**, 437.
29. Hirano,T, Yasukawa,K., Harada,H., Taga,T., Watanabe,Y., Matsuda,T., Kashiwamura,S.-i., Nakajima,K., Koyama,K., Iwamatsu,A., Tsunasawa,S., Sakiyama,F., Matsui,H., Takahara,Y., Taniguchi,T. and Kishimoto,T. (1986) *Nature*, **324**, 73.
30. Haegman,G., Content,J., Volckaert,G., Derynck,R., Tavernier,J. and Fiers,W. (1986) *Eur. J. Biochem.*, **159**, 625.
31. Van Damme,J., Opdenakker,G., Simpson,R.J., Rubiro, M.R., Cayphas,S., Vink,A., Billiau, A. and van Snick,J. (1987) *J. Exp. Med.*, **165**, 914.
32. Gery,I., Gershon,R.K. and Waksman,B.H. (1972) *J. Exp. Med.*, **136**, 128.
33. Auron,P.E., Webb,A.C., Rosenwasser,L.J., Mucci,S.F., Rich,A., Wolff,S.M. and Dinarello,C.A. (1984) *Proc. Natl. Acad. Sci. USA*, **81**, 7907.
34. March,C., Mosley,B., Larsen,A., Cerretti,D.P., Braedt,G., Price,V., Gillis,S., Henney,C.S., Kronheim,S.R., Grobstein,K., Conlon,P.J., Hopp,T.P. and Cosman,D. (1985) *Nature*, **315**, 641.
35. Lomedico,P.T., Gubler,U., Hellman,C.P., Dukovich,M., Giri,J.G., Pan,Y.-C., Collier,R.S., Chua,A.O. and Mizel,S.B. (1984) *Nature*, **312**, 458.
36. Gillis,S. and Mizel,S.B. (1981) *Proc. Natl. Acad. Sci. USA*, **78**, 1133.
37. Satsangi,J., Wolstencroft,R.A., Cason,J., Ainley,C.C., Dumonde,D.C. and Thompson,R.P.H. (1987) *Clin. Exp. Immunol.*, **67**, 594.
38. Morgan,D.A., Ruscetti,F.W. and Gallo,R.C. (1976) *Science*, **193**, 1007.
39. Matsui,H., Fujita,T., Nishi-Takaoka,C., Hamuro,J. and Taniguchi,T. (1986) In *Lymphokines*. Pick,E. and Landy,M. (eds), Academic Press Inc., London and New York, Vol. 12, p. 1.
40. Gillis,S., Ferm,M.M., Ou,W. and Smith,K.A. (1978) *J. Immunology*, **120**, 2027.
41. Tada,H., Shiho,O., Kuroshima,K., Koyama,M. and Tsukamoto,K. (1986) *J. Immunol. Methods*, **93**, 157.

42. Hamblin,A. (1981) In *Techniques in Clinical Immunology*. Thompson,R.A. (ed), Blackwell Scientific Publications, Oxford, p. 272.
43. Boylston,A.W., Anderson,R.L. and Haworth,A. (1981) *Clin. Exp. Immunol.*, **43**, 329.
44. Harbeck,R.J., Hoffman,A.A., Redecker,S., Biundo,T. and Kurnick,J. (1982) *Clin. Immunol. Immunopathol.*, **23**, 682.
45. Burgess,A.W., Camarkaris,J. and Metcalf,D. (1977) *J. Biol. Chem.*, **252**, 1998.
46. Howard,M., Burgess,A.W., McPhee,D. and Metcalf,D. (1980) *Cell*, **18**, 993.
47. Burgess,A.W., Metcalf,D., Russell,S.H.M. and Nicola,N.A. (1980) *Biochem. J.*, **185**, 301.
48. Lee,J.C., Hapel,A.J. and Ihle,J.N. (1982) *J. Immunol.*, **128**, 2393.
49. Ihle,J.N., Keller,J., Greenberger,J.S., Henderson,L., Yetter,R.A. and Morse,H.C. (1982) *J. Immunol.*, **129**, 1377.
50. Rennick,D.M., Lee,F.D., Yakota,T., Arai,K., Cantor,H. and Nabel,G.J. (1985) *J. Immunol.*, **134**, 910.
51. Yang,Y.C., Ciarletta,A.B., Temple,P.A., Cheng,M.P., Kovacic,S., Witek-Giannetti,J.A.S., Leary,A.C., Kriz,R., Donahue,R.E., Wong,G.G. and Clark,S.C. (1986) *Cell*, **47**, 3.
52. Nicola,N.A. and Vadas,M. (1984) *Immunol. Today*, **5**, 76.
53. Iscove,N.N., Roitsch,C. and Hirama,M. (1984) *Lymphokine Res.*, **3**, 67.
54. Schrader,J.W., Clark-Lewis,I., Crapper,R.M. and Wong,G.W. (1983) *Immunol. Rev.*, **76**, 79.
55. Gough,N.M., Gough,J., Metcalf,D., Kelso,A., Grail,D., Nicola,N.A., Burgess,A.W. and Dunn,A.R. (1984) *Nature*, **309**, 763.
56. Greenberger,J.S., Eckner,R., Ostertag,W., Colleta,B., Bashetti,S., Nagasawa,H., Karpas,A., Weicheselbaum,R. and Moloney,W. (1980) *Virology*, **105**, 425.
57. Dexter,T.M., Allen,T.D. and Teich,N.M. (1980) In *Experimental Haematology Today*. Baum,S.J., Ledney,G.D. and van Belckun,D.W. (eds), Karger, Basel, Switzerland, p. 145.
58. Ihle,J.N., Keller,J., Henderson,L., Klein,F. and Palaszynski,E. (1982) *J. Immunol.*, **129**, 2431.
59. Greenberger,J.S., Sakakeeny,M.A., Humphries,R.K., Eaves,C.J. and Eckner,R.J. (1983) *Proc. Natl. Acad. Sci. USA*, **80**, 2931.
60. Metcalf,D. (1970) *J. Cell. Physiol.*, **76**, 89.
61. Yokota,T., Otsuka,T., Mosmann,T., Banchereau,J., DeFrance,T., Blanchard,D., De Vries,J.E., Lee,F. and Arai,K. (1986) *Proc. Natl. Acad. Sci. USA*, **83**, 5894.
62. Azuma,C., Tanabe,T., Konishi,M., Kinashi,T., Noma,T., Matsuda,F., Yaoita,Y., Takatsu,K., Hammarstrom,L., Smith,C.I.E., Severinson,E. and Honjo,T. (1986) *Nucleic Acids Res.*, **14**, 9149.
63. Howard,M., Farrar,J., Hilfiker,M., Johnson,B., Kiyoshi,T., Takatsu,K., Hamaoka,T. and Paul,W.E. (1982) *J. Exp. Med.*, **155**, 914.
64. Yoshizaki,K., Nagagawa,T., Fukunaga,K., Kaieda,T., Maruyama,S., Kisimoto,S., Yamamura,Y. and Kishimoto,T. (1983) *J. Immunol.*, **130**, 1241.
65. Muraguchi,A., Kasahara,T., Oppenheim,J. and Fauci,A. (1982) *J. Immunol.*, **129**, 2486.
66. Maizel,A.L., Morgan,J.W., Mehta,S.R., Kouttab,N.M., Bator,N.M. and Sahasrabuddhe,C.S. (1983) *Proc. Natl. Acad. Sci. USA*, **80**, 5047.
67. Roehm,N.W., Leibson,H.J., Zlotnik,A., Kappler,J., Marrack,P. and Cambier,J.C. (1984) *J. Exp. Med.*, **160**, 679.
68. Noelle,R., Krammer,P.H., Ohara,J., Uhr,J.W. and Vitetta,E.S. (1984) *Proc. Natl. Acad. Sci. USA*, **81**, 6149.
69. O'Garra,A. and Sanderson,C.J. (1987) In *Lymphokines and Interferons — A Practical Approach*. Clemens,M.J., Morris,A.G. and Gearing,A.J.H. (eds), IRL Press, Oxford and Washington, DC, p.323.
70. Kung,J.T., Sharrow,S.O., Ahmed,A., Habbersett,R., Scher,I. and Paul,W.E. (1982) *J. Immunol.*, **128**, 2049.
71. Klaus,G.G.B., Hawrylowicz,C.M., Holman,M. and Keeler,K.D. (1984) *Immunology*, **53**, 693.
72. Coffman,R.L. and Carty,J. (1986) *J. Immunol.*, **136**, 949.
73. Nabel,G., Galli,S.J., Dvorak,A.M., Dvorak,H.F. and Cantor,H. (1981) *Nature*, **291**, 332.
74. Smith,C.A. and Rennick,D.M. (1986) *Proc. Natl. Acad. Sci. USA*, **83**, 1857.
75. Mossman,T.R. (1983) *J. Immunol. Methods*, **65**, 55.
76. Harada,N., Kikuchi,Y., Tominaga,A., Takaki,S. and Takatsu,K. (1985) *J. Immunol.*, **134**, 3944.
77. Gronowicz,E., Coutinho,A. and Melchers,F. (1976) *Eur. J. Immunol.*, **6**, 588.
78. Takatsu,K., Tanaka,K., Tominaga,A., Kumahara,Y. and Hamaoka,T. (1980) *J. Immunol.*, **125**, 2646.
79. Sanderson,C.J., Warren,D.J. and Strath,M. (1985) *J. Exp. Med.*, **162**, 60.
80. Strath,M. and Sanderson,C.J. (1985) *J. Cell Sci.*, **74**, 207.
81. Strath,M., Warren,D.J. and Sanderson,C.J. (1985) *J. Immunol. Methods*, **83**, 209.
82. Hirano,T., Taga,T., Nakano,N., Yasukawa,K., Kashiwamura,S., Shimizu,K., Nakajima,K., Pyun,K.H. and Kishimoto,T. (1985) *Proc. Natl. Acad. Sci. USA*, **82**, 5490.
83. Hirano,T., Teranishi,T., Toba,H., Sakaguchi,N., Fukukawa,T. and Tsuyuguchi,I. (1981) *J. Immunol.*, **126**, 517.

227

84. Hirano,T., Teranishi,T. and Onoue,K. (1984) *J. Immunol.*, **132**, 229.
85. Shimizu,K., Hirano,T., Ishibashi,K., Nakano,N., Taga,T., Sugamura,K., Yamamura,Y. and Kishimoto,T. (1985) *J. Immunol.*, **134**, 1728.
85. Rawle,F.C., Shields,J., Smith,S.H., Iliescu,V., Merkenschlager,M., Beverley,P.C.L. and Callard,R.E. (1986) *Eur. J. Immunol.*, **16**, 1017.
87. Kaplan,M.E., Woodson,M. and Clark,C. (1976) In *In Vitro Methods in Cell Mediated and Tumor Immunity*. Bloom,B.R. and David,J.R. (eds), Academic Press, New York, p. 83.
88. Goldsmith,P.K. (1987) *Anal. Biochem.*, **117**, 53.
89. Saiki,O. and Ralph,P. (1983) *Eur. J. Immunol.*, **13**, 31.
90. Muraguchi,A., Kishimoto,T., Miki,Y., Kuritani,T., Kaieda,T., Yoshizaki,K. and Yamamura,Y. (1981) *J. Immunol.*, **127**, 412.
91. Dumonde,D.C. and Papermaster,B.W. (1984) *Lymphokine Res.*, **3**, 193.
92. Hamblin,A.S., Zawisza,B., Shipton,U., Dumonde,D.C., den Hollander,F.C. and Verheul,H. (1982) *J. Immunol. Methods*, **59**, 317.
93. Dumonde,D.C. (1986) *Lymphokine Res.*, **5**, Supplement 1, 1.

CHAPTER 11

Biochemical characterization of lymphocyte surface antigens

ADELINA A.DAVIES and MARION H.BROWN

1. INTRODUCTION

The approach taken by cellular immunologists to characterize a lymphocyte surface antigen is usually to begin with an antibody. In the majority of cases the antibody has been raised by immunization with whole cells, that is against the native molecule as it occurs on the cell surface. If, on the other hand, the characterization of a lymphocyte surface antigen is to be approached from a knowledge of its DNA sequence, the antibody will most probably have been raised against a synthetic peptide. These antibodies are likely to have different reactivities with respect to unfolded versus native antigen in that they recognize the former but not necessarily the latter.

The initial biochemical questions asked by a cellular immunologist about an antigen include: What is its molecular weight? Does it consist of one chain or several linked by disulphide bonds? Is it glycosylated? Is it synthesized by the cells on which it appears? Is it phosphorylated? Is it different from previously identified antigens?

Two primary approaches are used to answer these questions depending on the properties of the antibody. The first, useful particularly with antibody binding to native protein, is to immunoprecipitate the antigen from cells labelled with a radioactive isotope and analyse it electrophoretically [e.g. by sodium dodecyl sulphate (SDS) polyacrylamide gel electrophoresis (PAGE) in one or two dimensions; isoelectric focusing (IEF), non-equilibrium pH gradient electrophoresis (NEPHGE), non-reducing/reducing two-dimensional gel electrophoresis].

The other approach employed, particularly if the antibody is against a synthetic peptide, is to use it to identify the unfolded antigen, for example denatured with SDS and immobilized on a membrane. This can be done using the technique of immunoblotting combined with SDS−PAGE. Recognition of denatured antigen is a useful property if the gene for the antigen is to be cloned. Thus, such antibody can be used to screen a λgt11 expression library.

The aim of this chapter is to present a straightforward approach to the biochemical characterization of lymphocyte surface antigens. The emphasis is on using an antibody and the techniques of immunoprecipitation and immunoblotting combined with SDS−PAGE to establish some of the more pertinent properties of the specific antigen.

2. IMMUNOPRECIPITATION

2.1 Introduction

Immunoprecipitation is a widely used method that, in combination with the use of radioactive isotopic labelling, allows characterization of an antigen biochemically, without having to purify large amounts of it. Specific antibody can be used to isolate detectable amounts of antigen from relatively few radiolabelled cells. For instance, 10^7 cells are ample for immunoprecipitation of the CD3 antigen which is expressed on the T cell surface at a density of 30 000 molecules per cell. The more antigen present, the lower the number of cells needed for immunoprecipitation. Characterization by immunoprecipitation is applicable when the epitope recognized by the antibody is exposed on the antigen either in its native form or after unfolding by denaturation.

The first step is to label the antigen with an appropriate radioactive isotope. The selective use of different isotopes makes it possible to gain a great deal of information about the nature and location of an antigen. There are two primary approaches to radioactive labelling: biosynthetic and *in situ* labelling of cell surface molecules. The most commonly used biosynthetic label is [^{35}S]methionine, as it has a high specific activity and is incorporated to a detectable amount by most proteins that are synthesized at a reasonable

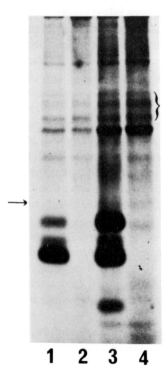

1   2   3   4

Figure 1. Immunoprecipitation of CD3 **(tracks 1 and 3)** and CD2 **(tracks 2 and 4)** from the human T leukaemia cell line J6 **(tracks 1 and 2)** and human T blasts **(tracks 3 and 4)** labelled with [^{35}S]methionine for 4 h. The arrow indicates the expected position of the CD3 γ chain (26 kd); the δ and ϵ chains can be clearly seen below this. The bracket shows the expected position of CD2, which is so weakly labelled that it is indistinguishable from 'background' bands (compare **tracks 3 and 4**).

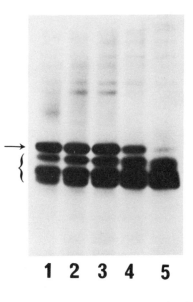

1 2 3 4 5

Figure 2. Immunoprecipitation of CD3 from human T blasts labelled for 10 min with [^{35}S]methionine and chased with cold methionine for 0 min **(track 1)**, 15 min **(track 2)**, 30 min **(track 3)**, 60 min **(track 4)** and 120 min **(track 5)**. The arrow indicates the immature form of CD3 γ chain (23 kd); the mature form is not visible. The bracket shows the positions of the CD3 δ and ϵ polypeptides and their precursors.

level ($\sim 10^4$ molecules/cell) and rate. However, even though a protein may contain methionine it may not label readily with the isotope, for example CD2 (*Figure 1*). The precursor form of the CD3γ chain (23 kd) labels well with [^{35}S]methionine, whereas the mature form (26 kd) is difficult to detect (*Figures 1 and 2*).

When a protein cannot be detected by incorporation of [^{35}S]methionine because, for example, it contains too few methionine residues, alternative biosynthetic labels are available, for example [^{35}S]cysteine, or [^{3}H] and [^{14}C]amino acid mixtures. Other properties of antigens, for instance acylation and glycosylation, can be investigated using [^{3}H]fatty acids such as palmitic acid (1), and [^{3}H]sugars such as mannose, respectively. Many surface proteins, particularly those that are receptors or receptor-associated, are phosphorylated. It is feasible to study the effects of activators or ligands on these antigens by labelling with ^{32}P. For example, exposure of T lymphocytes to phorbol esters, which activate protein kinase C, initiates the phosphorylation of the T3γ chain and hyper-phosphorylates the Class I antigen and transferrin receptor (*Figure 3*) (2).

Proteins that are exposed on the cell surface can be selectively labelled with ^{125}I in a carefully controlled reaction catalysed by lactoperoxidase. Immunoprecipitation from cells labelled in this way is a useful method for confirming the location of an antigen. As only a small percentage of total cellular proteins are labelled by lactoperoxidase-catalysed iodination, the number of labelled irrelevant proteins is reduced. If these are non-specifically immunoprecipitated they cause background on autoradiographs, often a problem with biosynthetic labelling. Proteins such as CD2 and the CD3γ chain that do not readily incorporate biosynthetic label may label well with [^{125}I]lactoperoxidase (*Figures 3 and 4*).

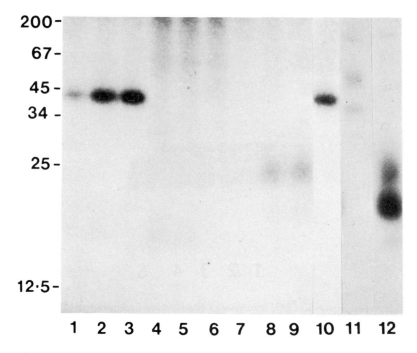

Figure 3. Phosphorylation of surface antigen induced by phorbol esters (2). Human peripheral blood acute lymphocytic leukaemia (HPBALL) cells, labelled for 3 h with ^{32}P, were treated with phorbol ester for 0 min **(tracks 1, 4, 7)**, 5 min **(tracks 2, 5, 8)** or 15 min **(tracks 3, 6, 9)** prior to immunoprecipitation with antibodies against Class I antigens **(tracks 1−3)**, T cell receptor (Ti) **(tracks 4−6)** or CD3 **(tracks 7−9)**. **Tracks 10−12** show immunoprecipitations of Class I, Ti and CD3, respectively, from [^{125}I]lactoperoxidase labelled HPBALL cells. Protein A−Sepharose was used as the immunoprecipitation method.

Immunoprecipitation of antigen from labelled cells requires the cells to be lysed and the antigen solubilized so that it can be selectively precipitated with antibody. Thus, the conditions used to lyse the labelled cells are important. Non-ionic [e.g. Nonidet P-40 (NP-40)] and weakly ionic (e.g. sodium deoxycholate) detergents are generally employed to solubilize and disperse antigens in their native state. Non-ionic detergents, such as Triton-X114, have been used to distinguish between hydrophilic proteins and integral membrane proteins which have an amphiphilic nature (3). Strongly ionic detergents, such as SDS, can be used to expose an epitope that is buried in the tertiary structure of the molecule.

Apart from the direct characterization of the specific antigen, immunoprecipitation can be used, by judicious choice of detergent, to identify molecules that are associated with an antigen. Solubilization with mild detergents, such as CHAPS (4), or digitonin (5), preserves macromolecular complexes, so that molecules associated with a particular antigen may be co-precipitated (*Figure 5*).

Immunoprecipitation can be used to determine if an antigen contains N-linked carbohydrate of the high mannose or complex type, and/or O-linked oligosaccharides. Antigen purified by immunoprecipitation can be enzymatically digested with a glycosidase of the appropriate specificity prior to analysis by SDS−PAGE. Removal of carbohydrate from the antigen by this means is detected as a reduction in apparent molecular weight.

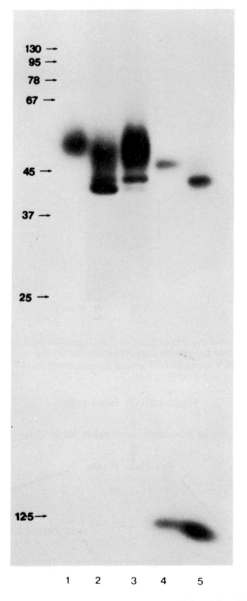

Figure 4. Endo F treatment of CD2 and Class I antigen immunoprecipitated from NP-40 lysates of the human T leukaemia cell line J6 labelled at the surface with ^{125}I (6): **track 1**, CD2; **track 2**, CD2 + 1.8 U Endo F; **track 3**, CD2 + 0.18 U Endo F; **track 4**, Class I; **track 5**, Class I + 1.8 U Endo F. β_2 microglobulin (12 500 mol. wt) is not glycosylated.

Alterations in glycosylation status of a protein during post-translational processing can be determined by assessing its sensitivity to different glycosidases with time. Deglycosylation permits an assessment of the molecular weight of the protein backbone of the molecule, for example that for CD2 is approximately 40 kd, represented by the band

233

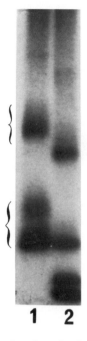

Figure 5. Immunoprecipitation of the CD3 antigen (lower brackets) showing co-precipitation of the antigen receptor (upper bracket). HPBALL cells were surface labelled with ^{125}I and immunoprecipitated using antibody coupled to beads. **Track 1** shows the CD3 antigen/receptor before Endo F treatment; **track 2** shows the effects of three treatments with 0.25 U of Endo F.

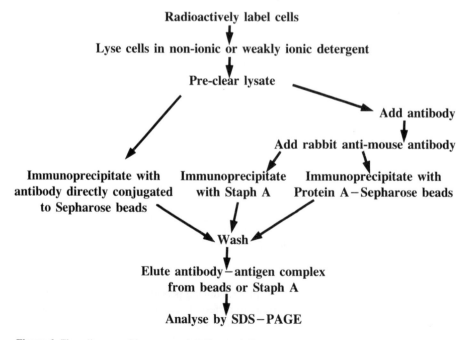

Figure 6. Flow diagram of immunoprecipitation procedure.

revealed after digestion of a CD2 immunoprecipitate with β-endo-glycosaminidase-F which removes both immature and mature N-linked oligosaccharides (*Figure 4*) (6). The effects of Endo F treatment of the CD3 antigen are shown in *Figure 5*.

A detailed protocol for immunoprecipitation is given below and outlined in *Figure 6*. Three radiolabelling methods are described, followed by details of immunoprecipitation using either *Staphylococcus aureus* (Staph A) or Protein A−Sepharose beads. In the final section there are some applications of the basic technique.

2.2 Radiolabelling of cells

2.2.1 *Cell surface iodination using lactoperoxidase (7)*

Lactoperoxidase cannot cross the plasma membrane of viable cells, and under the carefully controlled conditions described below, only proteins exposed on the cell surface are iodinated. It is important to use cells with a high viability ($>95\%$), to avoid labelling the intracellular proteins of dead cells. To maintain viability keep cells in phosphate-buffered saline (PBS) for as short a time as possible, and check that the viability does not decrease during the experiments. Another important parameter for ensuring vectorial labelling is the iodide concentration. This should always be lower than the lactoperoxidase concentration, so that all the iodide is bound to the enzyme and none is free to cross the plasma membrane and label intracellular proteins. Under the conditions described here the lactoperoxidase concentration is about 100-fold greater than the iodide concentration. Thus, the amount of iodide used to label the cells can safely be increased, if the need arises.

For safety reasons it is vital that the iodination is performed in a good fumehood.

(i) *Materials required.*

PBS, 10 mM sodium phosphate buffer pH 7.2, 0.17 M NaCl, 3 mM KCl
Cells in PBS
Lactoperoxidase (Sigma) (0.2 mg $\equiv$ 20 U/ml) in PBS (store in aliquots at $-70°C$)
Glucose oxidase (Sigma) (1 U/ml) in PBS
100 mM glucose in PBS
Sodium ^{125}iodide, carrier free (Amersham International: 100 mCi/ml)

(ii) *Method.*

(1)   Wash the cells quickly three times with PBS, by centrifugation. Count and adjust to 10^8/ml.
(2)   To 100 μl of cell suspension, add 10 μl of lactoperoxidase, 20 μl of glucose oxidase, 10 μl of glucose and 500 μCi ^{125}I (5 μl).
(3)   Cap the tube, mix and incubate for 10 min at 20°C.
(4)   Wash the cells three times with PBS.

2.2.2 *[^{35}S]Methionine biosynthetic labelling*

Two methods of biosynthetic labelling are described, the application of which depends on the number of molecules of a particular protein and their rate of turnover. The 4 h labelling gives good incorporation of [^{35}S]methionine into many proteins; however, those that are biosynthesized at a slow rate may need an overnight period of labelling.

T3γ chain is an exception to this, as it is only revealed by short labelling periods and disappears during long labelling procedures. The reason for this is not known, but it serves to illustrate that the best labelling conditions for a particular protein may need to be tested by experiment.

(i) *Materials required.*

Methionine-free RPMI 1640 medium
[^{35}S]Methionine (Amersham International: 15 mCi/ml)
Fetal calf serum (FCS) dialysed against PBS
Cells

(ii) *Method.*

(1)   Wash the cells three times with methionine-free medium by centrifugation. Count and adjust to 2×10^6 cells/ml in the same medium containing 10% FCS.
(2)   Incubate the cells for 45 min at 37°C.
(3)   Either (a) Add [^{35}S]methionine to a concentration of 20 μCi/ml. Label the cells overnight at 37°C.
     o r   (b) After incubation in the methionine-free medium, centrifuge the cells and resuspend at 10^8/ml in the same medium. Label the cells for 4 h at 37°C with [^{35}S]methionine at a concentration of 1 mCi/ml.

2.2.3 ^{32}P labelling

Most phosphoproteins are sufficiently labelled after 3 h. To increase the incorporation into a particular protein, label for a longer time and/or use a higher concentration of ^{32}Pi. If the cells are labelled for longer than 6 h the 'background' seen on the auto-radiographs of immunoprecipitates can be a problem.

(i) *Materials required.*

Phosphate-free Eagle's minimum essential medium
[^{32}P]orthophosphate (Amersham International: 10 mCi/ml)
FCS dialysed against saline
Cells

(ii) *Method.*

(1)   Wash the cells three times with phosphate-free medium by centrifugation. Count and adjust to 2×10^6 /ml in the same medium containing 10% FCS.
(2)   Incubate the cells for 45 min at 37°C, then add the ^{32}Pi to a concentration of 40 μCi/ml. Label the cells for 3−6 h at 37°C. Quiescent cells need to be labelled overnight.

2.3 Immunoprecipitation using *Staphylococcus aureus*

2.3.1 *Materials required*

The recipes for lysis buffer and other solutions required are given in *Table 1*. The methods for radioactively labelling cells are given in Section 2.2.

Table 1. Recipes for immunoprecipitation solutions.

1.	Lysis buffer = 10 mM Tris-HCl buffer pH 7.4, 1% NP-40 (w/v), 150 mM NaCl, 1 mM diethylenediamine tetraacetic acid (EDTA)
2.	Lysis buffer containing bovine serum albumin (BSA, 1 mg/ml)
3.	Wash buffer 1 = lysis buffer plus 0.5 M NaCl Wash buffer 2 = lysis buffer plus 0.1% SDS Wash buffer 3 = 10 mM Tris-HCl buffer pH 7.4, 0.1% NP-40
4.	3.5 M NaCl solution
5.	1 M phenylmethylsulphonyl fluoride (PMSF, Sigma) in acetone (care: poison)

Table 2. Protease inhibitors.

1.	20 mM iodoacetamide
2.	50 μg/ml soybean trypsin inhibitor
3.	2 μg/ml leupeptin

2.3.2 *Cell lysis*

(i) Wash the cells twice in RPMI 1640 by centrifugation.

(ii) Resuspend the cell pellet in 50 μl of PBS per 2 × 10^7 cells.

(iii) Add 1 ml of lysis buffer containing BSA, plus 1 μl of PMSF per 2 × 10^7 cells.

(iv) Mix gently and leave on ice for 30 min.

(v) Centrifuge at 400 g for 5 min to pellet the nuclei.

(vi) Remove the supernatant and centrifuge this at 100 000 g for 60 min at 4°C in an ultracentrifuge.

If time is short, centrifuging at 10 000 g for 15 min at 4°C in a microcentrifuge is adequate. The lysate may be stored at −70°C at this stage. 0.5 ml (10^7 cells) of lysate is used for each antibody/immunoprecipitation.

Various other protease inhibitors can be added to the lysis buffer if degradation is a problem (see *Table 2*). The lysates should always be kept cold because of this. If the cells have been labelled with ^{32}P then phosphatase inhibitors should be added. Vanadate (8) is specific for tyrosine phosphatases and sodium fluoride (50 mM) for threonine/serine phosphatases.

If the antibody recognizes an epitope that is only exposed when the antigen is unfolded, then the antigen must be treated with SDS prior to the immunoprecipitation.

(i) Add 1 ml of lysis buffer containing BSA per 2 × 10^8 cells.

(ii) Mix gently and leave on ice for 30 min.

(iii) Centrifuge at 400 g for 5 min at 4°C to pellet the nuclei.

(iv) Remove the supernatant and add SDS to this to a final concentration of 1%.

(v) Boil for 5 min and then dilute the supernatant 10-fold with lysis buffer plus BSA, plus 1 μl of PMSF/ml, so that the lysate is at an equivalent of 2 × 10^7 cells/ml and the SDS concentration is at a suitable level (0.1%) for antibody−antigen interaction.

(vi) Centrifuge at 100 000 g for 60 min at 4°C in an ultracentrifuge.

2.3.3 *Pre-clearing lysates*

(i)   Wash Staph A (9) twice in lysis buffer and resuspend as a 10% solution in lysis buffer plus BSA. Adjust the NaCl concentration to 0.5 M (to 1 ml of solution add 0.1 ml of 3.5 M NaCl).

(ii) Add 100 μl of washed Staph A per 1 ml of lysate (2×10^7 cells) and *rotate* for 60 min at room temperature or overnight at 4°C.

(iii) Spin at 10 000 g for 5 min at 4°C in a microcentrifuge to pellet the Staph A. This pre-clears the lysate of material that binds non-specifically to the Staph A.

(iv) Decant the supernatant and adjust the salt concentration to 0.5 M NaCl concentration (to 1 ml of pre-cleared lysate add 0.1 ml of 3.5 M NaCl).

2.3.4 *Immunoprecipitation*

(i)   Add 10 μg of purified antibody or 10 μl of ascites fluid or serum to 0.5 ml of pre-cleared lysate ($\equiv 10^7$ cells).

(ii) Incubate for 60 min at room temperature or overnight at 4°C if the antibody has a low affinity. The amount of antibody used may need to be titrated between 3 and 30 μg to obtain good precipitates. If a monoclonal antibody is used that is of an immunoglobulin class that does not bind Staph A (10), after the initial antibody incubation add rabbit anti-mouse immunoglobulin (2 μg/μg of monoclonal antibody) and incubate for 45 min on ice.

(iii) Add 50 μl of washed Staph A and rotate for 60 min at 4°C.

(iv) Spin at 10 000 g for 5 min at 4°C in a microcentrifuge. Remove the supernatant. This can be used again for immunoprecipitations with other antibodies (store at −70°C).

2.3.5 *Washing*

(i)   Add 1 ml of wash 1 to the Staph A pellet and resuspend *well*, using a pipette or a vortex mixer.

(ii) Centrifuge at 10 000 g for 5 min at 4°C in a microcentrifuge.

(iii) Discard the supernatant and wash the Staph A pellet with washes 2 and 3 as in steps (i) and (ii).

2.3.6 *Preparing for SDS−PAGE*

(i)   Resuspend the pellet in 50−100 μl of SDS sample buffer (see Section 4.2).

(ii) Boil for 4 min.

(iii) Spin at 10 000 g for 5 min at 4°C in a microcentrifuge.

(iv) Remove the supernatant and load onto an SDS−polyacrylamide gel for analysis. For quantitative recovery of antigen re-boil the Staph A with a further 50 μl of sample buffer, spin and combine this supernatant with the previous one. The eluted antigen can be stored at −20°C prior to analysis by SDS−PAGE. In this case re-boil the sample after thawing, before applying to the gel.

2.4 Immunoprecipitation using Protein A – Sepharose

2.4.1 *Preparing the Protein A – Sepharose (Pharmacia)*

Wash the beads in the same way as the Staph A (see Section 2.3.3). Resuspend as a 10% suspension.

2.4.2 *Immunoprecipitation*

(i)   Lyse the cells, pre-clear and add antibody in the same way as for Staph A (see Sections 2.3.2, 2.3.3 and 2.3.4).
(ii) Add 30 μl of washed Protein A – Sepharose beads to the lysate after incubation with the antibody. Rotate for 60 min at 4°C.

2.4.3 *Washing*

(i)   Centrifuge at 10 000 g for 30 sec at 4°C in a microcentrifuge.
(ii)   Carefully remove about 400 μl of the supernatant with a Pasteur pipette.
(iii)   Remove the rest of the supernatant with a special Hamilton syringe. This is a 100 μl syringe with a very narrow bore and blunt end (point style 3) that the beads are too large to enter. The beads resuspend very easily, so take care not to knock the tube.
(iv)   Add 100 μl of wash 1 to the beads and vortex for 5 sec.
(v)   Remove the solution with the Hamilton syringe.
(vi)   Add 100 μl of wash 2, carefully washing the beads back down the sides of the tubes: if some beads remain up the side of the tube, then centrifuge for 30 sec in the microcentrifuge. Vortex.
(vii)   Repeat (v) and (vi) with wash 3.

2.4.4 *Preparing for SDS – PAGE*

(i)   Add 50 – 100 μl of SDS sample buffer, boil for 4 min.
(ii)   Spin at 10 000 g for 30 sec in a microcentrifuge.
(iii)   Remove the supernatant with the Hamilton syringe and load onto an SDS – polyacrylamide gel.

2.5 Immunoprecipitation using antibody directly conjugated to Sepharose beads

A further improvement to using Protein A – Sepharose is to covalently bind the antibody directly to CNBr-activated Sepharose beads (Pharmacia). As little as 1 mg of antibody can adequately be bound to 1 ml of beads. Antibody – Sepharose is used in exactly the same way as the Protein A – Sepharose. The immunoprecipitation shown in *Figures 1* and *2* were performed using antibody coupled to beads.

2.6 Comparison of immunoprecipitation methods

The quickest immunoprecipitation method, and that which results in the lowest backgrounds on autoradiographs, is to use antibody directly coupled to beads. However, it is only worth the cost and effort of purifying and coupling the antibody if it is to be used regularly. If the quantity of antibody is low or only a few immunoprecipitations are required, then the use of Protein A−Sepharose is recommended. This is, however, expensive and the Staph A method may be adequate, as long as the antigen labels well, is abundant and the antibody is of high affinity. If the antigen−antibody does not meet these criteria, then high backgrounds on autoradiographs can be a problem. The Staph A method is more tedious, as it takes a longer time to resuspend the pellet during the washing procedures.

2.7 Immunoprecipitation applications

2.7.1 Glycosylation status

Antigens, that have been purified by immunoprecipitation, can be treated with various enzymes that cleave their different carbohydrate moieties, prior to SDS−PAGE analysis. Endo-β-N-acetylglucosaminidase F (Endo F) cleaves mature and immature N-linked carbohydrate moieties (see *Figures 4* and *5*) and Endo-α-N-acetylgalactosaminidase (O-glucanase) cleaves mature O-linked carbohydrate moieties from glycoproteins. Both these enzymes can be used to help estimate the molecular weight of the protein backbone of a glycoprotein. Endo-β-N-acetylglucosaminidase H (Endo H) cleaves immature, high mannose carbohydrate moieties and can be used to study the glycosylation processing of a protein in transit to the plasma membrane. Sialic acid attached to N- and O-linked carbohydrate moieties can be depleted with neuraminidase, thereby reducing the charge heterogeneity of an antigen and facilitating interpretation of 'spots' on two-dimensional gels.

Table 3 lists the buffers required for endoglycosidase treatment and a description of the protocols used for the endoglycosidases and neuraminidase treatment is given below. O-Glucanase is made by the Genzyme Corporation and can be obtained, along with the method of use, from Koch-Light Ltd.

(1)   Immunoprecipitate antigen using the methods described in Sections 2.3, 2.4 or 2.5. Lyse 10^7 cells in 0.5 ml for each immunoprecipitation.
(2)   Centrifuge the precipitates after the final wash 3, and discard the supernatants.
(3)   Add 10 μl of buffer A (*Table 3*) to the pellet of Staph A or Sepharose beads with the antigen bound to them. Boil for 5 min. Centrifuge and keep the supernatant.
(4)   Add another 10 μl of buffer A to the pellet and repeat step 3.

(i) Endo F treatment.

(1)   Combine the supernatants (20 μl) from step 3 above and add 80 μl of buffer B.
(2)   Add 1 μl of Endo F (250 U/ml, NEN Research Products) and 1 μl of PMSF (1 M in acetone) and incubate for 16 h at 37°C.
(3)   After 16 h and 24 h add a further 1 μl each of Endo F and PMSF.
(4)   Finally, after a total of 40 h add 100 μl of cold 25% trichloroacetic acid (TCA), leave 30 min on ice.
(5)   Centrifuge at 10 000 g for 5 min at 4°C in a microcentrifuge.
(6)   Carefully remove the supernatant and wash the pellet with 1 ml of cold acetone. Centrifuge at 10 000 g for 10 min at 4°C in a microcentrifuge and repeat the acetone wash of the pellet.

Table 3. Buffers required for endoglycosidase treatment.

A.	100 mM Tris-HCl buffer pH 7.4
	1% SDS
	1% β-mercaptoethanol
B.	0.1 M sodium phosphate buffer pH 6.1
	50 mM EDTA
	1% NP-40
	0.1% SDS
	1% β-mercaptoethanol
C.	150 mM sodium citrate buffer pH 5.5
D.	100 mM sodium acetate buffer pH 5.5
	0.3 M NaCl
	0.2% $CaCl_2$

(7)   Dry the tube.

(8)   Add SDS sample buffer, boil for 4 min, and analyse by SDS−PAGE and auto-radiography.

After the acetone washes, it is not always possible to see the pellet. Do not worry, it is just very small.

Some antigens are more resistant to Endo F than others and further treatment may be required to get good digestion.

(ii) *Endo H treatment.*

(1)   Combine the supernatants from step 3 above and add 80 μl of buffer C.

(2)   Add 1 μl of Endo H (45−74 μg/ml, NEN Research Products) and incubate for 16 h at 37°C.

(3)   Add 100 μl of cold 25% TCA and precipitate the antigen and wash it as described in the Endo F treatment.

(iii) *Neuraminidase treatment.*

(1)   Combine the supernatants from step 3 above and add 80 μl of buffer D.

(2)   Add 1 μl of neuraminidase (100 U/ml, Sigma) and 1 μl of PMSF (1 M in acetone), incubate for 16 h at 37°C.

(3)   Add 100 μl of cold 25% TCA and precipitate the antigen and wash it as described in the Endo F treatment.

2.7.2 Comparison with known antigens

The techniques of immunoprecipitation and immunoblotting can be modified to compare an unknown antigen with those previously characterized.

(i) *Sequential immunoprecipitation.* The principle of this technique is that if two antigens are identical, removal of one from a cell lysate will prevent subsequent precipitation of the other. The procedure depends upon the removal of all the first antigen from a labelled cell lysate which may take more than one cycle of immunoprecipitation. To ensure that a lysate is thoroughly depleted, wash the immunoprecipitates from each

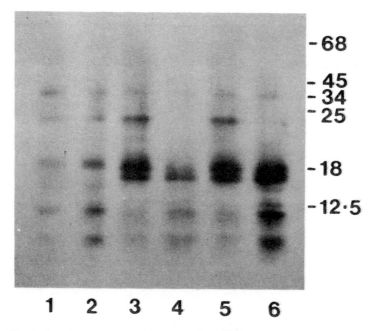

Figure 7. Cleveland peptide map of p36. NP-40 lysates from [^{35}S]methionine-labelled human BRI 8 lympho-blastoid cells **(tracks 1,2)**, mouse K2S lymphocytes **(tracks 3, 4)** and mouse 3T3 fibroblasts **(tracks 5, 6)** were immunoprecipated using rabbit anti-(p36) serum. The precipitated polypeptides were digested with either 1 μg/ml **(tracks 1, 3, 5)** or 10 μg/ml **(tracks 2, 4, 6)** of V8 protease. Peptides were visualized by fluorography.

Table 4. Materials required for Cleveland mapping.

1. Buffer A: 0.125 M Tris-HCl buffer pH 6.8 containing 0.1% SDS, 1 mM EDTA.
2. 20% glycerol in buffer A.
3. V8 protease (Sigma) — 1 mg/ml in 0.125 M Tris-HCl buffer pH 6.8. Store at −20°C.
4. 15% polyacrylamide gel with 1 mM EDTA added to the gel buffers and a 4 cm stack (see Section 4, *Table 6*)

cycle and analyse them by SDS−PAGE. Use the depleted lysate to attempt to immuno-precipitate the second antigen, and compare the result with a parallel immunoprecipitation on another undepleted aliquot of lysate as a control. If the depleted lysate has increased in volume, it is important to adjust the volume of the control lysate accordingly.

(ii) *Immunoblotting of immunoprecipitates.* The technique of sequential immunoprecipi-tation can be modified if one of the antibodies will bind to antigen on an immunoblot (Section 3). Prepare an immunoprecipitate with one antibody and blot it. Use the second antibody to probe the blot.

(iii) *Cleveland peptide mapping.* The Cleveland method of peptide mapping is useful for confirming the identity of a protein relative to a known protein or distinguishing between two proteins if they have similar molecular weights (11). The known and unknown antigens are isolated from radiolabelled cells by immunoprecipitation followed by SDS−PAGE. The gel slices containing the antigens are cut out, partially digested with a protease with restricted cleavage sites, and the resulting peptides compared on a second SDS−polyacrylamide gel. This method has been used to identify p36 (the major substrate for $pp60^{src}$) as a calcium binding protein associated with lymphocyte plasma membranes (*Figure 7*) (12). The materials required are given in *Table 4*.

(i)   Rapidly stain and de-stain the gel (Section 4.3) and identify the antigen by its molecular weight compared with markers. Cut out the gel slice containing the antigen and put in buffer A.

  Alternatively, rapidly stain and de-stain the gel and locate the antigen by autoradiography. Cut out the gel slice. Rehydrate the gel slice in buffer A, removing the paper if the gel has been dried down.

(ii)   Soak the gel slice for 30 min in buffer A. After this it can be stored at −20°C if necessary.

(iii)   Pour a 15% SDS−polyacrylamide gel with a 4 cm stacking gel at the top (Section 4).

(iv)   Push the gel slice into a slot at the top of the gel, using a spatula.

(v)   Overlay the gel with 20 μl of 20% glycerol in buffer A.

(vi)   Mix 5 μl of V8 protease with 95 μl buffer A and 100 μl 20% glycerol in buffer A.

(vii)   Add 50 μl of this enzyme solution (final concentration 25 μg/ml) to the gel slot.

(viii) Load sample buffer containing bromophenol blue in the tracks on either side of the one containing the gel slice. Run the gel until the blue dye reaches the interface between the stacking and running gels.

(ix)   Switch off the current and leave for 30 min for the digestion to take place.

(x)   Switch on again and run the gel as normal.

(xi)   Reveal the peptides by autoradiography or Coomassie blue staining.

(xii)   Compare the pattern of bands of known and unknown antigen to see if they are the same.

Try the V8 protease at several concentrations (between 1 and 25 μg/ml) to get various patterns of partial proteolysis. Other proteases are available and it may be worth trying several of them (12) to find the best one for a particular antigen.

3. IMMUNOBLOTTING

3.1 Introduction

Blotting is the term used for transferring molecules to a matrix on which they are immobilized. It was originally described by Southern (13) for DNA. Subsequently Towbin *et al.* (14) devised a protocol for the electrophoretic transfer of proteins from polyacrylamide gels to nitrocellulose sheets. The latter technique is commonly called electroblotting, Western blotting or, when employing a detection system involving antibody, immunoblotting.

  The principles, techniques and applications of protein blotting from different types of gels have been reviewed recently (15−17). The practicalities of immunoblotting

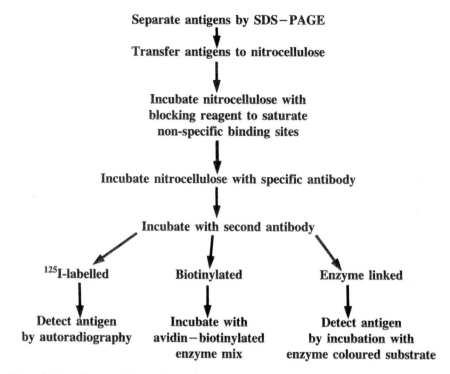

Figure 8. Flow diagram of immunoblotting procedure.

from SDS−PAGE are specifically addressed in this section. The principle of immuno-blotting is the same as for immunoprecipitation in that a specific antibody identifies its antigen in a crude antigen preparation. In the case of immunoblotting from SDS−PAGE the antigen is firstly denatured with SDS and the method is applicable in those instances where the antibody recognizes an epitope which survives SDS treatment. Equally well, epitopes which may not be accessible to antibodies on the native molecule are often exposed. The antigen to which the antibody binds is directly identified in immunoblotting, whereas in immunoprecipitation associated molecules may co-precipitate and make it difficult to tell which bears the relevant epitope.

3.2 Basic technique

Identification of antigen by immunoblotting requires the antigen to be immobilized on a membrane, where it is identified with a specific antibody. A crude antigen preparation such as a total cell lysate can be resolved by SDS−PAGE and the negatively charged proteins transferred from cathode to anode onto nitrocellulose. The nitrocellulose is then probed with a specific antibody which is localized using radioactively labelled antibody or an antibody-linked enzyme detection system. A protocol outlined in a flow diagram (*Figure 8*) for this approach to characterizing lymphocyte antigens is described in the following sections. Variations include transfer from other gel systems, such as two-dimensional gels, agarose gels and urea gels. The common matrix is nitrocellulose, but nylon membranes such as Hybond N (Amersham) can be used.

3.3 **Sample**

Crude samples can be used as antigen, for example whole cell lysates. Whole cell lysates can be prepared by solubilization directly in SDS sample buffer, as described below.

(i)   Wash the cells in PBS, pH 7.4 to remove proteins present in the culture medium.
(ii)   For efficient solubilization make sure the cell pellet is well dispersed; if necessary, add a small volume (e.g. ~ 10% of the final volume) of PBS.
(iii)   Add 4% SDS sample buffer (see Section 4.2) to a final concentration of 5 − 10 × 10⁷ cells/ml and boil for 10 min. Samples can be reduced by addition of 10% volume of 1 M dithiothreitol (DTT) before SDS − PAGE.

Alternatively, cells solubilized in 'lysis buffer' as for immunoprecipitation can be used (see Section 2.3.2). In this case, add an equal volume of 4% SDS sample buffer and boil for 10 min. As a general guideline as to how much antigen to load on a gel, the following example is given. A volume of lysate equivalent to $5 \times 10^5 - 10^6$ cells in a 0.5 cm track is adequate to detect CD2 in cells which express 150 000 molecules per cell.

Use of whole cell lysates when the antigen is present in low amounts can cause problems. So much cell lysate has to be loaded onto the gel that there is a loss of resolution and the increase in amount of irrelevant cellular proteins can cause non-specific background staining. Where a membrane protein is to be identified, the limitations of whole cell antigen preparations can be surmounted by preparing microsomes or plasma membrane. This is a crude way of increasing antigen concentration while preserving resolution and background. Blotting, using microsomes and the insoluble residues after solubilization of microsomes with detergent, enabled p36 to be identified as a component of lymphocyte plasma membrane, while blotting with whole cell lysates invariably failed to reveal the presence of p36 (*Figure 9*) (12).

Another example of blotting with microsomes is shown in *Figure 10*, in which CD2 is identified in a human T leukaemia cell line expressing 150 000 molecules per cell.

3.4 **Molecular weight standards**

Pre-stained molecular weight standards (e.g. from Amersham or BRL) are the ideal reagents to use. They are identified without the necessity for total protein staining of the nitrocellulose, which can alter its in size, making molecular weight comparisons with unstained nitrocellulose difficult. Transfer of pre-stained markers gives an immediate indication of blotting efficiency. They are also useful when the nitrocellulose has to be cut into several strips, as they can be used to mark the cutting line and to re-align strips. They are, however, expensive and, alternatively, unstained standards can be used and stained with amido black after transfer (see below).

3.5 **Gel**

The standard procedure described is transfer of proteins from a SDS − polyacrylamide gel at pH 8.3, that is with a negative charge. Where the same antigen is to be probed with different antibodies, use a large slot. If a number of different antigen preparations are to be used, load the samples to be probed with the same antibody next to each other to minimize the number of times the nitrocellulose must be cut. For large proteins use

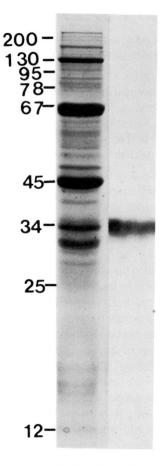

Figure 9. Identification of p36 as a component of the lymphocyte plasma membrane (12). Plasma membranes from the human B lymphoblastoid cell line BRI 8 were solubilized with 0.5% NP-40 and the detergent-'insoluble' residue (left hand track, stained with Coomassie blue) was immunoblotted and probed with rabbit anti-(p36) serum.

a low percentage SDS gel (see Section 4.1) as this aids the proteins' migration from the gel to the nitrocellulose. For example, myosin (200 kd) is mostly retained in a 12% gel but transfers well from a 5% gel.

3.6 Transfer of proteins

3.6.1 *Equipment*

Blotting tank
Scotchbrite scouring pads
Whatman 540 paper
Nitrocellulose sheets (0.1 μM)

Blotting tanks are commercially available. The basic apparatus consists of a tank which holds approximately 2.5 l of transfer buffer and contains platinum electrodes. The con-

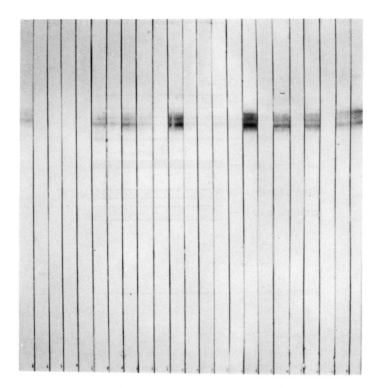

Figure 10. Immunoblotting of the CD2 antigen with monoclonal antibodies. Microsomes from the human T leukaemia cell line J6 were solubilized in 'lysis buffer' and an equal volume of 4% SDS sample buffer added before resolution on a 12% SDS−PAGE. Each 4 mm track contains approximately 2×10^6 cell equivalents. The blot was developed as described in Section 3.7. Transfer was performed in a Biorad Transblot cell at approximately 50 V with a current of approximately 150 mA for 16 h at 4°C. Each strip was incubated with a 1:50 dilution of ascites fluid, each containing a different anti-CD2 monoclonal antibody for 16 h at 4°C. The first three strips were incubated, respectively, with purified anti-CD2 (20 µg/ml), purified anti-CD3 (20 µg/ml), or no first antibody. Some CD2 antibodies reacted strongly with CD2 on the blots.

figuration of the platinum wire is designed to ensure a uniform electrical field between electrodes, for example the 'Transblot cell' (Biorad) has an S-shaped electrode whereas the 'Transphor cell' (Hoefer Scientific Instruments) has seven vertical platinum wires.

3.6.2 *Buffer*

The commonly used buffer for transfer from SDS gels is 25 mM Tris/192 mM glycine, pH 8.3, containing 20% (v/v) methanol. This buffer maintains the negative charge of SDS-bound proteins, whereas the methanol increases the binding capacity of nitro-cellulose. For large (>100 kd) proteins 0.05−0.1% SDS improves transfer. For small proteins (<50 kd) transfer in a carbonate buffer at pH 9.9 may be more efficacious (18). The buffer in the tank can be re-used three or four times.

3.6.3 *Preparation of sandwich (see Figure 11)*

(i)   Prepare the sandwich using running buffer without methanol (i.e. 25 mM Tris/ 192 mM glycine pH 8.3) as the methanol tends to fix the proteins.

247

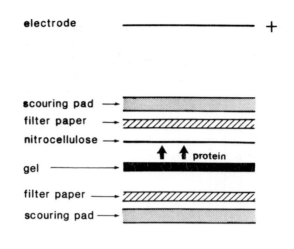

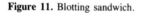

Figure 11. Blotting sandwich.

(ii)   Cut the nitrocellulose to the same size as the gel to be blotted. Wear gloves to avoid touching the nitrocellulose. Wet the nitrocellulose by dropping it flat onto buffer and soak for about 20 min.

(iii) When the gel is ready, soak it in buffer for about 20 min. Trim one corner of the gel for orientation purposes.

(iv)   Cut 2−4 pieces of Whatman no.540 paper (3MM will do, but 540 has better wet strength) the same size or slightly larger than the gel.

(v)   Soak one Scotchbrite pad in buffer. Wet 1−2 pieces of the no.540 paper and lay it on top of the pad.

(vi)   Place the gel on top of the filter paper.

(vii) Place the nitrocellulose on top of the gel, making sure there are no bubbles between the gel and nitrocellulose. Bubbles and excess moisture can be removed by rolling a pipette across the surface.

(viii) Complete the sandwich with the other two layers of no.540 paper and Scotchbrite pad.

(ix)   Make sure the whole sandwich is thoroughly saturated with buffer and place it in the carrier for the blot apparatus. Make sure it is a tight fit, without distorting the gel. Put extra Scotchbrite pads in, if necessary.

(x)   Submerge the holder in the blotting tank containing running buffer with methanol. For transfer from SDS gels at pH 8.3 the proteins are negatively charged and will travel to the positively charged anode. Therefore, *make sure the nitrocellulose is on the anode side.*

3.6.4 *Transfer conditions*

Transfer conditions will vary with the size of the protein: high molecular weight proteins transfer more slowly than lower ones. Transfer can be performed rapidly with a current of 350−500 mA and under these conditions 1−2 h is usually adequate to transfer proteins of less than 100 kd. It is often convenient to transfer overnight and in this case a lower voltage and current are used. Transfer for 16 h at 30−60 V with a current of approximately 150 mA in a Transblot cell (Biorad) gives satisfactory results for a protein (CD2) of approximately 50 kd. The blot shown in *Figure 10* was prepared in this way and good resolution of bands was maintained in the transfer. It is preferable to have the blotting tank in the cold room and to use a water cooling system, particularly for rapid transfer with high voltages. The apparatus can be placed on a magnetic stirrer to circulate the buffer.

3.7 Detection of antigen

The specific antibody is bound to the nitrocellulose and its location then visualized. Usually the sandwich method is employed in which a second antibody, with a label attached, binds to the first. The early description of immunoblotting by Towbin *et al.* (14) includes a detailed protocol for detecting antigen with a ^{125}I-labelled second antibody and autoradiography. Enzyme detection systems are now widely used. The second antibody is directly, for example horseradish peroxidase, or indirectly (biotin − avidin system), linked to an enzyme and antigen localized with a substrate that forms an insoluble reaction product. More recently, colloidal gold-labelled second antibodies have become available. The sensitivity of the enzyme detection systems and colloidal gold can be increased using silver to enhance the intensity of a reaction product (19). The emphasis in this chapter is on the use of the biotin−avidin system, which is sensitive and convenient to use. The second antibody is biotinylated and linked to a biotinylated enzyme via avidin, which has a high avidity for biotin.

An example of the detection of a lymphocyte surface antigen CD2 in cells expressing it at 150 000 molecules per cell, using the biotin−avidin method and monoclonal antibodies, is shown in *Figure 10*. CD3 (expressed at 30 000 molecules/cell) has also been detected by this method.

3.7.1 *Detection of protein*

(i)   After transfer, dismantle the sandwich. *Before* separating the gel from the nitrocellulose, make sure you know the orientation of the blot and which side has been in contact with the gel, the 'right side'. Cut off one corner of the nitrocellulose or label it with pencil.

(ii) Stain the gel with Coomassie blue to check the extent of transfer.

(iii) Wash the nitrocellulose in PBS. Cut off, if required, the strip containing markers, and a strip containing the antigen mixture, to stain with a general protein stain. To cut nitrocellulose, place it on a clean glass plate and use a sharp scalpel, preferably guided with a metal ruler.

(iv) Stain these strips with 0.55% amido black in methanol/acetic acid/water (1:5:1 by vol.) for 3 min. Wash in water for 3 min. De-stain with methanol/acetic acid/water (9:2:100 by vol.). Other stains can be used (17), including Coomassie blue, although backgrounds are high with the latter.

3.7.2 *Detection of specific antigen*

The nitrocellulose to be probed with specific antibody must first be incubated with a solution to saturate non-specific sites on the nitrocellulose. Irrelevant protein (e.g. BSA) can be used and/or detergent (e.g. Tween 20). The disadvantage of the latter is that it can eventually remove protein. BSA is commonly used and a cheaper product is dried skim milk powder. In Britain, Cadbury's Marvel is a useful blocking agent.

(i)   Block the nitrocellulose with PBS containing 2% BSA, 5% Marvel, 0.1% NaN_3 with optional 0.05% Tween 20 for 2 h at room temperature, with rocking. Longer blocking times are suggested for nylon membranes, for example 16 h at 4°C. Do not store this blocking solution for any length of time, as the Marvel tends to precipitate and becomes contaminated.

(ii)   Rinse the blot in PBS containing 0.05% Tween 20, twice, to remove excess protein.

(iii)   If appropriate, cut the nitrocellulose into strips.

(iv)   For incubation with specific antibody: dilute antibody in PBS containing 0.1% BSA, 0.01% NaN_3. For an initial experiment, a concentration of 10 µg/ml for purified antibody, or 1:100 dilution of ascites fluid are suitable. A volume of 250 µl is ample and even less than half this volume is sufficient for a 4 mm strip, if incubations are carried out in sealed plastic bags (made with a heat sealer).

(v)   Place the strips in the plastic, seal three sides and fill up with antibody solution. Remove air bubbles and seal the top. Incubations can be carried out in trays with individual troughs (e.g. Multipipet reservoir inserts; Dynatech). A 4 × 60 mm strip will fit comfortably into one trough, and 250−500 µl of antibody solution is sufficient to cover it.

(vi)   Incubate the strips with antibody solution for 1−2 h at room temperature. Backgrounds may be improved by incubation at 4°C and longer incubations may be effective (for example, overnight at 4°C) when no results are obtained with a 1 h incubation at room temperature. Antigen−antibody reactions can be accelerated by incubating at 37°C; however, this can result in higher backgrounds and increased fragility of the nitrocellulose.

(vii)   Wash the strips in PBS containing 0.05% Tween 20, with 3−5 changes over 15−30 min with rocking. Strips can be washed in individual troughs or all together, if there is sufficient agitation to keep them from sticking to each other.

(viii) For incubation with second antibody: biotinylated antibodies specific for various species of Ig and classes of mouse Ig are available commercially; for example, biotinylated horse anti-mouse Ig (Dakopatt). The manufacturers suggest a working concentration. If a new preparation is being used, it is preferable to titrate it to make sure it does not react with the blot directly. A control strip without first antibody should always be included in an experiment.

(ix)   Dilute the biotinylated antibody — usually 1:100−1:500 in PBS containing 0.1% BSA, 0.01% NaN_3; 1 ml is adequate for a nitrocellulose area of 10 cm^2. Place the strips together in a plastic bag. To prevent the strips overlapping one another, place a bulldog clip over the end of the bag. Use ^{125}I-labelled antibody (sp. act. ~1.5 µCi/µg of IgG) at a dilution of 10^6 c.p.m./ml (14).

(x)   Incubate the blot with biotinylated antibody for 1 h at room temperature. For
      ^{125}I-labelled antibodies longer incubations of 6−16 h are recommended.

(xi) Wash the strips as after incubation with the first antibody. At this stage blots
      probed with ^{125}I-labelled antibodies are dried. Air drying is preferable as heat
      makes the nitrocellulose brittle. Mount the nitrocellulose on filter paper, cover
      with Saran wrap and expose to X-ray film.

(xii) For development of blots with bound biotinylated antibody, the next step is to
      link it with the biotinylated enzyme via an avidin or, more recently, streptavidin
      bridge. These reagents are supplied separately, for example 'Vector stain' from
      Vector Laboratories, or as a pre-formed complex for high sensitivity (Amersham
      International). When using 'Vector stain' add 10 μl of (A)avidin and 10 μl of
      (B)biotinylated horseradish peroxidase to 1 ml of PBS, 0.1% BSA, 0.01%
      NaN_3. Add to the strips in a plastic bag, seal and incubate at 4°C for 1 h.

(xiii) Wash the strips twice in PBS without Tween 20. Tween 20 interferes with the
      colour reaction.

(xiv) Weigh out 25 mg of diaminobenzidine (be careful and wear gloves, as it is a
      'possible carcinogen') and dissolve it in 50 ml of 10 mM Tris pH 7.4. *Immediately*
      before pouring onto strips, add 100 μl of H_2O_2 (33% in water).

(xv) Allow the colour reaction to proceed. Colour development may be immediate,
      that is within 1 min of substrate addition. Sometimes it can take up to 15 min,
      but there is not usually any colour development after that. To stop the reaction,
      wash twice in distilled water and dry between two sheets of filter paper.

(xvi) Protect the strips from light to prevent fading.

4. SDS−POLYACRYLAMIDE GEL ELECTROPHORESIS (PAGE)

4.1 Introduction

SDS−PAGE is used extensively in the biochemical characterization of lymphocyte
surface antigens. One-dimensional SDS−PAGE is described briefly below. For a more
comprehensive description see *'Gel Electrophoresis of Proteins'* (20). For descriptions
of two-dimensional isoelectric focusing (IEF), non-equilibrium pH gradient electrophoresis (NEPHGE), and non-reducing/reducing two-dimensional gel electrophoresis,
see references 21, 22 and 23, respectively.

The percentage of the gel that is employed will depend on the molecular weight of
the proteins of interest. A 12.5% gel is suitable for proteins of molecular weight between
12 and 45 kd, but high molecular weight proteins will be difficult to distinguish. Alternatively a 7.5% gel would be ideal for proteins of molecular weight between 50 and
150 kd, but low molecular weight proteins would not be separated. Gradient gels can
be poured by mixing 5% with 15% acrylamide solutions using a gradient maker.

Boiling mixtures in sample buffer with or without the addition of reducing agent (DTT)
is a useful way of detecting if protein is composed of a single chain or several that
are disulphide linked. The presence of intra-disulphide linkages can be revealed by non-
reducing/reducing two-dimensional gel electrophoresis (23).

Table 5. Solutions for SDS−PAGE analysis.

1. Acrylamide solutions:	30 g of acrylamide and 0.8 g of bisacrylamide dissolved in 100 ml of water and filtered. Wear gloves and weigh out in fumehood.
2. 2% sample buffer[a]:	1 ml of 20% SDS (final conc. 2%) Mix and store at 1 ml of glycerol (final conc. 10%) room temperature 0.8 ml of 1 M Tris-HCl buffer pH 6.8 (final conc. 0.08 M) 7.2 ml of water 0.01% bromophenol blue Add 10 μl of 1 M DTT or β-mercaptoethanol to 100 μl of sample buffer for reducing conditions.
3. Running buffer:	0.025 M Tris base check pH 0.192 M glycine should be 8.3 0.1% SDS
4. Gel stain:	0.0125 g of Coomassie blue 52% water 41% methanol 7% acetic acid
5. Gel de-stain:	40% methanol 7% acetic acid 53% water

[a]To make 4% SDS sample buffer adjust the volume of 20% SDS to 2 ml and water to 6.2 ml.

Table 6. Recipes for acrylamide gels.

	Percentage acrylamide				
	5%	7.5%	10%	12.5%	15%
30%/0.8% acrylamide/bis acrylamide solution	5 ml	7.5 ml	10 ml	12.5 ml	15 ml
Water	13.7 ml	11.2 ml	8.7 ml	6.2 ml	3.7 ml
1 M Tris-HCl buffer pH 8.8	11.2 ml	11.2 ml	11.2 ml	11.2 ml	11.2 ml

4.2 Materials required

Table 5 describes the solutions and buffers required for SDS−PAGE. You will also need glass plates, spacers, combs and gel running tanks with power packs.

4.3 Method

(i)   Mix running gel to required percentage of acrylamide, as in *Table 6*, and de-gas.

(ii)   Add 150 μl of 20% SDS, 100 μl of 10% ammonium persulphate (made up fresh) and 20 μl of TEMED.

(iii) Pour the gel, overlay with water saturated dibutanol and allow to set (~30 min). Leave about a 2 cm space at the top for the stacking gel.

(iv) Tip off the dibutanol and add stacking gel (1.67 ml of 30% acrylamide/0.8% bisacrylamide solution, 1.25 ml of Tris-HCl buffer pH 6.8, 7.03 ml of water, de-gas, then add 50 μl of 20% SDS, 50 μl of 10% ammonium persulphate and 10 μl of TEMED).

(v)   Place the 'comb' into the stacking gel, making sure no bubbles are trapped in the sample wells, and leave to set (~15 min).

(vi)   Remove the comb and wash the sample wells with water.

(vii) Set up the gel in the gel apparatus, remembering to remove the bottom spacer.

(viii) Load the running buffer into the top and bottom of the apparatus. Remove bubbles that are trapped at the bottom of the gel.

(ix)   Load samples into the wells (50−150 µl depending on the size of wells). The amount of protein loaded depends on the number of proteins in the sample. If there is only one protein, then load about 5 µg. If a mixture of proteins is used, for example as in a membrane preparation or a cell lysate, then up to 200 µg of protein can be loaded. Samples which have been boiled in the sample buffer with 100 mM DTT added will contain no disulphide-bonded proteins.

(x)   Run the gels (towards the positive electrode) until the dye front reaches the bottom. This takes about 16 h at 35 V and 4 h at 140 V. The voltage can be adjusted for convenience but check that the current does not exceed 70 mA or the glass plates may crack.

(xi)   Stain the gel in Coomassie blue (2 h or overnight) and de-stain as appropriate. This will reveal molecular weight markers, etc.

(xii) Dry the gel down and locate radiolabelled antigens from immunoprecipitations by autoradiography.

5. ACKNOWLEDGEMENTS

We thank Mike Crumpton for his help in preparing this chapter, Neil Kirby for some useful references and Dorothy Fletcher for typing the manuscript.

6. REFERENCES

1. Omary,M.B. and Trowbridge,I.S. (1981) *J. Biol. Chem.*, **256**, 4715.
2. Cantrell,D.A., Davies,A.A. and Crumpton,M.J. (1985) *Proc. Natl. Acad. Sci. USA*, **82**, 8158.
3. Bordier,C. (1981) *J. Biol. Chem.*, **256**, 1604.
4. Samelson,L.E., Harford,J., Schwartz,R.H. and Klausner,R.D. (1985) *Proc. Natl. Acad. Sci. USA*, **82**, 1969.
5. Oettgen,H.C., Pettey,C.L., Maloy,W.F. and Terhorst,C. (1986) *Nature*, **320**, 272.
6. Brown,M.H., Krissansen,G.W., Totty,N.F., Sewell,W.A. and Crumpton,M.J. (1987) *Eur. J. Immunol.*, **17**, 15.
7. Hubbard,A.L. and Cohn,Z.A. (1976) In *Biochemical Analysis of Membranes*. Maddy,A.H. (ed.), Chapman and Hall, London, p. 427.
8. Swarup,G., Cohen,S. and Garbers,D.L. (1982) *Biochem. Biophys. Res. Commun.*, **107**, 1104.
9. Kessler,S.W. (1975) *J. Immunol.*, **115**, 1617.
10. Johnstone,A. and Thorpe,R. (1982) *Immunochemistry in Practice*. Blackwell Scientific Publications, Oxford, p. 210.
11. Cleveland,D.W., Fischer,S.G., Kirschner,M.W. and Laemmli,U.K. (1977) *J. Biol. Chem.*, **252**, 1102.
12. Davies,A.A. and Crumpton,M.J. (1985) *Biochem. Biophys. Res. Commun.*, **128**, 571.
13. Southern,E.M. (1975) *J. Mol. Biol.*, **98**, 503.
14. Towbin,H., Staehelin,T. and Gordon,J. (1979) *Proc. Natl. Acad. Sci. USA*, **76**, 4350.
15. Towbin,H. and Gordon,J. (1984) *J. Immunol. Methods*, **72**, 313.
16. Gershoni,J.M. and Palade,G.E. (1983) *Anal. Biochem.*, **131**, 1.
17. Beisiegel,U. (1986) *Electrophoresis*, **7**, 1.
18. Dunn,S.C. (1986) *Anal. Biochem.*, **157**, 144.
19. Moeremans,M., Daneels,G., Van Dÿck,A., Langanger,G. and Derney,J. (1984) *J. Immunol. Methods*, **74**, 253.
20. Hames,B.D. and Rickwood,D., eds (1981) *Gel Electrophoresis of Proteins − A Practical Approach*. IRL Press Ltd., Oxford and Washington, DC.
21. O'Farrell,P.H. (1975) *J. Biol. Chem.*, **250**, 4007.
22. O'Farrell,P.Z., Goodman,H.M. and O'Farrell,P.H. (1977) *Cell*, **12**, 1133.
23. Chilson,O.P., Boylston,A.W. and Crumpton,M.J. (1984) *EMBO J.*, **3**, 3239.

APPENDIX

Suppliers of specialist items

American Type Culture Collection, 12301 Parklawn Drive, Rockville, MD 20852, USA

Amersham International plc, White Lion Road, Amersham, Bucks HP7 9LL, UK

Amgen Biologicals Inc., 1900 Oak Terrace Lane, Thousand Oaks, CA 91320, USA

Becton Dickinson Immunocytometry Systems, PO Box 7375, Mountain View, CA 94039, USA

Bio-Rad Laboratories Ltd, Caxton Way, Watford Business Park, Watford, Herts WD1 8RP, UK

Cappel Laboratories, 237 Lacey Street, PO Box 37, West Chester, PA 19380, USA

Cedarlane Laboratories Ltd, 5516−8th Line, RR 2, Hornby ONT LOP 1E0, Canada

Cistron Biotechnology Inc., Pine Brook, NJ, USA

Coulter Electronics Ltd, Northwell Drive, Luton, Beds LU3 3RH, UK

Dakopatts A/S, Guldborgvei 22, DK-2000 F Copenhagen, Denmark

Difco Laboratories, PO Box 14B, Central Avenue, East Molesey, Surrey KT8 08E, UK

Dynal A/S, PO Box 158, Skoyen, N-0212 Oslo 2, Norway

Dynatech Diagnostics Inc., Inland Farm Drive, South Windham, ME 04082, USA

European Collection of Animal Cell Cultures, PHLS, Porton Down, Wilts SP4 0JG, UK

Flow Laboratories Ltd, PO Box 17, Second Avenue Industrial Estate, Irvine KA12 8NB, UK

FMC Bioproducts Europe, 1 Risingevej, DK-2665 Vallensbaek Strand, Denmark

Genzyme Corp., 75 Kneeland Street, Boston, MA 02111, USA

Gibco Europe Ltd, PO Box 35, Trident House, Renfrew Road, Paisley PA3 4EF, UK

Hendley Engineering Ltd, Loughton, Essex LG10 3TZ, UK

Hoechst UK Ltd, Hoechst House, Salisbury Road, Hounslow, Mddx TW4 6JH, UK

International Biotechnologies Inc., 275 Winchester Avenue, PO Box 1565, New Haven, CT 06505, USA

Jencons Scientific Ltd, Cherrycourt Way Industrial Estate, Stanbridge Road, Leighton Buzzard, Beds LU7 8UA, UK

L'Industrie Biologique Francaise, 35 Quai du Moulin de Cage, 92-Gennevilliers, France

Nordic Laboratories, Tukimustre 1, SF-90460 Oulunsalo, Finland

Northumbria Biologicals Ltd, South Nelson Industrial Estate, Cramlington, Northumberland NE23 9HL, UK

Nunclon (*see* Gibco Europe)

Nyegaard & Co., PO Box 4220, Torshov, Oslo 4, Norway

Ortho Diagnostic Systems Inc., Highway 202, Raritan, NJ 08869, USA

Pierce and Warriner Ltd, 44 Upper Northgate Street, Chester CH1 4EF, UK

Pharmacia Fine Chemicals, PO Box 175, S-754 04 Uppsala, Sweden

Sepratech Corp., PO Box 61, Wakefield, RI 02879, USA
Sera Lab Ltd, Hophurst Lane, Crawley Down, W. Sussex RH10 4FF, UK
Serotec Ltd, Bankside, Station Field Industrial Estate, Kidlington, Oxford OX5 1JD, UK
Sigma Chemical Co. Ltd, Fancy Road, Poole, Dorset BH17 7NH, UK
Southern Biotechnology Associates, PO Box 26221, Birmingham, AL 35226, USA
Sterilin Ltd, 43–45 Broad Street, Teddington, Mddx TW11 7NH, UK
Tissue Culture Services Ltd, 10 Henry Road, Slough, Berks SL1 2QL, UK
Vector Laboratories, 1429 Rollins Road, Burlingame, CA 94010, USA
Wellcome Diagnostics, Temple Hill, Dartford, Kent DA1 5AH, UK
J. Weiss & Son Ltd, 11 Wigmore Street, London W1, UK
Worthington Diagnostic Systems Inc., PO Box 650, Halls Mill Road, Freehold, NJ 07728, USA

INDEX

Accessory cells,
  for T cell lines and clones, 136
  heterogeneity, 4
Acquired immunodeficiency syndrome,
  diagnosis by flow cytometry, 83
Acute lymphocytic leukaemia,
  diagnosis, 81
Adherence,
  nylon wool, 28
  on columns, 28
  on plates, 27
Albumen,
  gradient separation, 25
Alkaline phosphatase, 100
Antibody,
  -complement lysis, 51
  conjugation with biotin, 43, 90
  conjugation with fluorescein, 42
  -forming cell assays, 109
  responses *in vitro*, 109, 114, 199
Antigens,
  for *in vitro* immunization, 112
APAAP,
  procedure on tissues, 100
Avidin, 41, 88, 90
Avidin−biotin system,
  use on sections, 103
  use in immunoblotting, 249

B cell,
  differentiation factor, *see* B cell-
    stimulatory factor-2
  differentiation scheme, 95
  growth factor II, *see* Interleukin 5
  preparation by panning, 48
  preparation of large, 221
  preparation of resting, 217
  preparation using magnetic beads, 61
  -stimulatory factor-1, *see* Interleukin 4
  -stimulatory factor-2, assays, 224
B lymphoblastoid cells,
  establishment, 149
  use for assay of B cell differentiation
    factors, 225
B lymphoblasts,
  preparation, 135
Beads, magnetic,
  coating with antibodies, 59
  use for cell depletion, 64
Biotin,
  conjugated antibodies, 41
  conjugation to antibodies, 43, 90
Blood lymphocytes,

antibody responses from, 116
  preparation, 9, 62, 69
Blotting,
  of proteins, *see* Immunoblotting
Bone marrow,
  cell preparation, 21, 69
  lymphocytes in, 1, 19
Bromodeoxyuridine,
  labelling cells with, 93
  use in suicide selection, 141
Bronchial lavage,
  for preparing macrophages, 16
Burkitt's lymphoma,
  cell lines, 151

Cannulation,
  thoracic duct, 11
Carbonyl iron,
  for macrophage depletion, 27
Cell,
  accessory, 4
  counting, 29
  CTLL, for T cell growth factor assays,
    213
  dead, removal of, 23
  dendritic, 5
  follicular dendritic, 7
  freezing, 157
  labelling, fluorescent antibody, 40
  labelling, ^{51}Cr, 144
  labelling, ^{125}I, 235
  labelling, with [^{32}P]orthophosphate, 236
  labelling, with [^{35}S]methionine, 236
  lysis, with detergents, 237
  peritoneal, 15
  pre-B, 1
  preparation of suspensions, 18, 22
  spleen, 16
  sorting, electronic, 35, 38
Cell lines,
  B cell, 149
  BCL$_1$, maintenance, 219
  CTLL, 213
  lymphoid, 3
  myelomonocytic, 7
  T cytotoxic, 138
  T helper, 138
Centrifugation,
  density gradient, 10, 24
Chromic chloride,
  for plaque assays, 121
  for rosetting, 44
Chromium labelling,